Bruno Kastler (Editor)

Interventional Radiology in Pain Treatment

(Editor)

Interventional Radiology in Pain Treatment

Bruno Kastler (Editor)

Fabrice-Guy Barral, Bernard Fergane, Philippe Pereira
(Co-editors)

Interventional Radiology in Pain Treatment

With contributions by

Hatem Boulahdour, Zakia Boulahdour, Philippe Brunner, Christophe Clair, Alain Czorny, Pierre Delassus, Olivia Delmer, Vincent Dousset, Patrick Eude, Blandine Kastler, Jean-Michel Lerais, Jean-François Litzler, Pierre-Yves Marcy, Jean-George Rohmer, Philippe Sarlieve

Foreword by Georges Salamon

With 159 Figures in 369 Separate Illustrations
and 6 Tables

Springer

Kastler, Bruno
Professor of Radiology and Head of Radiology
Service de Radiologie A et C
Centre Hospitalier et Universitaire Jean-Minjoz
Boulevard Fleming
Director of Laboratoire d'Imagerie et d'Ingénierie pour la Santé
Université de Franche-Comté
Besançon, France

ISBN-13 978-3-642-06394-7 e-ISBN-13 978-3-540-47199-8

Title of the Original French Edition:
Radiologie interventionnelle dans le traitement de la douleur

Springer-Verlag is a part of Springer Science+Business Media
springer.com

Editor: Dr. Ute Heilmann, Heidelberg
Desk Editor: Wilma McHugh, Heidelberg
Cover design: Frido Steinen-Broo, EStudio Calamar, Spain

Printed on acid-free paper 21/3100/YL 5 4 3 2 1 0

I dedicate this book to

- My children Tiphaine, Adrian and Florian
- My beloved wife Blandine (psychiatrist who made a contribution to this book)
- My parents Professor Daniel Kastler and Elisabeth Kastler Sander MD
- Nora, Poppi, Michel, Martha, Lucien and Mark
- My grandparents

- The patients from our daily consultations, who we hope to modestly relieve from their suffering with these techniques
- All my collaborators who work with me in every day's struggle
- Professor Auguste Wachenheim who convinced me to complete my training in radiology and tought me the basics in neuroradiology
- Andia Hashemizadeh for her drawings

Foreword

It is a great honor to present this magnificent book that Prof. Kastler and coworkers have dedicated to different modalities of pain treatment with the help of interventional radiology. Professor Kastler is a very well known French radiologist working at the University of Besancon, who has exceptional training in both medicine (internal medicine/cardiology) and physics (M.Sc.). His first textbook *Understanding MRI* was a great success (currently in its 6th edition) and was used by all students and teachers working in the field of MRI. This volume, his third book (the second was titled *MRI of Cardiovascular Malformations*), is devoted to a fascinating field that Kastler has explored for 15 years. I remember the impact of his first presentations in this field, when he was among the guest speakers at a meeting devoted to recent advances in radiology.

The reader will find all possibilities offered to patients in different areas involving facial, cranial and vertebral or paravertebral areas. But this book, written collaboratively by numerous specialists, is not limited only to the technical aspects of these different methods concerning nerves or bones. Great attention is paid to the psychological and psychiatric approach to patients with often-intractable pain. A special chapter is devoted to the metastasis of bones. It is an important message for every specialist in medicine or surgery to understand that in the hands of interventional radiologists with the collaboration of many other colleagues from pain therapy, psychiatry, anesthesiology and from scientific imaging laboratories, pain–benign or intractable–can be treated with exceptionally good results. I extend my best wishes for the great success of this textbook dealing with important developments in a field that has so many human implications.

Los Angeles, 4 May 2006

Georges Salamon M.D.
University of California at Los Angeles
Department of Radiological Sciences
Professor and Former Head of Neuroradiology
Centre Hospitalier Universitaire La Timone
Marseille France

Preface

Pain, a biopsychosocial model, is by definition multifactorial. Its treatment requires complementary medical and paramedical skills. However, this fact was only able to gain acceptance by the disruption of manifold customs and attitudes within established organ medicine, rooted in decades of tradition and whose undeniable successes gave rise to a degree of immobility, thereby guaranteeing and maintaining its power and territory.

Nonetheless attitudes are slowly changing. The French Ministry of Health for one, advised by pioneers in the field, often hospital doctors, became alerted to the fact that pain is first and foremost a human predicament before it is a social issue, and became intent on installing a new order. A pain control plan was established, backed up by a series of university and hospital decisions: introduction of a specific module in the graduate medical studies reform, university diplomas and the setting up of regional hospital pain management consultations, units and evaluation centres. Such structures have drawn attention to the wide-ranging scope of pain and its many components, the complexity of understanding pain, the difficulty of pain control from the patient's point of view and of relieving pain from the medical point of view. As a result of these consultations, the notion of transversal skills and horizontal know-how became apparent.

Therefore, although some were reticent at the outset and others enthusiastic, a variety of specialists met to share their knowledge and confront their respective points of view and indications. Anaesthetists, radiologists, surgeons, physiotherapists, neurologists, house physicians, psychiatrists and psychologists met together in the pain evaluation and control centre to attempt to provide a response, one which they considered best for the patient who expresses his or her pain and whom they listen to and believe.

Radiologists were quick to take an active role in this approach. Cutting-edge technology has transformed them into more than just "image readers", a role to which they were often relegated in the past. Thanks to ultrasound scans, scanners and MRI, they began to play a role in fields that until then had been reserved to surgeons and anaesthetists and have been able to make a contribution to the fight against pain.

This work is the fruit of the faultless collaboration of two doctors, in which the radiologist has played the major role, born out of their joint philosophical and humanist beliefs and their unfailing friendship. This book provides us with non-exhaustive insight into interventional radiological indications, indications proposed by therapists gathered together to study the files and interviews of patients, who are provided with all the necessary information. It is the proof that medical decisions in the field of pain control can no longer be made by a single therapist, but must be the fruit of a concerted study by all concerned parties. This requires the adoption of a team spirit, the relinquishment of medical power in terms of vertical disciplines, an open ear to everyone's voice beginning with that of the patient, trust from start to finish and the burning desire to relieve suffering from pain.

We are delighted that the success of the first edition has made it possible to update this work only two years later with a second edition and now an English version.

Bernard Fergane and Bruno Kastler

Contents

List of Contributors

Amoretti, Nicolas
Hôpital L'Archet
Centre Hospitalier Universitaire
Nice, France

Aubry, Régis
Service de Soins Palliatifs
Centre Hospitalier Universitaire Jean Minjoz
Besançon, France

Aubry, Sebastien
Service de Radiologie A et C
Centre Hospitalier Universitaire Jean Minjoz
Besançon, France

Barral, Fabrice-Guy
Professor of Radiology
and head of Service de Radiologie
Centre Hospitalier Universitaire
Hôpital-de-Bellevue
Saint-Étienne, France

Billon-Grand, Romain
Service de Neurochirurgie
Centre Hospitalier Universitaire Jean Minjoz
Besançon, France

Billiard, Jean-Sébastien
Service de Radiologie
Centre Hospitalier Universitaire
Hôpital de Bellevue
Saint-Étienne, France

Boulahdour, Hatem
Service de Médecine Nucléaire
Centre Hospitalier Universitaire Jean-Minjoz
Besançon, France

Boulahdour, Zakia
Service de Radiologie A et C
Centre Hospitalier Universitaire Jean Minjoz
Besançon, France

Brunner, Philippe
Département de Radiologie Vasculaire
Interventionelle
Hôpital Princesse-Grace
Monaco

Cadel, Gilles
Service de Radiologie A et C
Centre Hospitalier Universitaire Jean Minjoz
Besançon, France

Cazaux, Élodie
Département de Radiologie Vasculaire
Interventionnelle
Hôpital Princesse-Grace
Monaco

Cercueil, Jean-Pierre
Département de Radiolgie Imagerie Médicale
Hôpital du Bocage
Centre Hospitalier Universitaire
Dijon, France

Chevallier, Patrick
Hôpital L'Archet
Centre Hospitalier Universitaire
Nice, France

Clair, Christophe
Polyclinique de Franche-Comté
Service de Radiologie A et C
Centre Hospitalier Universitaire Jean-Minjoz
Besançon, France

Claussen, Claus D.
Professor of Radiology
and head of Department of Diagnostic Radiology
University Clinic Tübingen
Tübingen, Germany

Cornu, Jean-Yves
Centre d'Évaluation de Traitement de la Douleur
Centre Hospitalier Universitaire Jean-Minjoz
Besançon, France

Couvreur, Marc
Cabinet de Radiologie
Lens, France

Cucchi, Jean-Michel
Département de Radiologie Vasculaire
Interventionelle
Hôpital Princesse-Grace
Monaco

Czorny, Alain
Professor of Neurosurgery
and head of Service de Neurologie
Centre Hospitalier Universitaire Jean-Minjoz
Besançon, France

Delassus, Pierre
Département d'Anesthésie-Réanimation
Centre Hospitalier Universitaire
Côte-de-Nacre, Caen, France

Delmer, Olivia
Cabinet de Radiologie
Bayonne, France

De Billy, Benoît
Service de Chirurgie pédiatrique
Centre Hospitalier Universitaire Hôpital Saint Jacques
Besançon, France

De Billy, Marjolaine
Service de Radiologie A et C
Centre Hospitalier Universitaire Jean Minjoz
Besançon, France

De Peretti, Fernand
Service de Traumatologie-Orthopédie
Hôpital Saint-Roch
Nice, France

Dousset, Vincent
Professor of Radiology
and head of Service de Neuroradiologie
Hôpital Pellegrin,
Bordeaux, France

Eude, Ghislaine
Service de Radiologie
Hôpital Saint Roch
Nice, France

Eude, Patrick
Service de Radiologie
Hôpital Saint Roch
Nice, France

Fergane, Bernard
Service d'Évaluation de Traitement de la Douleur
Centre Hospitalier Universitaire Jean-Minjoz
Besançon, France

Fuerxer, Françoise
Département de Radiologie Vasculaire
Interventionnelle
Hôpital Princesse-Grace
Monaco

Fritz, Jan
Department of Diagnostic Radiology
University Clinic Tübingen
Tübingen, Germany

Haj Hussein, Hussein
Service de Radiologie A et C
Centre Hospitalier Universitaire Saint-Jaques
Besançon, France

Hadjidekov, George
Service de Radiolgie A et C
Centre Hospitalier Universitaire Jean-Minjoz
Boulevard Fleming
Besançon, France

Jacamon, Marie
Service de Radiologie A et C
Centre Hospitalier Universitarie Jean-Minjoz
Besançon, France

Kastler, Blandine
Service de Psychiatrie II
Hôpitaux Universitaires de Strasbourg
Strasbourg, France

Kastler, Bruno
Professor of Radiology
and head of Service de Radiologie
Centre Hospitalier Universitaire Jean-Minjoz
Boulevard Fleming
Director of Laboratoire D'Imagerie d'Ingénierie
pour la Santé
Université de Franche-Comté
Besançon, France

Klingelschmitt, Sébastien
Service de Médecine Nucléaire
Centre Hospitalier Universitaire Jean-Minjoz
Besançon, France

Kovacs, Robert
Service de Radiolgie A et C
Centre Hospitalier Universitaire Jean-Minjoz
Boulevard Fleming
Besançon, France

Krause, Denis
Professor of Radiology
and head of Service de Radiologie
Département de Radiologie Imagerie Médicale
Hôpital du Bocage
Centre Hospitalier Universitaire
Dijon, France

Laborie, Laurent
Service de Radiolgie A et C
Centre Hospitalier Universitaire Jean-Minjoz
Boulevard Fleming
Besançon, France

Lerais, Jean-Michel
Service de Radiologie A et C
Centre Hospitalier Universitaire Saint-Jacques
Besançon, France

Litzler, Jean-Francois
Service de Radiologie
Centre Hospitalier Universitaire Jean-Minjoz
Besançon, France

Marcy, Pierre-Yves
Service de Radiologie
Centre Antoine-Lacassagne
Nice, France

Manzoni, Philippe
Service de Radiologie
Centre Hospitalier Universitaire Jean-Minjoz
Besançon, France

Michalakis, Démosthènes
Service de Radiologie A et C
Centre Hospitalier Universitaire Jean-Minjoz
Besançon, France

Monnier, Guy
Professor of Radiology
and head of Service d'Anatomie
Faculté de Médecine
Besançon, France

Mourou, Michel-Yves
Département de Radiologie Vasculaire
Interventionelle
Hôpital Princesse-Grace
Monaco

Parmentier, Michel
Laboratoire d'Imagerie d'Ingénierie pour la Santé
Université de Franche-Comté
Besançon, France

Patay, Zoltan
Professor of Radiology
Faculty of Medicine
University of Tennessee
Head section of Neuroradiology
St. Jude Children's Research Hospital
Memphis, TN, USA

Pereira, Philippe L.
Professor of Radiology
Department of Diagnostic Radiology
University Clinic
Tübingen, Germany

Puget, Julien
Service de Radiolgie A et C
Centre Hospitalier Universitaire Jean-Minjoz
Boulevard Fleming
Besançon, France

Pousse, Annie
CR1-INSERM
Laboratoire d'Imagerie d'Ingénierie pour la Santé
Université de Franche-Comté
Besançon, France

Riboud Cyril
Service de Radiologie A et C
Centre Hositalier Universitaire Jean-Minjoz
Besançon, France

Rohmer Jean-Georges
Service de Psychiatrie II
Hôpitaux Universitaires de Strasbourg
Strasbourg, France

Russias, Benoît
Service de Radiologie
Clinique du Renaison
Roanne, France

Sailley, Nicolas
Service de Radiolgie A et C
Centre Hospitalier Universitaire Jean-Minjoz
Boulevard Fleming
Besançon, France

Sarliève, Philippe
Service de Radiologie A et C
Centre Hospitalier Universitarie Jean-Minjoz
Besançon, France

Schmutz, Gérard
Professor of Radiology
and head of Service de Radiologie
Centre Hospitalier Universitaire Sherbrook
Quebec, Canada

Sedat, Jack
Département de Radiologie Vasculaire
Interventionelle
Hôpital Princesse-Grace
Monaco

Tanji, Philippe
Service de Radiologie
Polyclinique des Minguettes
Vénissieux, France

Tiberghien-Chatelain, Florence
Hositalier Centre d'Évaluation de Traitement
de la Douleur
Centre Hospitalier Universitare Jean-Minjoz
Besançon, France

Evaluating and Managing Pain in a Pain Management Center

1

Bernard Fergane

Psychosomatic Approach to Pain

History

In very ancient times, pain and magic were one and the same. Pain was considered to be due to the presence of an evil spirit within the suffering man. It was then not uncommon to see a sorcerer inflict a wound on a suffering man in order to chase away the perturbing agent. These practices still exist nowadays in certain parts of Africa, conveyed by an animist philosophy.

Egyptians, Hebrews, ancient Greeks (Homer among them) still considered human pain to be a sign sent down by the gods. With his famous formula "Divine is the work of relieving pain," around 400 BC Hippocrates attempted to remove the sacred aura surrounding pain, asserting that it was a state out of step with natural Harmony.

Meanwhile, Aristotle and Plato kept seeing in it not a sensation, but an emotion.

Health to the Greeks was a fragile equilibrium that had to be protected for fear of disturbing Harmony. As expressed in his immortal Oath, Hippocrates of Cos (460–377 BC) had a lofty concept of the role of medicine, Prominent in his proposals were concerns with physicians' duties concepts of brotherliness among practitioners, equality of human beings in the face of sickness, protection of life, respect for medical secrecy – all leading to creation of a code of ethics.

Hippocrates' medical aphorisms are famous. Here are a few:

- Great aches call for great remedies.
- If two aches break out at once in different places, the stronger one obscures the weaker one.
- It is bad when stupor or delirium follow a blow to the head.

Galen and his Greco-Roman contemporaries located pain in the brain, center of all sensations. Galen was the first to look for means of fighting pain and sickness in pharmacology and surgery. Espousing a new vision of the role of the physician, his anatomic and physiological theories were to become a dogma that nobody dared challenge for almost 15 centuries. (With the efficient help of young king Louis XIV, Harvey eventually succeeded in such a rebellion.). In the Middle Ages (a thousand years of ignorance, misfortunes, wars, invasions, and epidemics), physicians, under the heel of the Church, did not seem to pay much attention to pain, even though analgesic plants were well known (opium, sage, ivy, mandrake).

A great name in both philosophy and medicine, Avicenna (Abû Ali-Husayn ibn-Abdullah Ibn-Sina; 980–1037) stood at the crossroads of eastern and western thought. His best known work in medicine was *The Canon of Medicine*, but it was not translated into Latin until 1491 (in Naples, then in Venice and Rome). It constitutes an exemplary synthesis of Hippocrates, Aristotle, and Galen.

He voiced a premonition of the role of rats in spreading plague, and of water and soil in certain other diseases. He wrote of the interaction of psyche and soma. He was the first to describe meningitis, the anatomy of the eye, and the symptomatology of diabetes.

An accomplished philosopher (whose teaching is still alive among Shiites), musician, poet, artist, humanist, he was the keeper of Greek tradition through very troubled times.

In the Renaissance, under the influence of Lorenzo de Medici and his Academy, the modern anatomic and physiological vision of pain appeared. It came to be regarded no longer as an emotion, but a sensation dealt with by the nervous system. Three great medical names of that time must be remembered: Vesalius, Paré, and Paracelsus.

Ambrose Paré (1509–1590) served four kings: Henry II; Francis II, Charles IX, and Henry III. (It must be anecdotally reported that King Henry II, wounded in a tournament, died in spite of the presence of both Paré and Vesalius.) Paré was the first to ligature blood vessels when amputating, a practice to remain the basis of the training of military physicians for centuries.

Famous for his orthopedic procedures, he is also considered as the father of French ophthalmology.

This legendary dialogue took place between Charles IX and Paré:

"I hope you are going to treat kings better than the poor?"

"No, Majesty, that's impossible."

"And why?"

"Because I treat them like kings."

Later, Descartes, as Paré had done, also looked into the mysterious problem of pain in the "ghost limb."

The 18th and the 19th centuries were important because of progress in pharmacology in general and the fight against pain in particular. Many physicians focused more and more on pain. This is evidenced by Marc-Antoine Petit's extraordinary *Discourse on Pain*, read aloud by way of a professional testament in front of his students and colleagues on 28 Brumaire of year VII (21 November 1799), at the opening of anatomy and surgery courses at the General Hospital for the Sick in Lyons, where he was the head surgeon.

Sydenham formulated laudanum in 1750. In Hanover, Sertuener began using morphine.

Discoveries were numerous: nitrogen dioxide was identified by Priestley in the 1770s and made use of by Davy in the 1840s; ether was described by Faraday in 1818 and used by Hickman in the 1830s; chloroform was simultaneously found by Von Liebig in Germany, Soubeiran in France, and Guthrie in the USA.

The first general anesthesia was performed by Morton on October 16, 1846, in Boston, MA, USA, (the word anesthesia having been suggested by Oliver Wendell Holmes). At first, Velpeau, Malgaigne did not support the notion of general anesthesia. Velpeau wrote in 1839: "Escaping pain during surgery is a chimerical dream that we may not entertain in our time. A sharp instrument and pain in surgical medicine are two concepts that never appear separately in the mind of the patient, and we, the surgeons, must accept their combination. Indeed, this evolution does not take place without the fanatical opposition of surgeons for whom pain is an integral and inevitable part of operations."

Magendie, for ethical reasons, considered the loss of consciousness as degrading and demeaning for any man with some courage. Surgeons of that day did not hesitate to say that the pain of patients on whom they operated did not do anything for the Academy of Medicine. This opposition quickly disappeared when they realized the enormous progress brought about by anesthesia.

The 20th century, with the development of analgesic techniques and of pharmacology, allowed man to imagine "a world without pain" for all time to come. The question remains whether that is possible and desirable. We cannot close this section without citing a few more great names.

W. Stewart Halsted (1852–1922), with precise technique and rigorous asepsis, furthered elegant surgery with as little mutilation as possible , and was the initiator of local anesthesia. He was the leader of a generation of surgeons who spread his humanist ideas. Like many surgeons of his time, he traveled in Austria and Germany, lodestars in medicine and surgery in the 19th century. Very impressed by Lister's work, Halsted advocated techniques of asepsis and founded subspecialties in orthopedics, urology, radiology, otorhinolaryngology, vascular surgery. He introduced rubber gloves into the OR (these were first made by Goodyear to take care of an eczema problem of his favorite assistant, miss Caroline Hampton, whom he ended up marrying).

René Leriche, one of his contemporaries; was a disciple of Poncet and Alexis Carrel. An organizer of military hospitals in the Paris area and a surgeon in the World War I, he ended the latter as "surgeon of *gueules cassées*" (facial injuries). Georges Duhamel testifies: "Leriche's patients were severely disabled, trephined, wounded in the thorax or the stomach. In order to treat them, to help them bear the torture of bandaging, Leriche had them put to sleep each time with ethyl chloride. He showed a great and admirable respect for suffering, in those very factories of industrial surgery. From the first day, I saw in him the future pain surgeon."

Leriche was the father of vascular surgery, publishing on juvenile obliterating arteritis, gastric ulcers, Volkmann's syndrome, painful stumps. He wrote *The Surgery of Pain*, which takes up 20 lessons taught at the Collège de France.

John Bonica, in the second half of the century, defined "pain clinics," the precursor of our centers for evaluating and treating pain. A Sicilian immigrant to the US, who had to support his family at age 15 by selling newspapers and shining shoes, still continued his studies in high school and university, where he proved to be a remarkable student in several ways. (For example, he followed his passion for wrestling to become the US collegiate champion in his weight class.) Still very young, in May of 1944, he was assigned as head anesthesiologist to the military hospital in Madigan, WA, USA, where he was struck by the pain that all too regularly accompanied war injuries. In 1960, he founded and ran the department of anesthesiology at Washington University in Seattle, where subsequently he advanced techniques in local anesthesia, in surgery, and in obstetrics. At the same time, he opened the first multidisciplinary pain clinic, which allowed for better interaction among medical personnel by calling on contributions and cooperation among surgeons, anesthesiologists, neurologists, psychiatrists, psychologists, and physical therapists.

Finally, in 1973 Bonica he founded the International Association for the Study of Pain (IASP).

Definition

The IASP defines the problem as follows: "Pain is an unpleasant sensory and emotional experience, connected with an existing or potential tissue lesion, or described in terms of such a lesion." This definition has two advantages:

- Pain is considered as a central neuro-physio-psychological event with a double dimension, a subjective, sensory one and an emotional one, whose unpleasant character can be assessed only by the sick person.
- It justifies the painful moan of a psychological disorder, as it stresses the possibility that pain-generating mechanisms may have a physical as well as a psychological basis.

Psychological Signs of Pain

Four components of pain are generally identified:

- The sensory component corresponds to the decoding of the sensory message in its quality, intensity, duration and localization characteristics. It is what the patient feels. Where? When? How long? What character (aching, sharp, electric, stabbing, etc.)??
- The emotional component comes into being if pain is prolonged, and consists of anguish and/or depression.
- The cognitive component corresponds to the place that the patient grants pain in his/her life; it calls on his/her educational, cultural, religious experience, the contents of which determine his/her way of treating the painful information in the brain. Continuing pain often causes cognitive alterations with erroneous, poorly suited, or catastrophist thoughts Elements of the relative importance that pain has come to have to a person, and the attention or lack of attention paid thereto, include: (a) attitudes in the cultural environment, (b) past experience, (c) situational context, (d) personal meaning of perceived pain.
- The behavioral component corresponds to the observable (objective) motor, verbal, and objective signs that pain determines,. If defined by the associated behavior, pain becomes a way of communicating with one's circle of friends and family, and has relational implications.

Pain and Identity

High-level sports activity not only demands thorough training, excellent physical shape, and a strong will, but also great resistance to pain and any temptation to slacken.

Many westerners with little qualification or natural ability for athletics embark on long and intense sports events in which a personal ability to fight off a steadily increased degree of suffering is the dominant feature (track racing, jogging, trekking, triathlon, etc.). It is not a matter of competing with another person, and the results are of secondary importance, having value only for oneself. It is as if the physical limit replaces a limit in meaning that is no longer provided by the social order. A symbolic reclaiming of one's life takes place.

A similar connection between pain and identity is seen in the way one relates to sickness. The emotional inequalities of childhood weigh generally three times more than social inequalities. A buried guilt weakens yet determines a resilient ability to suffer that rebounds after stress and allows life to continue. For some children, who have to relate to an uncommunicative mother, pain is the last trump to play in attracting her attention. One often notes that chronic pain sufferers had violent parents.

Some individuals escape their uneasiness, their feeling of not being loved, of not fitting into the family or other circle, by somehow acquiring a pain, which, if it makes their life less bearable, at least gives them the benefit of receiving care and attention. Pain, translated into a moan, is an identity abutment that allows them to keep their place. In fact, Man sometimes practices a progression of pain without which he could not live. In a relational system, pain can be an exchange currency. It allows one to stand a bit more straight in an unstable and threatened life. It is the poisoned gift of an unconscious relationship to a personal history.

Behind our perception of pain, which is so subjective, lies the whole memory of our past physical and psychological sufferings. Freud puts it thus: "Every affect is a repetition of old traumas" – which is to say, of every frustration, anguish, feeling of abandonment, of loneliness, of separation, of loss one has experienced.

Pain is incommunicable. It is at once a rape, a physical violence and a destruction of one's relationship to the world, in the sense that it invades everything and paralyses physical as well as intellectual activity. Withdrawn into him/herself, the sick person ends up tiring everybody because of his/her impatience, his/her irritability, his/her behavior, not to mention the apparent ceaselessness of his/her pains. His/her family circle sometimes ends up wondering and doubting, a reckoning ultimately unbearable to the patient.

Pain always puts language in check. It causes outbursts, crying spells, silence. It destroys speech, thoughts, and makes voice unrecognizable. It plunges us into an ocean of utter loneliness, drowns us in a world inaccessible to others. Man in pain is nothing but a scream nobody hears.

Living with pain is experiencing loneliness: "You don't share someone's pain, you only reach another person's pain in a roundabout way. You can't suffer like the other person, even when you love him/her, even when you would like to lighten his/her aching. There is something dreadful in pain in the sense that it locks up the person, reveals the weight of loneliness" (David Le Breton).

When pain is chronic and the patient, through his moan, seeks a relationship to others and to physicians, then subjective language becomes an act of speech.

Pain and Speech: Moaning

Screams and moans act as pain's outlet. Yelling prevents one from becoming mad with pain. A scream holds the fundamental touch of a motor discharge. It is also the echo of all our screams that were never heard but are only etched in our memory. Screams and moans serve other functions. When screaming, you are no longer passive, you are active. You try and control something that anguishes and eludes your attempt to capture.

On the palette of *moans* come words, with their meaning, their emotional tone, the intensity of their sound. They are full-fledged symptoms, signs of an inner life. It is through listening carefully to the moaning that ties can be established, little by little, allowing the patient to wonder, and subsequently perhaps to gauge, how much of his suffering is shown by pain. For moans appear to us as precisely the link between psyche and soma.

Moaning can become the expression of psychological as well as of physical suffering. Moaning allows one to inscribe suffering in a language, to name the inexpressible, the unbearable; thereby, it soothes anguish. Let us therefore not try to silence the moan. We have to accept it and accompany it, and to perceive the unsaid through the conscious speech, to seize the word, the mimic, the gesture which suddenly give another dimension to the speech. The moan can be a call for help, for appeasement, or it can be simply an expression of discontent. It can be a need to talk, an urgency to tell, a crisis that has to be put into words.

Pain is not only a physiological occurrence, it is above all an occurrence of life. It is not the body that is suffering, but the whole individual. In those cases, there is always a psychological component, a sometimes secondary suffering, that often reveals an older problem, unbeknownst to the patient. The painful moan then attests to things other than physical anomaly: to frustration, guilt, punishment, and separation, to name a few. It becomes an identifying landmark, narcissistic crutch; presence, which, in a hallucinatory manner, comes and fills an absence; it expresses the suffering of a past mistreatment; it is a locus of pleasure in a body that cannot be accepted as painful. It is therefore the body that is regularly denounced as the locus and cause of all aching. The difficulty in understanding these patients who come to lodge a complaint and ask for reparation is that they are the holders of a knowledge that runs against that of the physician, who is placed in the untenable position of being asked to do some repair work that he can't see as necessary.

Moaning bears multiple messages at various levels – unexpressed but implicit requests. The true request remains to be deciphered. The moan is the stage for the sick person's set of psychological problems. It can be begging, seductive, intrusive, aggressive, manipulative. The response will have to be in agreement.

The sick person is lodging a complaint. He/she is, in one way or another, asking for "compensation." Too often, the medical response stops at this highlighted set of problems. Moaning has a psychological dimension. It is intended for and expressed toward another person, modulated contingent on him/her, but he/she does not understand this call, he/she does not decipher it, he/she remains at the level of the physical moan without understanding that, behind this moan, there is a whole array of past frustrations. The response given is a part of the "secondary benefits," but it does not respond to the real need, which at bottom is to be recognized and loved for oneself.

There are some factors of positive reinforcement. "When I suffer, and only when I suffer, good things happen to me": medical care; rest; attention; financial or material compensation; concern of family, spouse. and physicians; analgesics, sedatives.

There are, however, some factors of negative reinforcement. "When I am hurting, bad things only increase the pain." Difficult situations, hard work, unpleasant discussions, responsibilities, emotional, and sexual relations are thus avoided.

Pain and its evoked moan allow one to take the cause outside of oneself. The guilty one, the scapegoat is the surgeon, the physician, the scientist; and there are others. Every attack on the body upsets the psychological balance of the person, who sometimes needs the pain in order to survive. One example of this not infrequently occurs with operative removal of some body part. The patient cannot make up his/her mind to say goodbye. "I want to live with what I no longer have," and pain comes to fill the void.

It is noteworthy that the nature and evolution of a pain is often conditioned by the situation in which it appeared. For instance, by such unpleasant circumstances as:

- Abrupt, thoughtless disclosure of cancer
- Removal of an organ without informed consent
- Premature and unprepared return home from hospital
- Treatment as an object by an examining team
- Endless time on a stretcher, at the back of a hallway with indifferent medical personnel passing through

Meaning and Pain

"Man is an animal that seeks meaning" (Camus)

Just as nature abhors a vacuum, so is man afraid of a lack of meaning. An effect without a visible cause brings into imagination all sorts of beliefs and claims that, according to the individual, have remained unheeded. A man tends to know full well that the cause of his pain is outside himself. It is a feeling, a vague impression, a form of malaise, a diffuse uneasiness.

But pain is not a punishment from God. It is rather a component of the human condition. Pain is not a value. Fighting it, under certain circumstances, as well as accepting it, can represent important values. It may allow opportunity for showing our resilience, our serenity, our hope.

Does pain have a meaning? If so, what? It is said that pain is critical as a warning signal, but this not always true; undeniable warning signals hunger and thirst are not painful at first. It is said that pain helps us locate sickness, but neither is this always true; coronary thrombosis and peritonitis in the elderly may be without pain, and many pains are projected to locations distant from the source.

Pain is a disruption of information, a mistranslation, a misinterpretation. The patient wants to be listened to, to be understood and wants a meaning to be given to this pain that is taking a hold of him/her, paralyzing him/her, altering him/her in every way. He or she comes to *be* pain, to be identified with it in such a way that he/she will only be free of it if it receives a meaning in his/her eyes.

The philosopher Nietzsche observed that what is revolting is not suffering itself but its lack of meaning. A certain conception of the idea of humanity incites us to intervene in order to limit the pain felt by man as far as possible as well as the total suffering that diminishes his personality at all levels.

More than any other field, pain therapy embodies a moral duty at the highest level of humanity, its desire and goal is to give back to man his uniqueness, to put back together in this disintegrated individual what has been scattered.

Life is what gives a meaning to pain; it is not pain that gives a meaning to life. We need to feel important in the eyes of others in order to live properly among them.

To be useful to a patient in pain, the physician must give up all feelings of power and be open to the outlook of the other.

Pain management is not so much a new medical specialty as it is a humanitarian attitude and a new responsibility of physicians toward their patients. In order to be worthwhile, the relationship between the patient and the physician (and vice versa) can only be from subject to subject, not from subject to object (or vice versa). It marks the reuniting of medicine with its primary aim, which is to put back together a man shattered by pain and sickness, to make him one again, to put him on his feet.

Pain Classification

Acute vs. Chronic

In an acute pain (that has appeared recently), the generating mechanism is often singular and somatic. It comes with neurovegetative and motor signs as well as a reactive anxiety. A somatic medical approach is often sufficient to come up with a diagnosis. An etiologically oriented cure is then offered.

In chronic pain (arbitrarily defined as a pain that has lasted for more than 6 months), pain can continue beyond the limit of recovery from trauma, come from a supposedly finalizing lesion (e.g., amputation, nerve ablation) or a progressive chronic disease (e.g., cancer, polyarthritis). Pain that is perpetuated ends up affecting the psyche and makes it more and more difficult to determine if the primary factor is somatic or psychological.

Physiopathology

Pains Due to an Excess of Nociperception

These result from a strong stimulation of the specific receptors of pain, without any lesion nor dysfunction of the peripheral or central nervous system. They stem from alterations of the viscera, the blood vessels, and/or the locomotor system. Such pain is the type found in cancer or rheumatism and can be soothed with peripheral or central analgesics, sometimes combined with co-analgesics.

Neurogenic Pain

These originate in lesions of peripheral nerves (e.g., stump pain, various neuropathies), in lesions of the radices (e.g., shingles, tearing of the brachial plexus), and in vascular or traumatic lesions of the central nervous system (e.g., cerebral vascular illness, brain tumor). A typical example here is the pain caused by shingles. These pains are not soothed by standard analgesics, but by an anti-epilepsy and anti-depression treatment. Transdermal nerve stimulation is also recommended.

Hysterical Pain

The diagnosis is based on the negative results of a meticulous organ checkup, a poor response to an analgesic treatment, and a-typical clinical picture consisting of evocative localizations, a particular description of pain, the presence of psychological signs, the particular way in which the patient relates to his/her circle of friends and family as well as to the physician, and his/her special ties to pain.

Treatment

Medicinal Treatment

Classification of Analgesics

The classification proposed by the WHO teaches us the concept of analgesic levels, an idea based on the strength of the various agents allowing a prescription corresponding to a simple scheme (weak pain: weak analgesic; strong pain: strong analgesic).

This classification replaced the old one, based on the dichotomy "central analgesics/peripheral analgesics". Pharmacology made this approach obsolete by showing the central action of acetaminophen, the "mixed" action of nonsteroidal anti-inflammatory drugs (NSAIDs; peripheral and central), and the action of opiates on specific receptors located outside the central nervous system.

The most logical classification is that according to mechanism(s) by which the agents at our disposal are effective (three mechanisms, three categories) [5]:

- Non-narcotic analgesics have an effect on non- specific receptors or on more or less complex enzymatic mechanisms.
- Narcotic analgesics have an effect on specific receptors located at central and peripheral levels.
- Mixed analgesics utilize both of these.

Local anesthetics are not a part of this classification.

Non-narcotic Analgesics

These are very numerous and most of them can be administered enterally. They can be classified in three groups depending on whether they have purely analgesic properties or those associated with anti-inflammatory and/or antipyretic effects:

Pure Analgesics

Floctafenine, clometacine, nefopam are three of these. This last molecule is becoming popular again in ambulatory and perioperative situations. Its mode of action is essentially central, inhibiting the recapture of sympathomimetic amines and serotonin.

Antipyretic Analgesics

Two of these are phenacetine and acetaminophen, amidopyrine and derivatives of noramidopyrine are being progressively withdrawn from distribution.

Anti-inflammatory and Antipyretic Analgesics or NSAIDs

These are ranked highly and find routine use in the treatment of many acute or chronic painful syndromes.

Narcotic Analgesics

These work on receptors that are physiologically activated by the endogenous ligands called endorphins. There are three categories of receptors: OP1 (μ), OP2 (d), and OP3 (k). The analgesic strength depends on their intrinsic activity, wrongly linked to the strength, and on the affinity of the receptors for these agents [1,5].

Agonists

Morphine is the agent of reference. This group comprises weak agonists, such as codeine and dextropropoxyphene and strong agonists, such as meperidine, morphine, fentanyl, and morphine/fentanyl derivatives. Strength is always expressed by reference to morphine whose analgesic coefficient is 1.

Partial Agonists

Here the connection with receptors sets off effects that are lower than the maximum biological effect. An example is buprenorphine.

Agonists–Antagonists

These have a varied actions on the different types of receptors; pentazocine and nalbuphine are examples.

Antagonists

These compete with agonists for receptors for which the affinity is strong. An example is naloxone, which antagonizes the effects of all morphinic medicines, with the exception of buprenorphine. These antagonists can cause a weaning syndrome in dependent subjects.

Administering Narcotic Medicines

There are several routes for giving narcotics, including oral, intravenous, subcutaneous, peridural, intrathecal, and transdermal. Oral administration should be the preferred method. Intravenous administration is used when quick titration is desirable before switching to oral delivery.

Other methods are acceptable when it is impossible to administer orally(e.g., dysphagia, vomiting, somnolence) or when side effects are too strong.

The technique of analgesic control by the patient (PCA), first introduced for treatment of postoperative pain, has now been applied to cancer pain, by either intravenous or subcutaneous route.

The coefficients of conversion for proper dosage of morphine are: oral or rectal = 1; subcutaneous = 1/2, intravenous = 1/3, peridural = 1/10, intrathecal= 1/100.

Undesirable Effects of Narcotics

- Constipation, the treatment for which rests on the prescription of laxatives, physical exercise, and appropriate diet
- Nausea, vomiting (30 to 40% at the beginning), which can be neutralized with metoclopramide (Reglan, Wyeth, Madison, NJ, USA; Motilium)
- Sedation and somnolence, properly treatable only by reducing the dosage
- Urinary retention, requiring catheterization and treatment with an anticholinesterase agent
- Respiratory depression is exceptional, but requires appropriate ventilatory therapy, often accompanied by a trial of naloxone

Mixed Analgesics

These substances work at once through morphine-like mechanisms and on the other systems of transmission and pain control. For instance,. tramadol works both like a weak μ agonist and like an inhibitor of the serotonin recapture.

Co-analgesics

Psychotropic medicines (such as anxiolytics, neuroleptics, and tricyclical antidepressants), antihistamines, and corticosteroids are often included in the treatment of acute or chronic pain in order to decrease the dosage of analgesics [1].

Neuroleptics

These medicines have a limited use in the treatment of pain, even in cases where a sedative treatment and an anti-emetic treatment are desirable.

Anticonvulsants

Carbamazepine (Tegretol) is a treatment used for pains of deafferentation with algic paroxysms, such as neuralgia of the trifacial nerve and post-shingles pain.

Gabapentin (Neurontin) seems to work on neuropathic pains, particularly in the case of allodynia to cold.

Clonazepam (Klonopin, Roche, Basel; Rivotril) is used in the treatment of neuropathic pains without paroxysm (drops are easier to modulate and are preferred for the elderly).

Benzodiazepines

These are the group of tranquillizers characterized by their anxiolytic, myorelaxant, and anticonvulsive as well as hypnosedative action. The use of benzodiazepines is justified as a treatment for the anxious component and/or an attempt to effect myorelaxation.

Antidepressants

These are used to break the vicious circle: pain-anxiety-depression-increased pain. And they have specific analgesic properties that appear faster than the antidepressant effect (3 to 5 days or less instead of 14 to 21 days). This analgesic effect is due to a reduction in the recapture of serotonin, dopamine and noradrenaline.

Antidepressants are particularly prescribed in neuropathic pains, in small doses.

Corticosteroids

In cancers, corticoids reduce edema and peri-tumoral inflammation, and consequently the compression of connected structures. In spite of their anti-inflammatory action, they are less effectual than NSAID on bone pain. They often stimulate the appetite and give a feeling of well-being, and sometimes of euphoria.

They are appropriate in advanced cancer in high doses, especially for a medullar compression, a blockage of the vena cava, a blockage of respiratory tracts, carcinomatous lymphangitis (for instance, 240 mg of solumedrol per day for a week, slowly decreasing). They are co-analgesic in pains due to intracranial hypertension, nerve compression, hepatomegaly, pelvic tumors, articulatory metastases, and malignant pleural invasion.

Myorelaxants

Spasms of the skeletal muscle sometimes occur due to nerve complications or direct irritation from a tumor. An effective medicine is diazepam (Valium 2, 5, 10 mg), but somnolence, sometimes due to build-up of the drug because of faulty elimination, must be guarded against.

A New Concept: Rotating Opioids

Definition

In the case of certain stubborn pains, morphine, even in increasing doses, seems to become ineffectual and/or to bring about some unacceptable side effects (deliria, hallucinations, somnolence, myoclonia). After having eliminated the metabolic causes, the secondary localizations (metastases), the way of administering is generally changed, but the molecule itself can also be changed. One can replace an opioid by another, then come back to the previous one before side effects appear. Such is the definition of the rotation of opioids.

Pharmacological Basis

As with any other product, responses to the various opioids differ among patients as well as in one patient over time. Two hypotheses are offered to explain the advantages of the rotation strategy:

- One rests on the belief that each opioid molecule has a different intrinsic activity on each receptor among the various families of μ receptors.
- The other rests on the idea that an accumulation of the metabolites of morphine is significant in the appearance of, among other undesirable effects, myoclonia.

Products

These are the agonists of morphine, including meperidine (phetidine), hydromorphone, methadone, fentanyl, oxycodone, and hydrocodone. In France, we are in the process of making up lost time regarding the prescription of these products for pain. Fentanyl patches are not that recent and, with the exception of a few limited centers, methadone is only prescribed in substitution treatment for drug addicts.

The index of conversion is the following: 1 mg of hydromorphone = 7.5 mg of morphine; 1 mg of oxycodone = 2 mg of morphine; 25 μg/ per hour of transdermal fentanyl = 40 to 80 mg of morphine.

Conclusion

When oral administration is preferred, rotating opioids is a therapeutic alternative in the treatment of cancer pain that, for one reason or another, responds poorly to morphine alone.

Non-medicinal Therapies

Peripheral Analgesic Stimulations

These are symptomatic, not etiological treatments of pain. The techniques were developed from the gate-control, or inhibiting control theory; they are techniques of counterstimulation. The methods are external, non-invasive and simple. [4]

Transcutaneous Neurostimulation

Notable in this technique is the miniaturization of the equipment, allowing a continuous stimulation. It is appropriate for:

- Neurological pains such as those accompanying or following lesions of peripheral nerves, which include amputation sequelae as well as shingles, peripheral neuropathologies, postsurgical sciatica.
- Non-neurological pains such as posttraumatic and chronic rheumatic pains.

Factors that favor a good prognosis for this technique:

- Pain that is topographically limited
- Fixed, nonradiating pain
- Pain with limited intensity
- Good cooperation of the patient

Acupuncture

There are two models for acupuncture. The classical model uses the Chinese points and meridians, the yin and the yang. The modern reflexotherapeutic model uses the cutaneous, subcutaneous, muscular painful points, and the nerve course (projected pains).

Treatment modalities are varied: simple puncture, manual stimulation of the needles, electro-acupuncture.

Physical Techniques

Cryotherapy, thermotherapy, vibrotherapy, electrotherapy, massage, immobilization, and settings, tractions, and manipulations of vertebrae are among the techniques used.

Pain Surgery

Techniques that Break into the Paths of Pain

A direct surgical approach has progressively been replaced by less invasive as well as more selective techniques:

- Percutaneous neurolyses and sympatholyses (destruction of skeletal and sympathetic nerve fibers) done under ultrasonography, scanography, or stereotaxy:
  - Local anesthesia required
  - Patient cooperation needed in locating the target
  - Neurolytic agent pure alcohol
- Thermocoagulation allowing neurolysis with the heat induced by an electrode in contact with the target nerve
- Posterior rhizotomy, the oldest (1889) and least-used technique
- Anterolateral cordotomy

Techniques of Retro-pain Control

These rest on the neurostimulation of peripheral nerves, the spinal chord, or sensory cerebral nuclei through surgical implantation of a stimulator. Indications are:

- Incomplete posttraumatic peripheral nerve lesions
- Partial lesions of the brachial plexus
- Amputation pain
- Pain due to incomplete paraplegia
- Thalamic syndrome with a painful anesthesia (deep cerebral stimulation)

Intracerebral and Intrarachnoid Narcotic Therapy

This treatment is appropriate for chronic pains that don't respond to major analgesics dispensed in a traditional manner.

Interventional Radiology

Thanks to the progress of technology, there are now many indications for use of these techniques, the main ones being:

- Infiltration and neurolysis of the sphenopalatinal ganglion
- Neurolysis of the mandibular nerve
- Neurolysis of the stellate ganglion
- Thoracic sympatholysis
- Neurolysis of the celiac plexus
- Neurolysis of the sympathetic interiliac plexus and of the unpaired plexus
- Infiltration of the pudendal nerve
- Infiltration, block, or ablation of a nerve root
- Treatment under TDM control of osteoid osteoma
- Radiofrequency ablation or tumoral alcoholization
- Acrylic cementoplasty under scanographic control

Cognitivobehavioral Approach to Chronic Pain

Concept

This is an analysis of the role of various psychosocial factors, having in mind a modification of the behavior they determine:

- Appreciating the various components of the painful behavior
- Evidencing how such behavior is fostered or increased by environmental or personal factors
- Investigating techniques of relaxation, biofeedback, systematic desensitization, stress management, modification possibilities for reinforcement activity, behavioral approach
- Modifying maladapted mental processes, factors involved in an increase in the perception of pain and of its affective-emotional concomitants (anxiety and depression): cognitive approach

Indications

These are twofold:

- When behavioral manifestations are exaggerated in comparison with the somatic data
- When psychological factors play a determining role in the genesis or the continuation of a pain (i.e., chronic sciatica, stress cephalgia)

Evaluation

This rests on the use of behavioral scales.

Techniques

As in every psychotherapeutic approach, the patient must be the main one directing the process; therefore it is advisable to:

- Strengthen his/her motivation (reformulating representation(s) of pain)
- Set precise, realistic, and limited goals
- Establish a therapeutic contract between the patient and the therapist (stop seeking other opinions, carry through the prescribed tasks)
- Start techniques of relaxation (e.g., Jacobson, Schultz, biofeedback, hypnosis), the objective being a relaxation response to the established patterns of "sensation of pain/loss of control," "stress/painful response"

- Insure a control over important factors: reinforcing behaviors adaptive to pain, avoiding stress, fighting inactiveness, facilitating a return to work
- Integrate the family circle in the therapy

Pain Centers

History of Pain Centers

Industrialized countries have been taking an interest in pain for almost six decades; but for economic rather than ethical or philanthropic reasons. Dozens of millions of dollars were dropped each year in the USA and in Japan because of lost work days due to lumbago and other chronic illnesses. Treating only the sensory dimension of pain was a failure. As described earlier, John Bonica was the founder of the first Pain Clinic [4]

Motivation

Financial Aspect; Insurance Companies

In the United States in around 1934–1936, chronic pain became a center of interest for the financial groups behind insurance companies. They came up early on with the idea of sponsoring physicians in order to get involved in fighting these chronic pains, whose benefit payments were significantly penalizing. They quickly realized the validity of their approach when they noticed that they were recovering their outlay; their expenses for sick leave had gone down by 50 to 90%.

Technical Progress

In the 1960s, Wall and Melzack (1965) formulated a theory on pain, regarding its propagation through nerves as well as inhibiting medullar controls. This theory (which for the most part proves today to be accurate) finally allowed a better understanding of the physiology of pain.

In the 1970s, neurochemistry advances, particularly those of Guillemin, allowed discovery of the receptors of morphine (which had been known for many years, but not their mode of action).

In the 1980s, the moral aspect appeared: the "right to health" and the "refusal to suffer" are slogans that carry sufficient social weight to pose a real problem.

Pain Physicians

Traditionally, pain physicians have come to disturb the organization of medicine; by defining chronic pain as an entity, they introduce a "transverse break" in the order of traditionally vertical specialties and question the current distribution of recognized clinical conditions, and therefore of the patients. It has remained for these practitioners to convince the medical milieu of the new clinical approach. [3]

Not sure of how to present pain as the subject of their efforts, they begin by talking about the management of cancer pain, though it is far from being the main part of their practice. But cancer pain can easily take the role of a legitimizing tool. Every hospital has become aware of their "claim of usefulness."

That is how pain doctors were, and still are, variously heard, depending on the degree of seriousness enjoyed by their original departments and on that they've been able to acquire personally. Whether the development of pain consultation as part of the more or less routine evaluation and treatment of patients is to become recognized depends a lot on the tenacity and (at least in the first generation) the status of the initiators of such a plan. Pain centers are thus both very progressively and very slowly being put in place in hospitals, a niche that is all the more limited in that the occupying physicians play only a modest role in the function of the institution.

As far back as 1951, John Bonica, a resuscitator and anesthesiologist, faced with the pains of wounded GIs, and working together with John White, a neurosurgeon, brought various specialists into a multidisciplinary organization, thus founding the first Pain Clinic in Seattle. The multidisciplinary approach was set as a requirement from the start and has since become a kind of dogma. In a specific management structure, pain does not belong to a specialty, whatever might be considered the regular practice of medicine. This notion had already been put forward by Leriche, who was too far ahead of his time to be lastingly effective. John Bonica solidified the goal he envisioned by founding the International Association for the Study of Pain (IASP) in 1974, which gathered researchers and physicians, as well as psychologists who were not physicians, around the study of pain. A year later he founded the magazine *Pain*, which to this day remains the voice of the IASP.

The Situation in France

The bill of June 1997 specifies that it is necessary to identify these pain-treatment structures. It defines three organizational levels according to the following criteria:

- The general practitioner of a patient with chronic pain must supply a consultation request to the pain-management unit
- The unit must have at its disposal qualified, competent medical personnel with appropriate technical equipment
- Besides the physical means of and care offered by the unit, a management center must exist with its own hospital beds(or some put at its disposal) and the wherewithal to provide teaching and research [4]

This bill establishes the mission of an institution, with its reference team and their relationship with professionals as well as with the whole population in the area they serve. Structures labeled as pain centers must act as moderators of a network they form with other teams in the area. Authorities at the state level make the last decision as to what funds will be allotted to the various substructures (pain related or others).

In each institution, an elected medical commission must have a committee for pain management put in place. Pain management must also be included in the clauses of the contracts signed jointly by the institutions and the State Hospital Agencies, stating the means and objectives pertaining to the quality and safety of health care.

Initial Consultation

The patient must be referred by his family doctor or by a hospital department. It is fundamental to be able to have at one's disposal clinical and para-clinical elements, to be used as elements of basic knowledge and comparison.

The essential contact with the patient is established on the first appointment. The physician must also receive a letter from the family doctor, with whom he should be in touch on a regular basis. The pain physician becomes the patient's personal doctor, in charge of coordinating all aspects of his care.

The consulting physician will become the coordinator of the medical file. His role will be:

- To re-evaluate the diagnosis
- To perform a complete History and Physical Examination and to become thoroughly familiar with the medical record
- To confirm the organicity or non-organicity of the pain
- To track down existing claims, the possibility of a material compensation, the functional character of the pain, all the while knowing that the aching moan can be modified by anxiety, anguish or by ethnic factors;
- To assess behavioral repercussions while taking socio-cultural factors into account that can play the role of a filter or of an enlarger
- To re-evaluate treatment already given
- To evaluate the intensity of the pain (essential) as well as the relief brought by the pain management already established

The consulting physician is not to take the place of the family doctor or to multiply existing specialized consultations. We have at our disposal subjective measuring tools that use one-dimensional scales (visual analogical scale, simple verbal scale, numeric scale) and questionnaires covering the sensory-discriminatory, affective-emotional, and cognitive components of pain.

Possible Perverse Effects of These Centers

These centers can be a part of other specialized networks, in particular those dealing with cancer and palliative care [2].

A first mistake is to think that these structures must handle all aspects of pain management within the institutions. The media, as well as political and administrative decision makers often disregard the idea that acute pain management does not have to depend exclusively on pain management structures.

A second mistake is to let ideological reasons or insufficient multidisciplinary means lead to dealing with pain according to a single pattern. Pain management requires more from physicians that just listening or being available.

A third mistake is to favor therapeutic empiricism. Structures must therefore undergo an ongoing evaluation. This evaluation must compare therapeutic actions, measure objective and subjective changes in the patient, and analyze the financial impact; these structures, however, must refuse to be judged solely on their profitability.

A fourth mistake is to deal with chronic pain solely within pain structures. These can only be efficient if they work together with various medical specialists as well as have their own specialists trained in pain management. Ideally such a structure includes an anesthesiologist, a rheumatologist, a psychiatrist, a neurologist, a physical therapist, a radiologist, and a neuro-surgeon.

Pain centers must be acknowledged by other specialists. They share a common ethical goal, which consists in thinking that medicine must relieve a man's suffering, not fix a body. If medicine is the science of the body (of a certain body), it is, unfortunately, not always the science of human beings.

A Government Plan

Supervising authorities must publish a list of institutions, to be followed by an identification of structures. This identification is an integral part of the French government's tri-annual plan for the fight against pain. This plan was a real progress. It was followed by a quadrennial plan, which expanded the original one and came up with these precise goals: improving pain management after surgery, managing pain in children, and treating migraine.

Some significant shortcomings are still present in spite of the progress made over the last 10 years. Summit meetings on pain are therefore held to raise the awareness of professionals and citizens in favor of a pain management plan better suited to the needs of the population and to sensitize public opinion to the national program for the fight against pain.

This project is supposed to spark off nation- and state-wide actions aimed at rallying the various actors within the health care system. It must also involve local and state authorities through debates sensitizing them to the fight against pain in order to bring together all the actors from civil society and to rally local communities.

France used to have a lot of ground to make up in the area of pain management, but it has largely caught up: a comparative study of 15 Western European countries shows it to be the only one to implement government plans, and the only one to make the teaching of pain management a mandatory part of a physician's initial training.

Broadening the Set of Problems

While the Pain and Palliative Care clinic may do a good job of managing end-of-life suffering, it might not do so for, e.g., pains subsequent to shingles, for stubborn rheumatological pains, for disabling cephalgia of ten-years duration, for algodystrophia after a routine operation or everyday accident, for recurring postoperative sciatica, for disabling cervico-brachial neuralgia, for paraplegic pain, or for a vascular facial pain.

As life expectancy increases it can be expected that in upcoming years more and more pains of the senior patient will have to be dealt with. Nosocomial and iatrogenic pains, often unavoidable in operations and therapeutics, can also be expected to require increased attention in the future.

It is likely that the consideration given all these pains will change once the number of wasted days, of consultations, of physical therapy sessions, of additional examinations, of trips by ambulance, of disability rates, and of grievances and trials are tallied.

Conclusion

"What's new today?" the attending physician asked the intern. "Oh, nothing," the younger man answered, "but, oh yes, by the way, that malingerer died last night."

Medicine has too often reduced suffering to a physical occurrence by focusing on a function or an organ. This reduction has undoubtedly been a effective for certain problems. But we cannot forget that man is immersed in a cultural group (reference and value system) and a social group (way of life, life system, ecology, etc.), not to mention the imaginary dimension that binds any group and any relationship of an individual to the world. Moreover, we live in a multicultural society in which numerous social groups coalesce. An individual is not interchangeable among such groups, but lives within a particular system of meanings, values, and representations.

Managing pain requires the combination of an act of faith, an act of listening, and an act of discernment. Pain tests the relationship between the patient and the physician. That relationship is made up, above all, of belief, trust, and loyalty. Does the physician believe the patient when he (or she) says he is in pain? Isn't there a suspicion of exaggeration when the claim is made that, in spite of treatment, the pain still exists?

Since pain doesn't follow "Pasteurian" reasoning (given pain, given cause, given treatment), does the physician reconsider the diagnosis and ask himself or herself what might lie behind the "I'm hurting"?

The ability of the physician to extricate the patient from pain and from his or her customary share of anxiety and depression depends on his way of identifying, reading, and interpreting it. For that purpose there is only one avenue to follow: to listen. Not to be heard is to be negated in one's identity, in everything that is built within oneself for oneself and for others. It is a retreat to square one; it is to be left without a defense or an answer. The patient may have seen his claim to pain negated. That offence must be admitted by the physician before he can try and fix his body.

References

Fergane B, Collin E, Krakowski I, Pichard-Leandri E (2001) Stratégie face à une douleur cancereux, in Douleurs aigues, douleurs chroniques, soins paliatifs CNEUD, CNMD, SFAP. Module Med Line 6:209–230

Lauren B, Boureau F, Krakowski I (2002) Les structures d'evaluation et de traitement de la douleur chronique rebelle. Douleurs 3:267–275

Lefay A (1992) La douleur. Approches pluridisciplinaires. L'Harmattan, Paris, pp 143–155

Serrie A (2002) Organisation de la prise en charge de la douleur, in La douleur en pratique quotidienne. Diagnostic et traitements. Ed. Arnette, pp 1–29

Viel E, Classification of Analgesic Agents. Correspondances en Médecine No 2, vol 3, pp. 52–54

Pain and Psyche

Clinical and Therapeutic Aspects

2

Blandine Kastler, Jean-Georges Rohmer

"If I could moan like dogs, I would go off into a wide plain or deep into the forest and I would howl for hours; I think it would be a relief." (Guy de Maupassant)

Introduction

Pain is an integral part of medicine with its philosophical notions, its scientific ventures. It has a cultural, a religious, a social and a political dimension. Chronic pain is a major public health problem, as 20% of the people in the general population suffer from it. The terms of suffering are very restrictive to express pain, whatever forms it has, be it exquisite, sharp, acute, chronic, mental, organic, or functional.

Pain is defined as a physical or mental suffering (Larousse dictionary), a painful sensation in some part of the body (Robert), a physical suffering, or a suffering which is to the soul what physical suffering is to the body (Littré), suffering being defined by this last author as a painful sensation that goes from a simple feeling of discomfort to pain. The definition of pain has become international. The International Association for the Study of Pain (IASP) has adopted Merskey's: Pain is an unpleasant sensory and emotional experience, associated with a real or virtual tissue damage or described in terms of such a damage.

By this definition, pain is no longer defined from the perspective of the physician, but from that of the patient. The physician no longer needs to use his knowledge in order to look for an organ or a tissue lesion. He must listen to the moan and to what the patient says about it. This definition is important because it does away with the differences between an organic, a functional or a psychogenic origin. It restores the psyche and the human moan, forcing the radiologist, the surgeon, the pain specialist to ask him/herself a question that is simple but has an authentic clinical meaning: "Where does it hurt?"

We psychiatrists don't know pain, we only know the words that express it: "I am hurting, it is horrible, I can't do anything any more, I am apprehensive, I am suffering, do something, help me, nobody can do anything about it any more, etc."

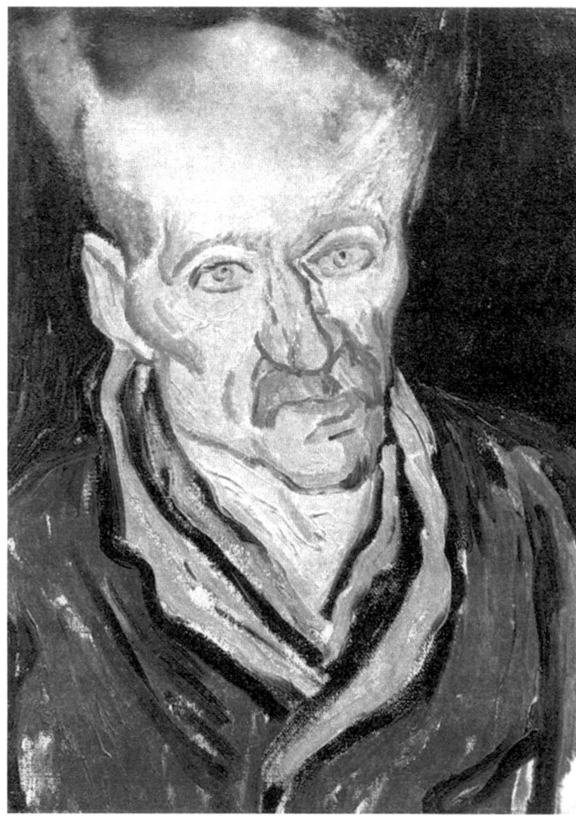

Fig. 2.1. Van Gogh, portrait of a sick person at the Saint-Vincent Hospice, 1889

The only pain we relieve each day is psychological pain, mental pain, madness with its hallucinations and its painful anguish (Fig. 2.1).

Currently there are two trends in the response to pain as it is defined by the IASP.

- The first refers to American material, with a therapeutic option, and which is mostly cognitive and behavioral: it essentially addresses stress factors and the socio-familial context. Intra-psychological conflicts are ignored in favor of environmental factors.

Table 2.1. Diagnostic criteria of "F 45.4. Pain disorder" (DSM IV R)

A pain in one or several anatomical localizations is at the center of the clinical picture, and this pain is intense enough to justify a clinical exam. The pain is at the root of a clinically significant suffering or of an alteration of a patient's functioning in a social, professional or any other significant area. Psychological factors are considered to play a significant role in the setting off, the intensity, the worsening or the persistence of the pain. The symptom or the deficit is not produced intentionally or feigned (as in a fake disorder or in simulation). Pain cannot be better explained by a mood disorder, an anxious disorder or a psychotic disorder and does not correspond to the criteria of dyspareunia. Specify the type: [307.80] Pain disorder associated with psychological factors: it is considered that psychological factors play a major role in the setting off, the intensity, the worsening or the persistence of the pain (if there is a concomitant general medical affection, it may not play a major role in the setting off, the intensity, the worsening or the persistence of the pain). One does not make a diagnosis of this type of pain disorders if the criteria of a somatization disorder are also present. Specify whether: [307.89] Pain disorder associated with psychological factors as well as with a general medical condition: it is considered that psychological factors and a general medical condition play a major role in the setting off, the intensity, the worsening and the persistence of the pain. Code the associated medical condition or the anatomical localization of the pain on axis III (see below). Specify whether: Acute: lasting less than 6 months. Chronic: lasting 6 months or longer.

- The second refers to psychoanalytical concepts that rely on more European material and address psychopathology in the light of psychodynamic function.

However, beyond petty quarrels and in spite of completely dissimilar approaches and investigations, some common points appear, even though described with different words.

Current Nosologic Aspects

The diagnostic and statistical handbook of mental disorders (the "Bible" of American psychiatrists) preferred the word pain disorder in its latest version (DSM IV R; Table 2.1), abandoning the words psychogenic or somatoform pain of previous editions (DSM III R)

Pain disorder is a broad diagnostic category, devoid of precise clinical elements. All chronic sufferers can belong to this diagnostic category from the moment that pain can be blamed for "a clinically significant suffering or for an alteration in functioning." The presence of a psychological component in every chronic pain can no longer be questioned.

These chronic pains are generally low back pain, abdominal or pelvic pains, cephalgias, or diffuse muscular pains. In the US, low back pain is the number one cause of visits to the general practitioner's office and the number two cause of sick leave.

There are few correlations between the felt intensity of a pain and its physiology. If we look at lumbar MRIs done on subjects free of all pain-filled moan (please see Chap. 1 for a discussion of "moan"), we find significant lesions in 30 to 40 % of the cases. Conversely, we find few discal or vertebral lesions that can explain the intense pain felt by chronic lumbar pain sufferers and that have serious repercussions in their daily life. Diagnosing a psychogenic pain remains difficult and subjective.

Chronic Pain Syndrome

I will use the definition given by F. Bourreau (1988, 72): "We will use the term chronic pain syndrome (CPS) to describe the set of physiological, psychological, behavioral and social symptoms which tend to make us look at persistent pain, regardless of its original etiology, more as a 'sickness in itself' rather than as the mere sign of an underlying physiopathological disorder. This syndrome can be observed in various degrees in pains with a different initial etiology: migraines, lumbar pains, neurological ailments and sine materia psychogenic pains, etc. There is no doubt that the symptoms of CPS include disparate and still imperfectly compiled physiopathogenies. The advantage of referring to such a syndrome is, above all, due to its operative worth in common practice."

The option of treating a syndrome without worrying about etiology is not a standard practice in medicine. The more common thinking is that we then run a risk of making erroneous evaluations that can lead to therapeutic errors. Acute and chronic pains are quite different entities that cannot be addressed in similar ways, and although we are limiting ourselves to chronic pains here, let us point out that in the case of acute pains differentiation between organic and psychogenic etiologies is quite common.

The psychological repercussions of a pain with an organic etiology or a pain with a psychogenic etiology, even if there is a local irritative spot, cannot be confused; they come under essentially different psychopathological mechanisms. How can we confuse the psychological dimension of a cancer pain, the thorny problem of lumbar pain, the sensory hallucination of the hypochondriac and the spasmic pain attacks of prepsychotic illnesses?

These different pathologies must be addressed separately, and, even if there are certain common points in how they are dealt with therapeutically, one will have to decipher the meaning of each patient's pain-filled message and its specific function in relation to the underlying psychopathology.

This approach leads to dealing with the person as a whole as well as to a multidimensional element amounting to a criticism of classical medical management as insufficient and classical psychiatric management as inappropriate. Indeed, managing chronic pain sufferers as well as all psychosomatic patients requires an adjustment of the therapeutic approach in which neither the body nor the psyche are neglected, and in which one must agree to start from the symptom in order to proceed.

In conclusion, I will say that not taking factual and environmental factors in the chronic pain sufferer into account is certainly an error, but not taking the psychopathology and the intrapsychological factors into account is one as well. I think one cannot avoid taking the etiological dimension into account, even if it must be qualified by reinforcement factors.

In order to keep the advantages introduced by the notion of the chronic pain syndrome while limiting its disadvantages, I suggest that we distinguish two big groups:

- A chronic pain syndrome with a dominant organic component
- A chronic pain syndrome with a dominant psychological component

Chronic Pain Syndrome with a Dominant Organic Component

Either in the course of a serious illness or of surgical or other traumatic aftereffects, a strong organic pain if not relieved can lead the patient to withdraw, reducing his/her involvement, and finally making him/her freeze into an antalgic withdrawal attitude. The anxious patient is on the lookout for the painful attack, the over-invested painful zone becomes his/her only concern; the anxiodepressive context takes precedence. Life stops and is only punctuated by painful attacks – any plans, any anticipation become impossible. The subject becomes anxious and depressed because of hurting in his or her body.

We physicians find ourselves confronted with death anguish within the context of palliative care. Besides organic pain, another mechanism can generate anguish and depression.

Indeed, at the time of any serious illness, the patient perceives a change in the markers defining one's course through life. The picture one has of oneself, one's place, one's role are suddenly called into question. The individual must sometimes adapt to a new cerebral body diagram, and beyond that the body picture is changed, too. The various factors on which one's identity is based are disturbed, as are relationships to family and friends and to reactions to events. Destabilized, the subject is no longer him or her self. This more or less sudden break causes anxiety and sometimes depression.

Psychological assistance will help the patient find new markers on which to lean; it will help this individual mobilize the resources inside in order to rebuild a new, hopefully more accurate picture of himself or herself. Destabilizing factors will also have to be pinpointed and formulated. Adapting to the illness or the handicap, restoring the psyche will thus need to be fully worked through, a process we've come to call "working out sickness."

The patient will have to progressively reinvent this modified body that is betraying him/her in order to make it one's own again, to formulate one's anguish, to put one's experience into words and to express one's suffering. For, if this suffering remains impossible to express, to formulate, it will manifest itself in other ways, in particular in pains, but now of a psychological kind. Now, the patient experiences pain because he or she is anxious and depressed. Thus, with an organic pathology, the moan can indicate:

- An organic pain that requires the use of analgesics
- A psychological pain due to facing illness or is a manifestation of a reactionary depression and requires a psychological approach, as medicine cannot fill the need for words and reassurance
- An anxious call for help directed at the medical team, and in which the request for pain relief can become the favored means for communicating in place of expressing the anguish

The physician will therefore have to be able, at the time of each moan, to evaluate where the request is coming from and not to respond systematically by prescribing analgesics under the assumption that the cause is organic. A patient is sometimes seen who is receiving large doses of medicine but still without effect; the temptation may be to keep increasing the dose. However, if the psychological dimension were better heard, not only might the patient be calmed down but the original doses reduced – provided of course that the organic pain is properly evaluated (overafferentation or deafferentation) and treated.

The patient can naturally be expected to face each attack with his or her own personality, reactions, and way of relating, giving the pain-filled moan its specific aspects, but that does not change the principle etiological factors.

A favorable evolution will allow restoration of oneself after an attack, a redefinition of place and role with one's new, modified body. But the evolution can also drift toward a worsening and a psychological decompensation. The original somatic pathology will then serve as a fixation point, as a mnesic trace upon which the anguish will be unloaded. The body symptom will remain a point of emphasis, but it will be understood in this case that the problem lies elsewhere. The physician must decode the hidden suffering, the conflict that cannot be verbalized and allow the subject to finally express that which can't be put into words, but inscribes itself in the body.

The symptom(s) can be functional or associated with a lesion at the time of somatization; in the two cases the underlying psychological aspects will be different. In all cases, however, it is no longer the pain itself that is on the front burner, but the way in which the patient talks about it and presents it. The relational dimension of the pain is what must be taken into account before anything else.

Chronic Pain Syndrome with a Dominant Psychological Component

In this type of pain syndrome, we can distinguish two different populations of patients, those who have:

- Centrifugal pains, a means of expression intended for others that penetrates relational exchanges and permeates family life, that encourages everything in the environment to revolve around it. Suffering becomes a way of being in the world that translates into a call for help, that cannot be formulated differently, as well as a subconscious way of manipulating or tyrannizing one's family circle. This relational type can naturally only exist with the conscious or unconscious complicity of relatives and friends, who often also find it perversely beneficial even as they denounce the situation and seem to suffer from it. In fact, they often contribute to reinforcing it. The social and familial place of the subject can be defined by his/her pain.
- Centripetal pains, which are no longer really a means of expression intended for others, even though the pain is omnipresent. It, too, is a way of being in the world, but now in the dynamics of a narcissistic withdrawal. Suffering shown this way functions as a support for a feeling in the subject that existence is faltering. Pain comes and eases the unspeakable suffering of failing to be, and helps one to survive.

Naturally, these two types of population require different forms of management.

Let us now see whether it is possible to distinguish specific clinical entities. It is classically acknowledged that all personality types can be encountered, from ordinary neurosis to psychotic decompensation, through psychosomatic patients. Everything can indeed be encountered. However, some characteristic profiles appear more frequently than others. First of all, the association of pain and depression is unanimously recognized, but in the context of organicity depression is the consequence of pain, while with these patients it is its cause. In certain cases, it appears quite obvious that the depressive aspect, presented as secondary, has in fact preceded the outbreak of the symptom, without having been identified or named as such by the patient.

When the thymic side of depression does not come out clearly, pain is a "depressive equivalent," a "masked depression." One can encounter reactionary as well as essential, melancholic, or other depressions. And yet even though the association is very common, there are pain-filled chronic patients who exhibit no depressive syndrome.

Let us now distinguish in the history of the patient the way in which the illness has appeared.

Pains Within the Context of a Factual Crisis

At the time of the first consultations, in telling his or her story the patient refers, consciously or not, to an event or a series of events perceived as traumatic. What is important is the way in which the patient describes the event, the emotional reactions or, conversely, lack of reaction and the fact that a spontaneous connection is made between the event and the pain. Three types of circumstances are encountered particularly frequently.

Reactional Depressions

Here, the intensity of the event does not allow the subject to face it. The suffering cannot be formulated and manifests itself in the body. The somatic dimension often predominates and the subject is not necessarily aware of a depressive state; the functional pain testifies to the depression. The person can be relatively well balanced without a clear psychopathology. In this type of pain, the prognosis is usually good, and short treatments are a good course of therapy.

Pathologies of Bereavement

Complicated bereavements have given rise to numerous articles, and it is surprising that this type of pathology is quoted so seldom by pain specialists, considering how very frequent it is. Depression again predominates, even if it is hidden, but now the psychopathology is always present. However, the intensity of the regression and of the underlying disorder varies, going from neurosis to melancholy.

In all cases, pain has a defensive function in relation to the task of mourning and protects against a true suffering. Therapeutic work will consist in allowing the task of mourning and the formulating of this pain into a suffering. It is precisely the opportunity to express this suffering, to share it, which will allow one to free the enclosed object and to start the act of representation anew.

Let us not forget that there is not necessarily a parallel between the significance of the loss and the magnitude of the reaction. The latter depends rather on how much the patient is invested in the object or the situation. Some event, apparently benign to an outside observer, can be a source of major decompensation; a typical example is the death of a pet dog for some persons who live alone.

Post-Accident Pains

Other frequently encountered pains are those appearing after physical injury, often referred to a post-traumatic illness. There is no parallel between the significance of the trauma and the magnitude of the reaction; some accidents out of which the subject comes unharmed can lead to catastrophic decompensations. The decompensation has nothing to do with the event that set it off, even if it refers to it. The event that is truly important is different from the one that can be detected in the words; it is older and connected to the emotional history of the subject.

In the specific case of the low back pain sufferer, a subject who is often hyperactive, and who decompensates after a trauma, even if it is a mild one, one notices that the hyper-investment in the painful zone replaces the hyper-investment in activity. It shows that these patients establish narcissistic relationships. Sometimes decompensations appear through mere immobility, made necessary by the accident, as the patient is unable to fight a rising anguish over the lost usual hyperactivity.

Here we encounter some post-traumatic neuroses and pessimisms with a paranoid decompensation structured around a claim in a persecutory context, but also some true traumatic neuroses.

Thus, the pain specialist may not fail to acknowledge that, at the time of certain accidents that appear as the organic cause par excellence, psychological etiology is present, that it sometimes precedes the accident, and that the painful aftereffects, picking up the psychological aspects, will be a part of the logical continuation of the evolution. Such a scenario is almost predictable, and from the first an appropriate management should include systematic preventive treatment aimed at avoiding decompensations, and which would incidentally have a definite impact on overall cost of treatment.

Pains Within the Context of a Progressive Worsening

These include chiefly hysteria and hypochondria, both of which can be accompanied by a depressive state, but not necessarily; most of the time anguish is the dominant factor. We have already talked about pains as depressive manifestations; different mechanisms are paramount here.

Pain and Hysterical Neurosis

In his studies on hysteria, Freud showed that physical pain takes the place of mental pain. Pain expresses in the body what cannot be expressed otherwise, in the form of either anguish or depression. Moans, psychogenic algias, hysterical conversions are functional pathologies that affect the relational life and the locomotor system. Paresthesias, hyperesthesias, various spasms lead to functional pains associated with handicaps. Painful hypertonias can be significant. These manifestations can be accompanied by other manifestations that are specific to a typical hysterical personality with hyperemotionalism, theatricality, and eroticization of the relationship.

Here, the symptom that is connected with the intrapsychological conflict is given a meaning in an oedipal aspects. However, we must not forget that symptoms with a hysterical appearance can be encountered in other personality structures.

The body manifestations of anguish, the various algias, are usually located in the visceral areas and accompany other neuro-vegetative reactions: oppressions, cardiac, and respiratory functional disturbances. These pictures can also be encountered in hysteria, as well as in anguish neurosis and many anxious disorders.

Pain and Hypochondria

Hypochondriac manifestations are real sensory hallucinations that preferentially affect the deep areas of the body. Anguish takes over the cenesthesia ("body sense"), which becomes painful, thence to mobilize the patient's full attention. The problematics here is more narcissistic and challenges the body. These states can be encountered in neuroses, but they also take on a more delirious aspect in borderline states or psychoses, particularly in the well known Cotard syndrome.

Within the context of these functional pains, we cannot fail to mention pain as an alternative to pleasure and masochistic problematics in which aggressiveness and guilt are meeting. If some patients describe horrible pains with a radiant face from which pleasure is scarcely missing, we also hear incredible accounts of the skills and style of persecuting each other, as a couple or as a family.

In pain treatment, we see many couples that function in a sadomasochistic mode. Pains and moans are inexhaustible, but the steadfastness in perpetuating the unhappy union is unshakable. Let us not forget, however, that even if we are irritated by such a patient's ceaseless moans, we are dealing with real suffering with which the subject is struggling the best (s)he can. Within this context, we also see failure neuroses in which the subject persists, quite unconsciously, in ruining his/her life.

Pains and Somatization

These are sometimes likened to each other, and some authors mention a psychosomatic personality within the context of chronic pains. Currently, theories regarding somatizations are not unanimously approved, and yet archaic problematics are always brought into play. In an existential approach, it is thought that pain lets us know our body through the body experience (in accord with the existential reality of a presence and of an actualization of oneself).

Pain and Psychoses

Psychoses also can express themselves through algias. More specifically, in identity and undelineated body image disorders, in almost noiseless schizophrenic dissassociative psychoses, and in paranoids who structure themselves around a claim within a persecutive context; and let's not forget melancholia.

It is consequently very difficult to define the population of chronic pain sufferers. (In France, for example, no serious epidemiological survey has been undertaken. Not to mention the way in which the patients are usually recruited, which completely distorts statistics.)

Indeed, some consultations come directly from a medical specialty (rheumatology and neurosurgery come first to mind), and such specialists may treat one single type of pathology (center for the treatment of migraine) and draw specific populations.

The more general centers have their own specificities, too. They generally select seriously ill patients, those who have trouble healing. Others are treated upstream by GPs and other specialists; they never get to us, having already recovered.

Moreover, some centers preselect their patients and do not admit those whose psychological dimensions are either too significant or obviously psychiatric. These patients are directly referred to psychiatrists and do not show up in the statistics of pain management centers.

Conclusion

How can we suppose that hurting can bring benefits? And yet … As we've seen, a psychogenic pain can be the expression of a wound and it sometimes protects from more menacing suffering. Thus, as opposed to what some say, chronic pain sometimes performs a defense function with real protective worth for the subject. That does not, however, mean that it should not be relieved. One must simply be careful and not try to make it go away; the use of morphinic drugs in such a case is disastrous, for it increases the psychological disorder. Moreover, besides the primary benefits that caused the symptom, pain often allows secondary benefits of a psychological nature. These include:

- Obtaining rewards that cannot be expressed, particularly in the case of a dependence
- Giving shortcomings and consciously unacceptable claims a respectable excuse
- Creating a living space for oneself, sheltered from an invasion of privacy
- Letting go of one's social mask without being a failure
- Allowing an avoidance, the handicap offering a shield from certain situations that cannot be taken on

Finally, the characteristics that are specific to the psychopathology of chronic pain sufferers do not prevent us from finding certain common traits:

- A never-filled need for attention
- An immaturity and an excessive dependence on the family circle, even if this regressive need is sometimes denied, pain then becoming the "alibi" that explains everything
- An underlying aggressiveness that can be significant
- A particularly frequent separation anguish
- The presence of a narcissistic flaw where pain acts as a personal and relational support (in fragile patients)

Early emotional deficiencies are found in high proportion in the population of chronic pain sufferers (corroborated in epidemiological surveys) as are antecedents of bodily violence (by accident or abuse), a lack of physical reward, and a lack of pleasure-causing enjoyable sensations.

All these characteristics will give the therapeutic relationship a particular tinge, occasionally causing some relational difficulties in which the defense mechanisms of the patient as well as of the physician can work toward perpetuating the disorder.

Decoding what is happening when the painful moan is heard, thwarting unconscious manipulations, aggressive or seductive attitudes, is then fundamental. The therapist will also have to take into account the relational role of pain in the couple or the family, if one does not want the next-of-kin to engage in an unconscious sabotage as soon as a symptomatic improvement occurs.

We still have to mention patients putting us in check by telling us right away that they have consulted the greatest professors and even the most expensive ones and that none of them has been able to relieve their pain. Then, don't even go trying, it's a lost cause! The only possibility here may be to play the game of therapeutic non-intervention and to use a few consultations to analyze these failures. But that is already doing psychotherapeutic work. Almost invariably, the patient manages to say at some point that medicine is incapable of treating him/her and that no relief is expected by having taken this step. It is then sometimes possible to change the course of things by bringing the patient to ask him or herself what is actually being sought. What drives you to come here anyway?

In all cases, to be a pain specialist is to offer the chronic pain sufferer an attentive ear to the moan, consultation after consultation, even while putting us in check. Of course, there can always be some mixed cases in which organicity and psychopathology are equally significant. It will suffice, in fact, to treat one and the other at the same time; which still does not mean confusing them.

Psychiatric Co-morbidity and Chronic Pains

Classic psychiatry considers the psychological aspects of chronic pain in terms of co-morbidity: it studies the presence or absence of psychiatric disorders defined by diagnostic criteria.

Major depression seems to occur in subjects suffering from chronic pain with a frequency of between 15 and 55%. Dependence on alcohol or on another psychoactive substance occurs in 15 to 23% of the cases, anxious disorders in 7 to 63% of the cases.

There also seems to be a strong co-morbidity between the disorders of axis II of the DSM-IV-R and chronic pain. Chronic pain sufferers are often histrionic, dependent, narcissistic, or borderline personalities.

Depressive symptoms are the psychological symptoms most often associated with chronic pain. A consensus establishes the prevalence of a major depressive episode at about one third of the chronic pain sufferers coming to consultation. The model of psychogenic pain as a depressive equivalent rests on the idea that chronic pain belongs in the spectrum of emotional disorders.

Psychotherapeutic Treatment

The various forms of psychotherapeutic treatment depend on the theoretical approach of the practitioner but also on the patient's request. Forms of psychotherapy include:

- Cognitivo-behavioral therapy
- Body therapy (Schultz's autogenous training, relaxation)
- Couple, family, and group therapy
- Biofeedback
- Psychotherapy with a psychoanalytical inspiration
- Support psychotherapy

These therapies were studied by Americans, who wanted to objectivize the improvement of the results obtained by the various psychotherapeutic techniques, in order to insure their coverage by private insurance companies.

Pain appears to be a psychosomatic symptom par excellence: it requires the whole person to be addressed, and is aimed at calming pain as well as hearing and relieving suffering. It is necessary to allow the person to express him or her self, with his/her means at the time, under accessible conditions and to lead the way to formulation of a true request.

Patient management should occur within a unit of time, of location and that of a team thus avoiding the body/psyche dichotomy. The body dimension should never be neglected even if the etiology is psychological. If we are to maintain trust, the patient must feel from the beginning that the somatic complaint is being fully acknowledged.

A multidisciplinary approach allows a refining of the diagnosis. The various specialists, shedding different lights, allow us to better grasp the various components of the patient's distress. Moreover, considering the complexity of some diagnoses, such a plan protects against an always possible therapeutic error. It is then much less likely, for example, to impose psychotherapy on a patient with a purely organic problem. Hence, psychiatric diagnosis must be undertaken on precise elements whose investigation runs parallel to the organic diagnosis and treatment, and not after failure of medical therapy (made then, for instance, as a diagnosis of exclusion).

Most of the time, a psychiatric consultation brought in as a last resort reinforces the defenses of the patient who feels misunderstood and rejected, perhaps rightly so, and compromises the psychotherapeutic approach. Trust can be brutally broken by the fateful phrase, "There is nothing wrong with you." Of course there is something wrong with this patient, but this "something" often does not interest medicine.

Way too many patients get lost between medicine, which rejects them, and psychiatrists, who are inaccessible to them. That leads us into a therapeutic impasse. We should direct ourselves to avoiding the traps of medical outbidding, as well as to the struggle of the patient between somaticians and psychiatrists, who sometimes send him or her back and forth without organizing any coherent treatment. Adding a psychological approach from the beginning need not cause any split with the somatician.

Finally, all the while looking for the etiology, the probing of pain does not have to be done according to a linear pattern of understanding. And it is necessary at once to address:

- The synchronic dimension, looking for both the offsetting and the aggravating factors in the current situation
- The diachronic dimension, looking for the factors of vulnerability in the subject's history

As a first step, a nonspecific psychological approach must be introduced by the pain specialist from the first consultation on, regardless of the type of pain. This will greatly help in averting the body/psyche dichotomy and the subsequent resistance on the part of the patient to consulting the psychological team. The role of the psychiatrist in the multidisciplinary team should be:

- To avoid diagnostic or therapeutic medical outbidding, as well as iatrogenic risk
- To listen to the moan and hold the anguish in check
- To reveal the main factors that are found at the forefront
- To insure a psychological accompaniment for organic patients, when it can be done without any particular difficulty

Chemotherapeutic Treatment

Psychotropic drugs (antidepressants, neuroleptics, benzodiazepines, thymic regulators such as lithium carbonate) have proved effective in the treatment of both acute and chronic pain.

Antidepressants and Pain

As we have seen, depression and pain often go hand in hand and the prescribing of antidepressants has a very positive effect on the depressive syndrome as well as on the pain itself.

A recent meta-analysis of 39 studies controlled against a placebo yielded objective statistical data. The conclusion was that antidepressants were efficient antalgics, showing that 74% of the patients treated with these products for light chronic pains experienced an improvement, as compared to the placebo.

Rules for Prescribing Psychotropic Drugs

- Inform the patient about the prescribed drug, its indications, its dose, its side effects, and the effectiveness that can be expected.
- Treat with an effective doses for a sufficient period of time (antidepressants).
- Respect monotherapy as far as possible.
- Exercise caution and watch out for side effects.
- Recognize the great importance of individual receptibility.

Products in Use

Imipramine (Tofranyl), the first antidepressant to be commercialized, was offered in the treatment of pain syndromes two years after the interest of using it for depressive syndromes had been evidenced. Since then, other tricyclical antidepressants (in particular amitriptyline) have been used by numerous practitioners in order to treat patients with chronic pain syndromes of either a benign or malignant origin.

Main Indications

- Neurological pains, in particular pain of peripheral neuropathy: diabetic and other neuropathy, post-shingles neuropathy, phantom pain
- Cephalgias: migraine, stress headache, psychogenic headache
- Facial algias
- Rheumatological pain:, rheumatoid polyarthritis, ankylosing spondyloarthropathy, and rachidian pain, chronic lumbar and other back pain
- Neoplastic pains
- Pains in gastroduodenal ulcers

One will also have to take into account the presence of:

- Depressive syndromes
- Anxious conditions, panic attacks
- Social phobias
- Obsessive-compulsive disorders (OCDs)

Five positive aspects are recognized in the co-prescribing of antidepressants: an increase in the effectiveness of the other prescribed analgesics, a decrease in their dosage, a delayed use of opiates, and an improvement of the psychological condition.

Table 2.2. Antidepressants used in the treatment of pain

Medicine	Initial Dose mg	Maintenance Dose (mg/day)	Indications for use	Therapeutic Concentration (ng/ml)
amitryptiline	25 × 1 or 2 daily	50–300	Depression, chronic pain, migraine, sleep disorders	60–200[a]
amoxapine 1>	50 × 2 or 3/daily	100–600	Depression	180–600[a]
bupropion	50–75 × 2 daily	300–450	Depression, attention deficit	50–100[a]
clomipramine	25 × 3 daily	100–250	Depression, compulsive obsessive disorder, panic disorder	200–300[a]
desipramine	25 × 1 to 3 daily	50–300	Depression, panic, attention deficit	125–250[b]
doxepine	25 × 1 or 2 daily	75–300	Depression, chronic pain, gastroduodenal ulcer, irritable colon syndrome, sleep disorders	110–250
fluoxetine	20 × 1 daily	10–80	Depression, eating and compulsive obsessive disorders, panic disorder	–
fluvoxamine	50–100 × 1 daily	100–300	Obsessive compulsive disorder, depression, panic disorder	–
imipramine	25 × 1 to 3 daily	50–300	Depression, panic disorder	>180,[a], [b]**
maprotiline	25 × 1 to 3 daily	50–225	Depression	200–400[a]*
nefazodone	100 × 3 daily	100–600	Depression, compulsive, obsessive disorder [c]***	–

[a] Parent molecule and metabolite
[b] Well established monitoring of the drug treatment
[c] Little clinical data available

Mechanism

The effectiveness of antidepressants is related to their analgesic property, the mechanism of which remains to be defined; but which seems to due, among other possibilities, to a combination of monoaminergic and opioidic actions.

The analgesic effect could be explained as a thymoanaleptic or a sedative action, but also as specifically antalgic. A survey of studies on antidepressants revealed that 56% of them reported an anti-nociceptive in animals, which is considered to be experimental proof of antalgia. However, the mechanisms through which antidepressants might be likely to modify the pain-filled message have yet to be elucidated. The probable role of serotonin, which has a part in the inhibiting control of nociceptive messages and in depression, has been demonstrated. It is supposed to have a part in the potentiation of morphinic effects and in diffuse analgesic systems. It is understood that there are some mechanisms common to depression and pain, and considering also that serotonin and noradrenaline have roles in the mechanisms of analgesia, all antidepressants may be potentially analgesic and should be studied.

Therapeutic Modalities

Tricyclical antidepressants: amitryptiline (Elavil, Zeneca, London; Laroxyl), clomipramine (Anafranil), are currently the most widely used. Non-tricyclic antidepressants: mirtazapine (Norset), fluoxetine (Prozac), fluvoxamine (Luvox, Solvay, Brussels; Floxyfral) and other antidepressants that inhibit the recapturing of serotonin (SRI) are also potent and, above all, manageable; see Table 2.2.

For tricyclical antidepressants, whose leaders, again, are clomipramine and amitryptiline, the common dose is 10 to 15 mg at first, then a progressive increase in stages up to 150 mg. It can take up to 4 weeks for one of these drugs to become effective.. Treatment can therefore be stopped as ineffective only after this period of time.

Monitoring the treatment is particularly justified for tricyclical antidepressants whose most common undesirable effects (dry mouth, constipation, orthostatic hypotension, shaking) can lead the patient to stop the treatment. More serious problems, particularly coagulation problems and urinary difficulties, can result in necessary discontinuation.

The inhibitors of the recapturing of serotonin paroxetine (Paxil, SmithKline Beecham, Brentford, UK; Deroxat), fluoxetine, fluvoxamine and (sèropram (Celexa, Forest, New York) are easy to use and don't evidence the contraindications of the "old" (tricyclic) antidepressants, or their side effects. They can be prescribed at the rate of 1 to 3 pills per day, with daily doses usually beginning at 20 mg.

Neuroleptics and Pain

Neuroleptics were discovered in 1957 and were defined by their anti-psychotic action and their extrapyramidal effects. As is well known, they are mainly used in psychotic conditions, particularly schizophrenia. Classic phenothiazine neuroleptics chlorpromazine (Thorazine, SmithKline Beecham; Largactyl), thioridazine (Melleril), and levomepromazine (Nozinan) have shown some antalgic power and thus are occasionally used in chronic pains. Fowley recommends combining morphine and one of the phenothiazines in the treatment of cancer pains. These old neuroleptics, however, have serious undesirable effects, principally extrapyramidal, that limit their use to minimal doses. Currently, a new class of neuroleptics has appeared on the market, referred to as "atypical antipsychotics," that have nothing in common with the phenothiazines. They are olanzapine (Zyprexa), rispéridone (Risperdal), clozapine (Leponex), but no study of them pertaining to pain has been reported yet.

Tranquilizers and Pain

These are mainly benzodiazepines known for their anxiolytic, hypnotic, myorelaxing properties. They have been frequently prescribed by GPs for various reasons, but no study has shown them as significant in the management of chronic pain syndromes, although they work essentially on anxiety, often associated with this type of pathology. They have several drawbacks, self-medication, with a risk of dependence, of causing disorders of memory when prescribed over a long period of time, of an alteration of slow deep sleep, and above all a significant withdrawal syndrome when stopped suddenly.

We recommend, if they have to be given in order to control anxiety, that they be prescribed on a short term basis, informing the patient of the limits of the prescription. We prefer using non-benzodiazepine anxiolytics such as bromazepam (Lexomil) and alprazolam (Xanax).

Hypnotics and Pain

It is sometimes judicious to prescribe hypnotics (sleeping pills) in a selective and limited manner in order to help people sleep. They are always prescribed on a short term basis, while waiting for the regulating effect of antidepressants on sleep disorders, and they can be quite effective at the beginning of the treatment. The best currently appear to be zolpidem (Ambien, Sanofi, New York; Stilnox) and zopiclone (Imovane). Their advantage over others is a reduced predisposition to dependence and withdrawal syndrome.

Anticonvulsants and Pain

The searing component of some pain syndromes is similar to the epileptiform discharge of nociceptive neurons recorded in animals. In this regard, the anticonvulsant carbamazepine (Tegretol; Novartis Pharma SA, Paris) has been found to have undeniable effect in acute pain syndromes of a neuralgic kind. Effectiveness of anti-epileptics has likewise been seen in various deafferentation pains, e.g., post-shingles pain, painful neuropathy, painful aftermath of medullar lesions. Tegretol seems more effective and is much better tolerated than lithium. Sodium valproate (Dekapine; Depacon, Abbott, Chicago) and clonazepam (Klonopin, Roche, Basel; Rivotril, Roche) have been subjects of studies regarding acute and chronic pain syndromes. These molecules have also been offered for the treatment of cancer pains and in the long term treatment of vascular cephalgia.

This type of compound must be used with caution and monitored since effectiveness has yet to be fully explored, drug interactions have been reported, and other side effects have been seen.

Sociotherapeutic Treatment

Before ending this chapter, emphasis must be placed on the quality of life of these patients, and on society's obligation to acknowledge their suffering. This is where the prescription of a cure at a spa comes in, which will surprise some, but in difficult cases can offer certain advantages:

- Isolation from the family circle
- Atmosphere of relaxation and rest
- Multiple and regressive body treatments, baths, massages
- Significant therapy on a daily basis

With good psychological preparation at the start, there are sometimes spectacular improvements, even when the prognosis is gloomy.

Compensation in the case of post-traumatic pains due to accidents at the workplace. comes within the scope of a reparation, which is often therapeutic for the patient. It also may avoid "iatrogenization" of pain disorders, since multiple consultations can sometimes lead to an endless claim, perhaps a trial in court.

- Physical therapy offers either verification or refutation of the painful body syndrome. PT allows a better knowledge of the body and its limits, of muscle tensions, of painful spots; and it offers, via a medium of bodily sensations, an approach to psychotherapy.

- Programs and courses (called "back pain schools" in France) directed toward chronic pain can teach patients the physical actions and postures to be adopted in order to minimize pain; such education can thus provide help and support for improving the quality of each day's life.
- "Parallel" pain management strategies such as acupuncture and mesotherapy, to name but two modes, may also bring awareness of the psychological component of pain disorders.

References

1. Blumer D, Heilbronn M (1982) Chronic pain as a variant of depressive desease: the painprone disorder. J Nerv Ment Dis 170:425–428
2. Bonica JS (1990) The management of pain, vol I and II. Lea and Fehiger
3. Fischbain DA (1999) Approaches to treatment decisions for psychiatric comorbidity in the management of the chronic pain patient. Med Clin North Am 83:737–760
4. Fischbain DA, Cutler RB, Rosomoff HL et al (1997) Chronic pain associated depression antecedent or consequence of chronic pain a review. Clin J Pain 13:116–137
5. Kaplan HI, Sodock BJ (1990) Synopsis de psychiatrie. Masson, Paris
6. Senon JL, Sechter D, Herrmann RD (1995) Thérapeutique psychiatrique

Computertomography-guided Percutaneous Interventions

General Information, Tips and Hints for Optimization of Guidance Techniques

Bruno Kastler, Marc Couvreur,
Jan Fritz, Philippe L. Pereira

3

Introduction

As magnetic resonance (MR) imaging is not yet widely available for interventional purposes (see chapter 20), computertomography (CT) represents at present the best imaging guidance technique in numerous interventional procedures [1–5].

The precise anatomic delineation is one advantage of CT that allows excellent distinction between musculoskeletal structures, fat, soft tissue, and vascular structures fairly easy. In addition, using CT the placement of interventional devices can be visualized and guided step by step leading to increased precision. Furthermore, the risk of traumatizing sensible structures such as vessels, nerves, lung and pleura, gut, or bone that may be identified on the needle pathway can be minimized.

Owing to the high spatial resolution and the good tissue contrast, it is possible to place precisely and safely needle and trocar tips on target, and lytic agents or anti-inflammatory drugs can be delivered with high reliability. This results in significantly reduced morbidity (lower than 2.5% out of 756 interventions [6]) and improves the effectiveness of the various interventional procedures. In certain procedures where real-time imaging is necessary a combination of CT and X-ray fluoroscopy may be interesting [7].

In this chapter the general approach of CT-guided interventions will be described and *proven* strategies and guidance techniques for successful interventional procedures are discussed [1, 2].

Patient Preparation

All interventional procedures are obligatorily preceded by a consultation a few days prior to the procedure (at least 24 hours). Detailed patient history is necessary to rule out contraindications to the procedure. It also helps to establish patient's confidence through individual clear and simple explanation of the course of the procedure. The patient is informed on the possible rare complications of the procedure and consent should be obtained[1)]. Prior to the procedure intravenous access is obtained, and as for any CT examination that includes injection of iodinated contrast media, physiological saline solution is connected in parallel during the entire procedure. The patient is placed on the examination table of the CT-Scanner by the technician in the most comfortable and technically optimal position for the particular procedure. The CT-scan table is set at its lowest level (in order to allow positioning of instruments in the gantry opening). Prior to the intervention it is mandatory to recheck the general precautions.

A review of the patient's complete blood count and blood chemistry is necessary. Special attention is given to the hemostasis parameters thromboplastin time (international normalized ratio; INR), partial thromboplastin time, and platelet count to rule out bleeding disorders. Contraindications for percutaneous procedures are: platelet count below 100,000/mm^3, thromboplastin time below 60%, and an INR of 1.4 or below. To ensure sufficient renal function blood creatinine is assessed. In case of hypersensitivity, anti-allergic premedication may be appropriate. The administration of hydroxyzine one day and one hour prior to the procedure proved to be efficacious in our institutions. It is important that the patient does not eat for a minimum of four hours prior to the intervention. In our experience a preliminary empathic conversation makes an important contribution to optimal cooperation of the patient and usually (except in particularly anxioux patients) no prior prescription of anxiolytic medication is necessary.

Intervention Room Preparation

Prior to each intervention, all surfaces (such as the CT-scan table and gantry) as well as the floor is to be cleaned and disinfected using aldehyde agents. The

1) Written consent should be obtained if applicable, depending on such regulations as may exist (not mandatory for France). We believe that written statements have a risk of negatively altering the patient–doctor mutual confidence relationship.

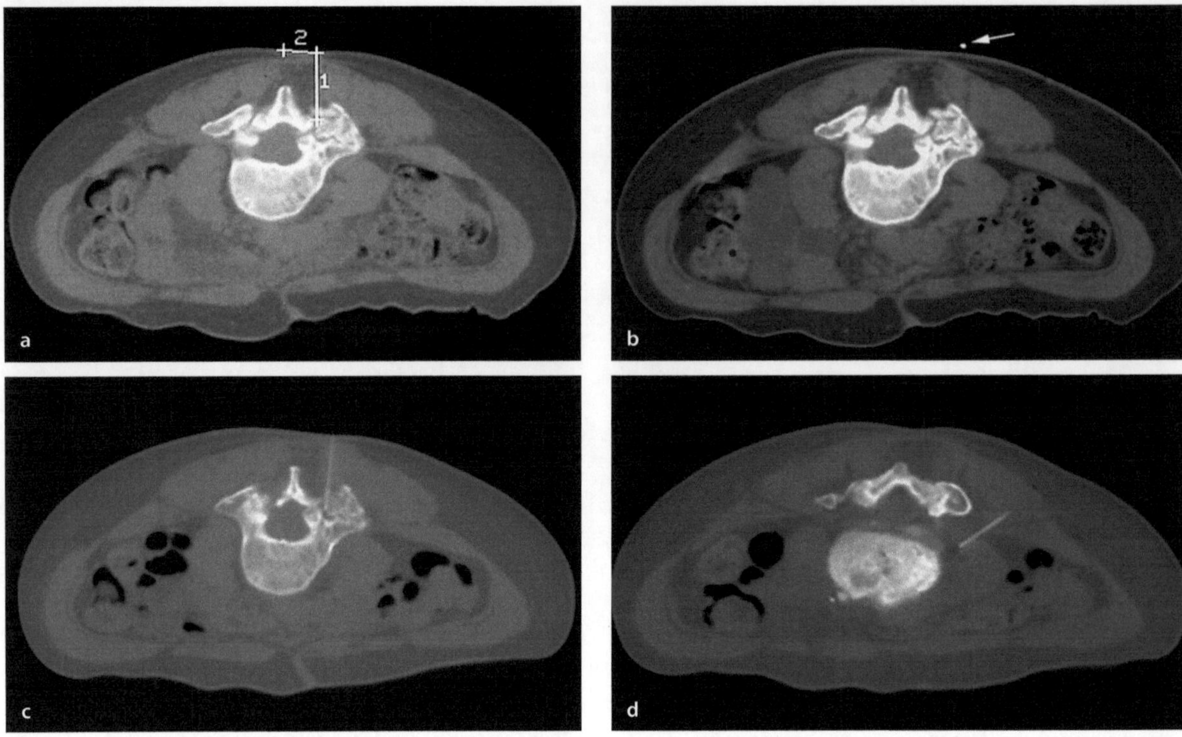

Fig. 3.1 a–d. Spondylolysis infiltration in a patient presenting with lumbar pain irradiating to the right side (also refer to chapter 5). **a** The distance between the midline (spinous process) and the skin entry point is measured on the monitor. The puncture point is determined manually by measuring the distance of line *2* starting from the palpable spine (spinous process). **b** A self-adhesive hyperdense marker (*arrow*) is used to visualize the point. **c** Using the marked point the needle can be safely placed. **d** Here a periradicular infiltration is also performed (also refer to chapter 4)

mobile stainless steel instrument table is covered with sterile sheets. The following items should be available:

- Syringes (2 ml, 5 ml, 10 ml and 20 ml)
- Hypodermic needle for local anesthesia
- Saline solution, anesthetics, and different volumes of ionized contrast medium. In addition to clear labeling, it is advised that a fixed arrangement be used in order to avoid confusion.
- Sterile pads
- A set of sterile sheets for interventional purposes
- Flexible or rigid 20 gauge therapy needles (22 gauge for neurolysis)
- Absolute (dehydrated) alcohol, long-acting corticosteroids, and/or possibly other agents, trocards or specific needles, according to the procedure.

Preprocedural Imaging and Planning of Percutaneous Approach

For procedure planning, images of a recent examination can be used. To increase the precision of navigation and to obtain specific orientation we, however, prefer to acquire an additional set of contrast-enhanced images of the anatomical area of interest at the beginning of the intervention.

Image acquisition with a slice thickness of 3 to 7 mm in the region of interest is sufficient. On the additional acquired image set the reference slice, assuring that the safest and shortest needle pathway is determined. It is materialized by drawing a line on the patient's skin with a felt pen along the projection of the laser light of the CT-Scanner. The skin entry point, the puncture angle, and the skin–target distance can be easily drawn, measured, and calculated on the workstation of the scanner (Fig. 3.1a). In the determination of the skin entry point, the spine is an invaluable reference because it can be palpated and lies in a median position in the majority of patients. Originating from the spinous process of the vertebra, a horizontal line of the predefined length gives one the skin entry point, which then can be visualized by sticking a self-adhesive hyperdense (see Fig. 3.1b) marker on the patient's skin. It is also possible to use the central laser pointer, which corresponds to the central line of the reference grid displayed on the image by the workstation. The correct puncture point is finally confirmed by the hyperdense signal of the needle centered to the skin entry point (see Fig. 3.1c, d).

Following careful surgical washing of hands and forearms the physician or technician ("interventionalist" shall be used hereafter) gets dressed with grown and surgical gloves. Betadine or some other disinfectant is used to clean the puncture site three times. Following sterile draping, local anesthesia is generously instilled at the skin entry point and presumed initial pathway.

Despite preprocedural imaging and the accurate visualization of the virtual needle pathway, in certain cases obstacles such as osseous structures may obstruct access to the target. Foremost, when passing body cavities the interposition of structures that imperatively need to be avoided (gut, vessels, nervous tissue, etc.) often do not allow an axial approach. Beside the possibilities of digital reconstruction and the inclination of the gantry, axial imaging represents an inherited limitation of computed tomography. In this situation MR imaging with its multiplanar imaging capabilities, easily allowing non-axial guidance, may be considered (see chapter 20).

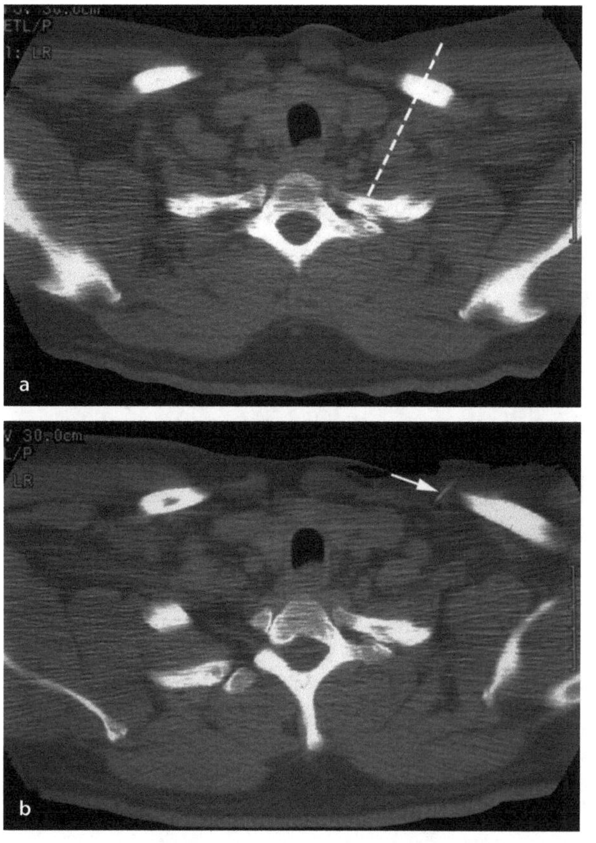

Fig. 3.2 a, b. Neurolysis of the right stellate ganglion (at T1 level), (also refer to chapter 10): **a** The interposition of the right clavicle prevents needle access (*dotted line*) between the cutaneous puncture point and the 1st rib. **b** The lowering of the ipsilateral arm and shoulder causes a caudal movement of the clavicle allowing the preferred needle path to be used without osseous interposition

Patient Positioning for Optimal Access

In addition to supine, lateral, and prone patient positions, which depend on the practiced routine in certain procedures, it can be useful to modify patient position in order to optimize access:

- In the prone position a cushion can be placed under the belly to reduce lumbar lordosis or to avoid the interposition of pleura.
- In the supine position a cushion can be placed under the thorax to widen intercostal spaces.
- In neck procedures the head turned to the opposed side allows better access to the puncture site, and lowering the patient's shoulder and arm avoids the interposition of the clavicle (Fig. 3.2)

Gantry Tilting

The craniocaudal or caudocranial inclination of the gantry enables para-axial image acquisition within a small range. It can particularly be helpful in cases of an initially obstructed needle pathway (Fig. 3.3) by uncovering a para-axial needle pathway that was invisible on initial strict axial images.

In a dyspneic patient referred for celiac neurolysis preprocedural axial images revealed the interposition of pleura preventing the posterior access to the epigastric plexus (see Fig. 3.3a, b). The inclination of the gantry finally enables a safe approach without traumatizing pleuro-pulmonary parenchyma (see Fig. 3.3c, e), and to carry out uneventful neurolysis (see Fig. 3.3d).

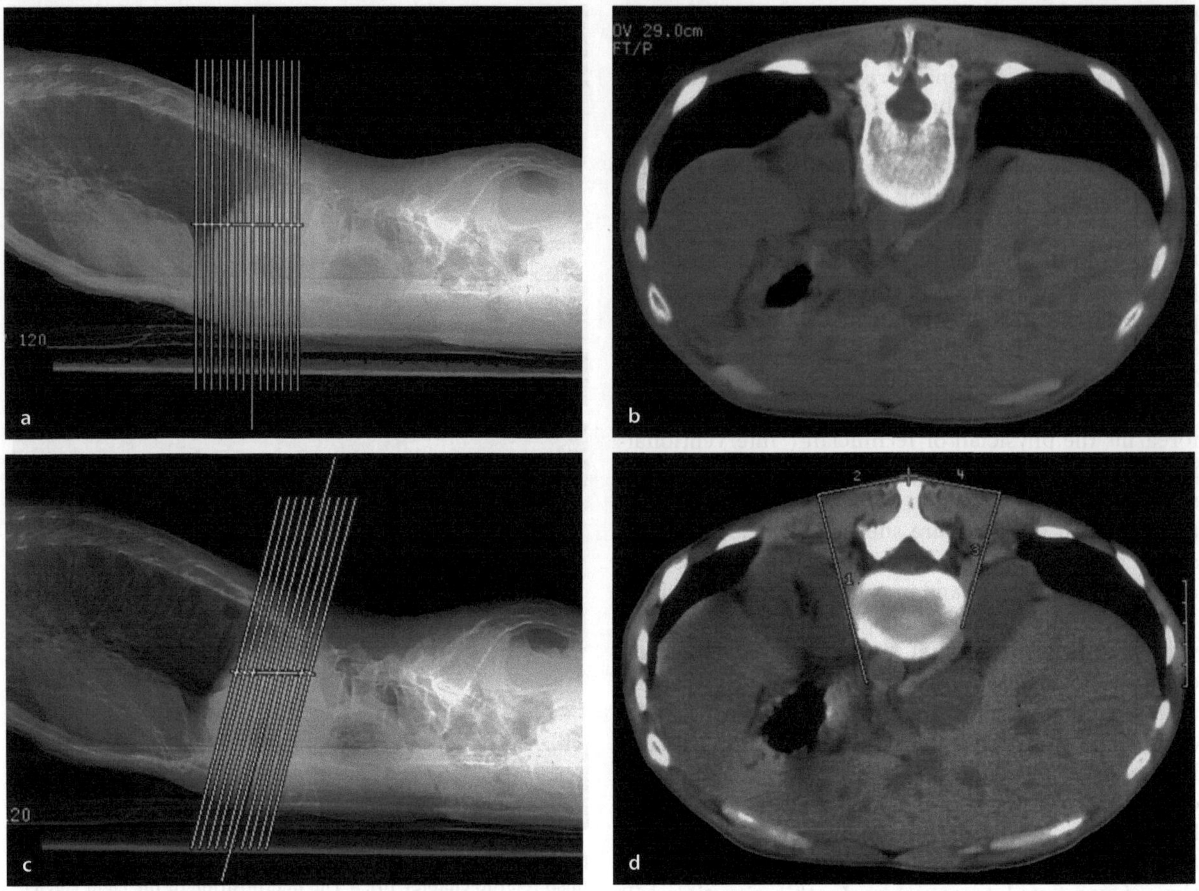

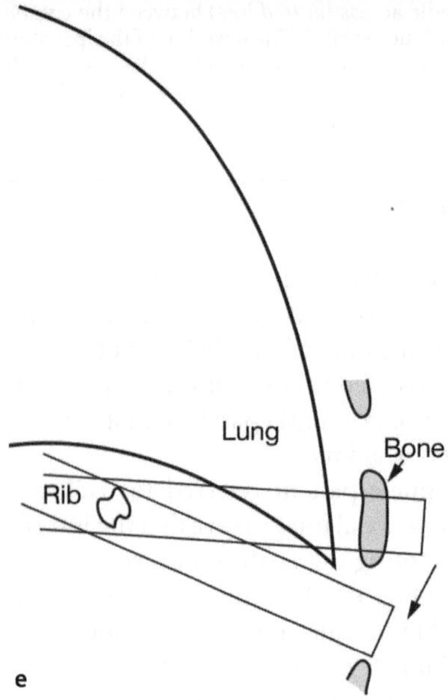

Fig. 3.3 a–e. Splanchnic and celiac neurolysis in a dyspneic patient (also refer to chapter 1): **a** Sagittal topogram: the strict axial orientated slices pass through the pleural space. **b** Corresponding axial CT image of interest through the origin of the celiac trunk: The presence of pleural cavity prevents the posterior access. **c** Sagittal topogram: the craniocaudal inclination of the gantry makes it possible to avoid the medial part of the pleural cavity. **d** Corresponding angulated CT image: The posterior access is now bilaterally possible without risk of perforating the pleural cavity. **e** Diagram clarifying the maneuver: The inclination of the gantry makes it possible to avoid the rib (*Bone*) and the pleural cavity (*Lung*) allowing safe access to the target (*Rib*)

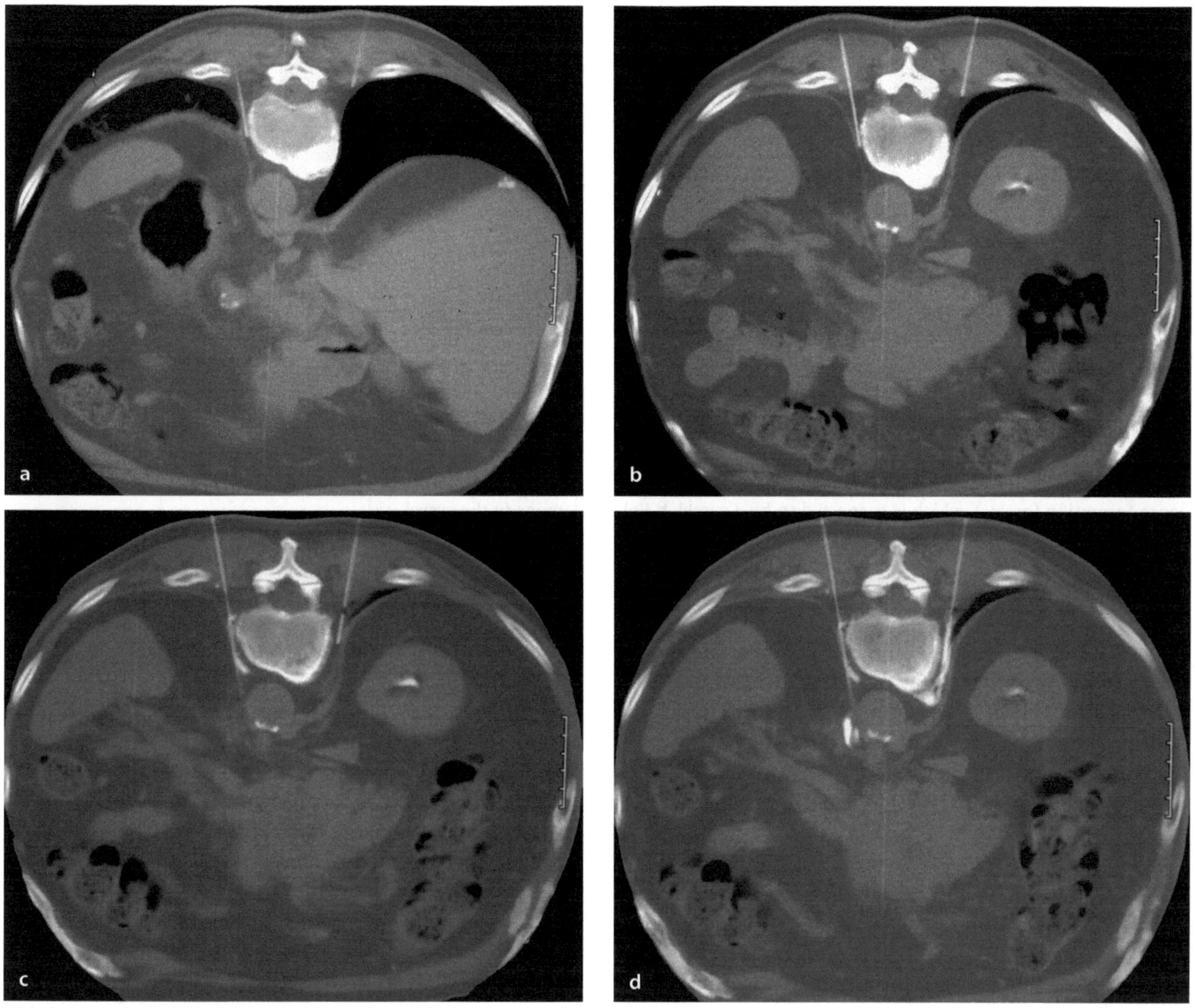

Fig. 3.4 a–d. Splanchnic and celiac neurolysis in prone position (also refer to chapter 11). **a** End inspiratory axial CT image. To get to the target, the needle pathway would in this case pass through both pleural cavities (more obvious on the right side). **b** Axial CT images in end expiratory apnea demonstrate the disappearance of the pleural recess (completely on the left side, and incompletely on the right side). Injection of physiological saline on the right side in order to widen the paravertebral region for a safer needle course. **c** Both needles go through the paravertebral region with no risk to injure the pleuropulmonary space. **d** The neurolysis is performed without complication

Utilization of Breathing

As known from diagnostic imaging. breathing of the patient can negatively influence image acquisition. The same is true for interventional imaging, however in certain cases an inspiratory or expiratory breath hold is an excellent maneuver to facilitate access to certain areas (if the patient is cooperative). Breathing maneuvers play an important role in pulmonary and abdominal punctures and are especially useful in some CT-guided neurolysis. Figure 3.4 demonstrates the dorsal needle placement for splanchnic neurolysis in end-expiratory apnea.

Target Localization and Visualization of the Needle Tip

Identification of Vessels

The potential presence of vessels on the needle pathway requires their exact preinterventional identification. For this reason repeated acquisitions of additional contrast-enhanced CT images may be useful. This is illustrated in the case of a neurolysis of the left stellar ganglion (at the level of C7; Fig. 3.5). The needle tip (identified by the tip artefact – see further on), is in the vicinity of a

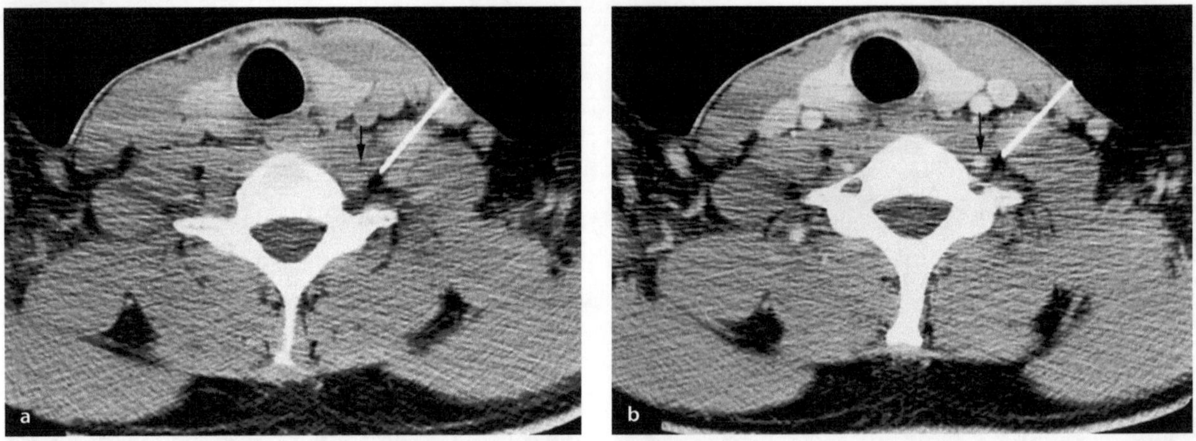

Fig. 3.5 a, b. Neurolysis of the left stellate ganglion in C7 (also refer to chapter 10). **a** the needle tip is in contact with a round hypodense formation (*arrow*), which is suspected to be a vessel. **b** Following the re-injection of contrast, the hyperdense signal of the structure nicely confirms the ipsilateral vertebral artery. Subsequently the position of the needle is modified in order to avoid damage to the vessel

structure similar to a vessel (Fig. 3.5a). Injection of contrast medium confirms that this structure corresponds to the ipsilateral vertebral artery (Fig. 3.5b). The needle pathway has to be reevaluated in order to position the instrument to avoid this vessel. This example illustrates how important it is to exactly visualize vascular structures.

Cross Reference Mark Localization Technique

Another possibility for locating crucial structures such as arteries is to permanently mark the structure on initial contrast enhanced images for comparison. This method is potentially less accurate but has the advantage of requiring no further contrast administration for imaging.

With this technique it is possible to locate target structure although it is not visible on axial CT images. The localization of invisible structures is estimated using anatomical structures (bone, muscles, or vessels) as landmarks. The lumbar sympathetic chain, for example, can be located anterolaterally to the vertebral bodies by the surrounding anatomic structures. Anatomical variations from one slice to the other, however, can sometimes impede this technique. Additional contrast images with dissimilar inclination may be helpful in accurately determining the location of the structure by comparing different views.

Neurolysis of the Mandibular Nerve (CN V_3)

For the neurolysis of cranial nerve V_3 (mandibular nerve) an axial transpterygoidal approach can be used (Fig. 3.6) with the patient's head turned to the contralateral side. The nerve is located inferiorly to the foramen ovale where it leaves the base of the skull. On this level, however, the foramen ovale is not visible anymore on axial images and thus does not serve as a reference mark. To achieve a permanent reference mark a digital permanent cross can be placed at the foramen ovale on the respective axial images (Fig. 3.6a). On inferior images the persistent cross can now be used for orientation. The needle tip can now be placed using a true axial approach (Fig. 3.6b).

Celiac Neurolysis

For celiac neurolysis, the target cross is positioned on the first CT examination, with contrast medium anterior to the abdominal aorta on the right side of the origin of the celiac artery. This region represents the most constant relationship to the celiac plexus. Contrast enhanced CT images are necessary to accurately demonstrate the vascular situation (Fig. 3.7a). In the case of reduced visibility during placement of the needle tip, the reference mark enables localization of the target structure without the additional application of contrast medium (see Fig. 3.7b). Thus, the procedure is not delayed and the renal function of the patient is not compromised by the injection of a large quantity of contrast medium.

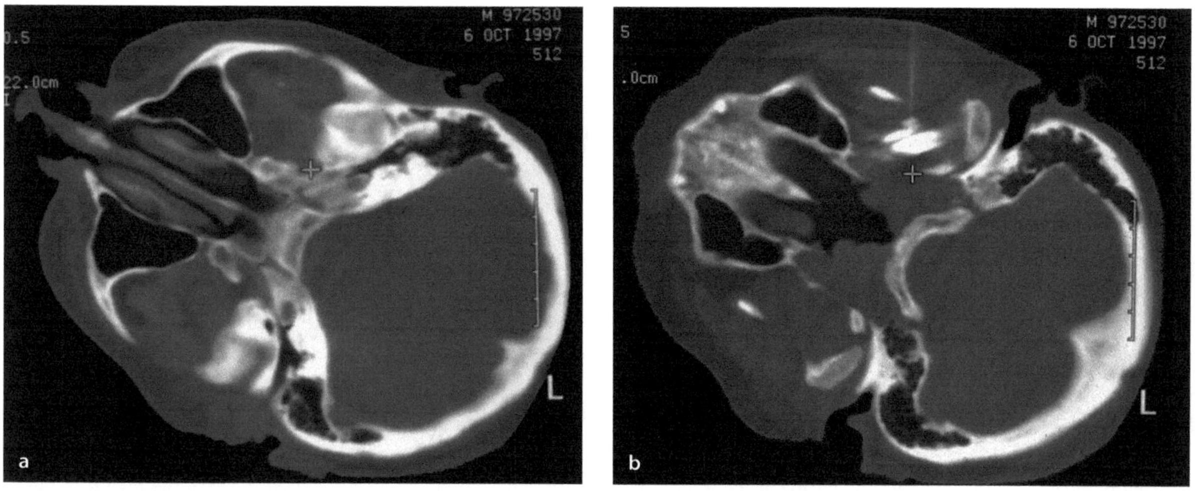

Fig. 3.6 a, b. Neurolysis of the right mandibular nerve (CN V_3). **a** Placement of the reference mark (*white cross*) at the foramen ovale. **b** The *cross* again indicates the location of the foramen ovale on an inferior image at which the needle tip is aimed

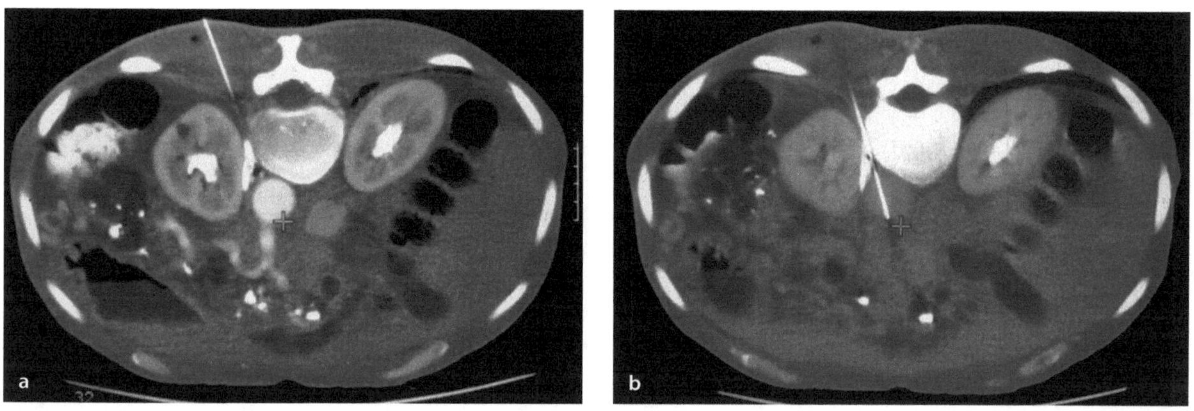

Fig. 3.7 a, b. Neurolysis of the celiac plexus (also refer to chapter 11). **a** Placement of a reference extravascular mark at the anteriolateral border of the abdominal aorta during arterial opacification: The *white cross* serves for orientation on images with less clearly visualized vessels (contrast media flushed away). **b** The reference mark at the identical level allowing to position needle tip anterior to the aorta at the celiac emergence. Note that a left splanchnic neurolysis was also carried out before penetrating the aorta (hyperdense mixture signal)

Needle-Target Pathway Angulation

The hypodermic needle used for local anesthesia can be used to estimate and verify the optimal angle of the *therapy* needle. After injection of the anesthetic agent toward the target, this anesthesia needle remains in place during further imaging. With this data the interventionalist gains relevant information regarding the puncture angle, the direction and the distance to the target. With this method less correction of needle position is necessary, which potentially leads to a straight and tissue-sparing puncture.

A hypodermic needle used for local anesthesia prior to neurolysis of the sympathetic chain at the L2 level can also be used as a guide. It is sufficient to introduce the therapy needle in parallel to reach the target located in the angle between the vertebral body (L2) and the psoas muscle (Fig. 3.8a). At the L4 level the therapy needle is introduced at a certain determined angle with respect to the anesthesia needle for access to the right anterolateral angle on, a more medial needle pathway (see Fig. 3.8b).

In addition, a reference line from the needle inserted at the skin level toward the target can be drawn on the monitor to estimate the orientation of the needle. This line serves as an extension that projects the needle tip according to the initial direction.Thus inapropriate needle orientation can be detected in advance and required corrections performed more easily (Fig. 3.9).

A coaxial technique represents an alternative approach that makes it possible to use a preadjusted puncture angle. Initially a large-bore needle used for local anesthesia is introduced with an exact direction to the

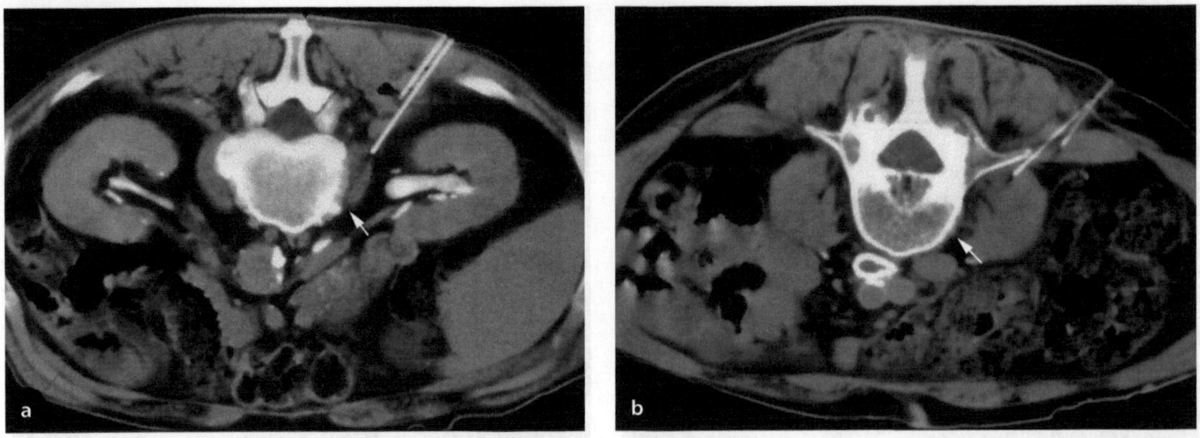

Fig. 3.8 a, b. Right lumbar sympatholysis. **a** A therapy needle is oriented parallel to a short hypodermic needle at the level of L2. The hypodermic needle was left in place to guide the therapy needle to the target: the anterolateral region of the vertebral body (*arrow*). **b** At the L4 level at a certain angle correction with respect to the anesthesia needle is required to reach the region of interest (*arrow*). This moreover allows to circumvent the transverse process

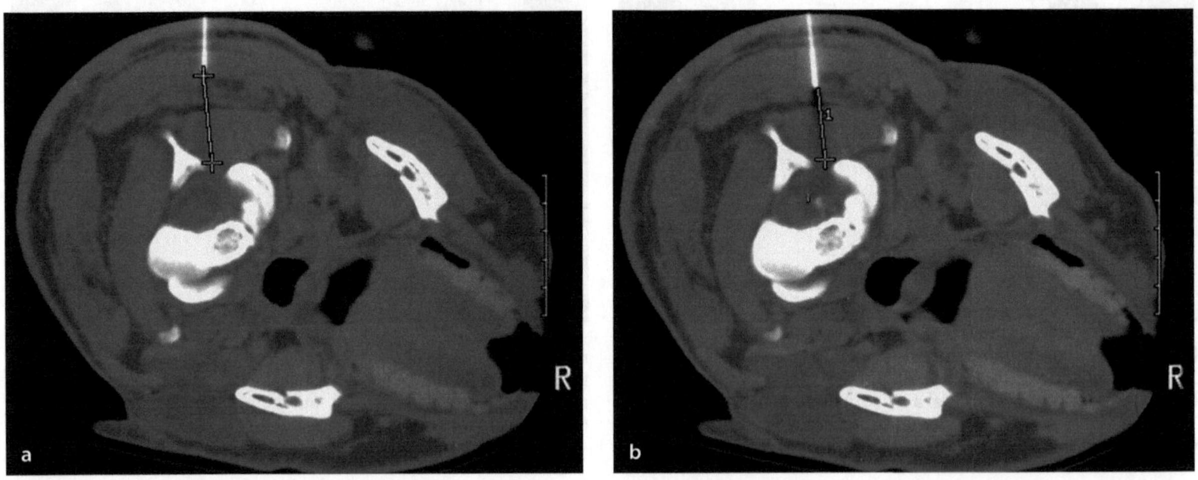

Fig. 3.9 a, b. Infiltration of the right nerve of Arnold (also refer to chapter 8). **a** The line connecting the needle tip and the reference mark (*white cross*) shows an imprecise approach, and allows a rectification of the previously calculated angle. **b** After altering the approach of the therapy needle the reference line indicates a correct orientated needle path toward to the origin of the nerve, near intervertebral joint of C1 and C2 in the area of the posterior arch of the atlas

target. Following local anesthetic delivery, the large-bore needle can be used as a guide. The therapy needle (smaller gauge) is introduced into the large bore needle and follows the predefined direction to the target (Fig. 3.10).

Exact Positioning of the Needle Tip

It is essential to exactly localize the needle tip to ensure safety and accuracy. For this reason precise localization of the needle tip during placement is a basic requirement. In the sequential mode, three adjacent strict axial slices with same thickness are used. The central slice is placed exactly at the skin entry point of the needle. When the needle pathway is exactly axial, the needle remains within the range of the central image plane, and is completely visualized. The needle tip can be easily identified by its dark shadow. This phenomenon called tip artifact is due to the *attenuation* of the x-ray beam (Fig. 3.11b).

If the needle pathway is not perfectly parallel to the image plane, the needle tip will exit the central plane and cannot be visualized anymore. The disappearance

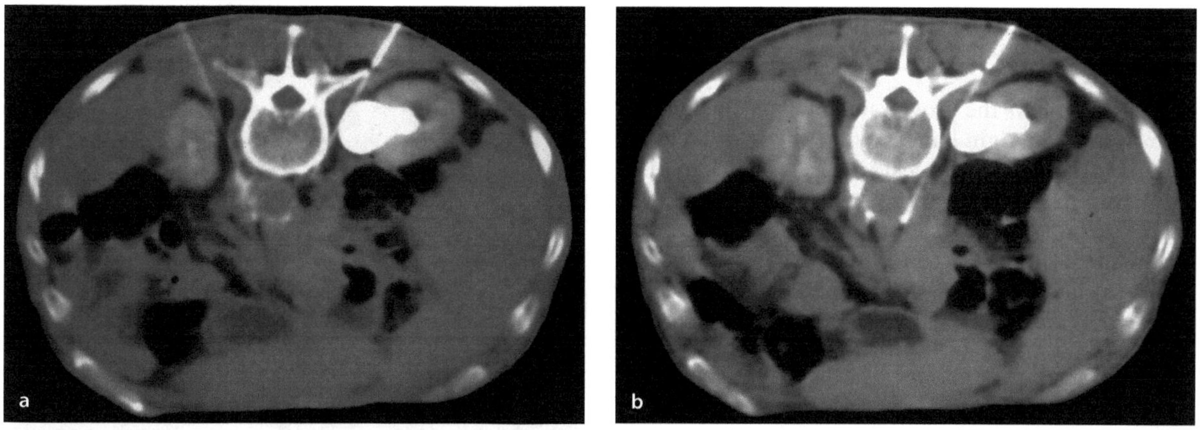

Fig. 3.10 a, b. Celiac neurolysis (also refer to chapter 11). **a** On the left side a short rigid 18 gauge needle for superficial local anesthesia is introduced in the exact direction of the splanchnic nerve and left celiac ganglia located anterolateral to the abdominal aorta. Following anesthesia of lower layers a second flexible 22 G needle is introduced step by step on the right side. The smaller needle follows the direction of the large-bore needle to the target structure. At the transverse process the tip of the needle bevel is rotated (180°) to the opposed side in order to pass this obstacle. **b** The same maneuver is repeated to pass the dilated right renal pelvis (the space was distended by injection of physiological saline solution) and to pass the lateral periosteum of the vertebral body. The first neurolysis is carried out here to destroy the splanchnic nerve. The needle is then placed anterolateral to the abdominal aorta to allow alcoholization of the celiac plexus

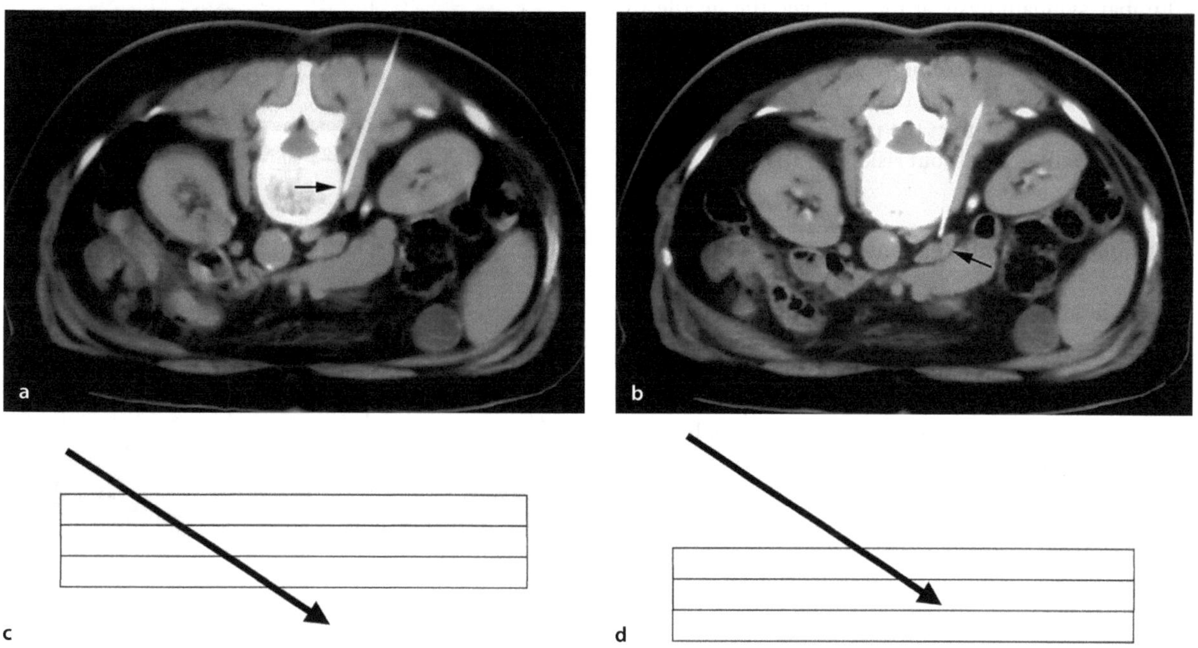

Fig. 3.11 a–d. Lumbar sympatholysis (also refer to chapter 12). **a** In this first image the needle tip appears to be located in contact with the right lateral aspect of the vertebral body (in fact the needle tip drops out of this slice). **b** A more caudal image, however, reveals the exact location of the needle tip, which is in fact in concact with the inferior vena cava. **c** Diagram clarifying the maneuver. Owing to a non-axial needle path (not parallel to slice), the needle was not completely displayed on the central image, falsely imitating a needle tip (as seen in **a**). **d** The needle tip is in fact located on another plane, as is recognized on a deeper slice (as seen in **b**).

of the needle exiting the slice may thus be mistaken for the needle tip. If the direction to target is still satisfactory, a parallel shift of the stack of image slices should be used to get the needle back into the central slice to ensure continuous tracking of the needle tip (in the central slice). A partial visualization of the needle can be misleading on the actual position of the needle tip and lead to dangerous complications This requires special attention in CT-guided punctures (see Fig. 3.11). In spiral mode, this technique follows the same principles.

Instead of the three image planes corresponding acquired volumes are used that corresponds to the three planes.

Figure 11 shows the progression of a needle during a neurolysis of the right lumbar sympathetic chain at the level of L2. During needle positioning, the stack of three slices was apparently not properly shifted to keep the needle tip on the central slice. In this case, the needle tip is not in the psoas/vertebra angle where the needle seems to end. The needle tip cannot be identified since it drops out the slices (see Fig. 3.11a). In fact, the needle tip is already in contact with the inferior vena cava (Fig. 3.11b).

Localization of the Needle

In order to avoid partial volume effects it is important to adapt the slice thickness to the size of the structures that need to be distinguished. Additional thinner slices may be necessary during needle placement, particularly when approaching the target or any small structures. In a lumbar sympatholysis at the L4 level, the needle tip seems to be in close proximity to the ureter, and penetration of the ureter cannot be excluded. The situation appears much clearer on thinner slices. Actually, the needle tip does not affect the ureter and the procedure could be continued without risk (Fig. 3.12).

Techniques for Needle Guidance

A straight and accurate placement of the needle tip via the shortest possible safe pathway is aimed at avoiding multiple withdrawals and changes of needle orientation at deeper tissue levels. For exact needle placement a guidance technique allowing early corrections by step-by-step imaging control is necessary. Other important factors are flexibility vs. rigidity of the needle and the shape of its tip. Special maneuvers can be used to circumvent certain obstacles or to improve access to areas hard to reach.

"Tutor" Technique

A quite useful technique for placing large bore needles is to use a thinner needle as a "tutor" (Fig. 3.13). The thin needle is placed first with precise orientation toward the target. During placement local anesthesia can be carried out in superficial regions and at lower levels through this needle on the presumed pathway. Finally, the large bore needle is introduced with close contact and parallel to the small bore needle ("tutor") allowing guidance to the target lesion in procedures such as biopsy or cementoplasty.

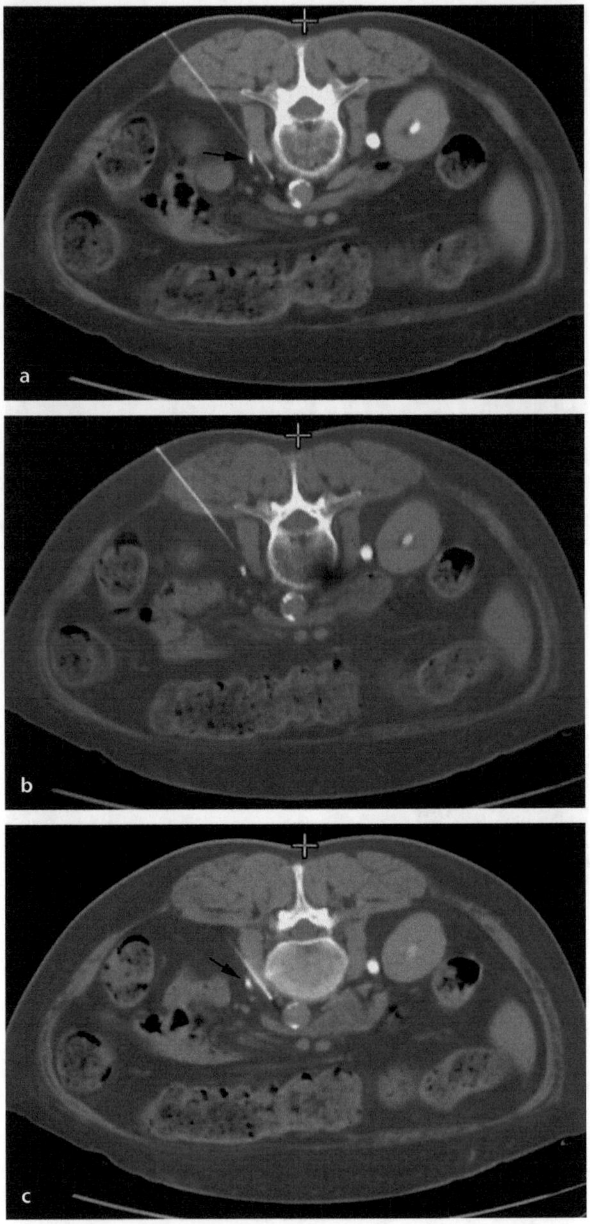

Fig. 3.12 a–c. Lumbar sympatholysis (also refer to chapter 12). **a** On this CT image (slice thickness = 7 mm) the needle is suspected to be in contact with the ureter (*arrow*). Penetration cannot be excluded. **b** and **c** Images with 3 mm slice thickness clearly demonstrate the needle medially to the ureter. On image **c** the needle tip can be identified by the needle tip artifact, which is only seen on images **a** and **c**

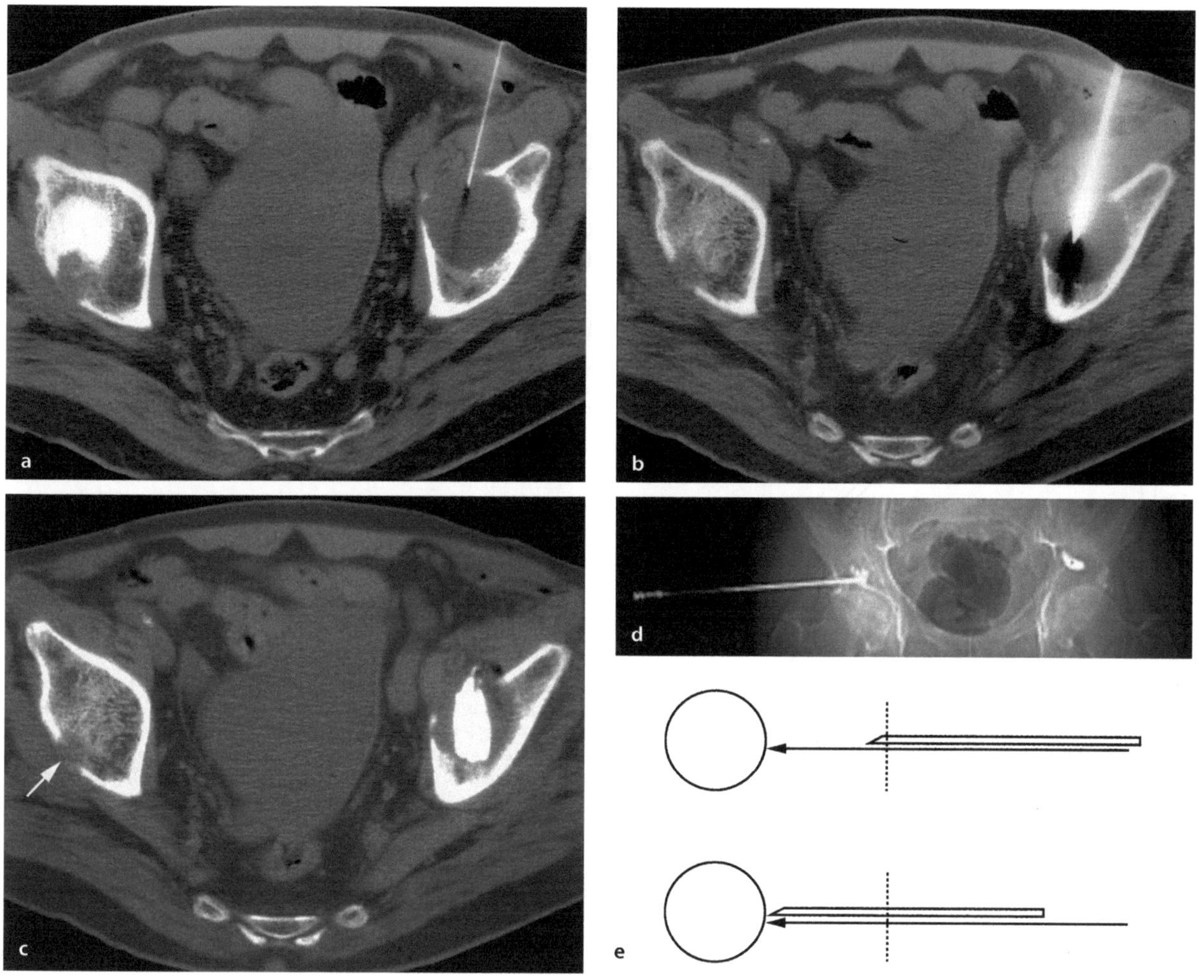

Fig. 3.13 a–e. Cementoplasty (also refer to chapter 15). Painful lytic metastasis of the left acetabulum. Patient could not bear weight on his left leg because of pain. **a** Introduction of a 22 gauge spinal needle for superficial and deep anesthesia. Following placement this needle serves as a guide ("tutor") for the insertion of a large-bore needle in contact and parallel to it. **b.** CT image of the correctly placed 15 G trocar within the lesion prior to the injection of the cement. **c** CT image following cementoplasty. **d** Second cementoplasty treating the other lytic metastasis on the right side (*arrow* on image **c**). **e** Diagram clarifying the maneuver

Needle "Steering"

Flexible needles can be used to circumvent obstacles in certain procedures. The relative flexibility of the needle allows alternating straight and curved needle pathways during needle tip progression, which can even be modified (curved course) in deeper regions. This technique permits one to avoid obstacles located on the needle pathway at different levels (Fig. 3.14).

For the neurolysis of the lumbar sympathetic chain such a flexible needle (superior to 20 gauge) may be used. In this posterior approach the vertebral body is located on the needle pathway as can be seen on the acquired series of three slices. With rigid needles the sympathetic chain may not be accessible because it is located in the blind angle behind the vertebral body (see Fig. 3.14a). As opposed to a rigid needle that may have to be removed and another approach attempted, a flexible one is capable of skirting the vertebral body. Although such a needle may not have an optimal position originally, it only needs to be withdrawn a few centimeters; the tip of its bevel re-directed away from the vertebral body, and a curved trajectory applied for the subsequent advance[2)] (see Fig. 3.14b). With the trajectory thus changed, the needle tip can be placed posterior to the aorta or posterior to the inferior vena cava, according to the side to which the neurolytic substance needs to be delivered.

2) The obstacle is avoided as when skiing over a bump!

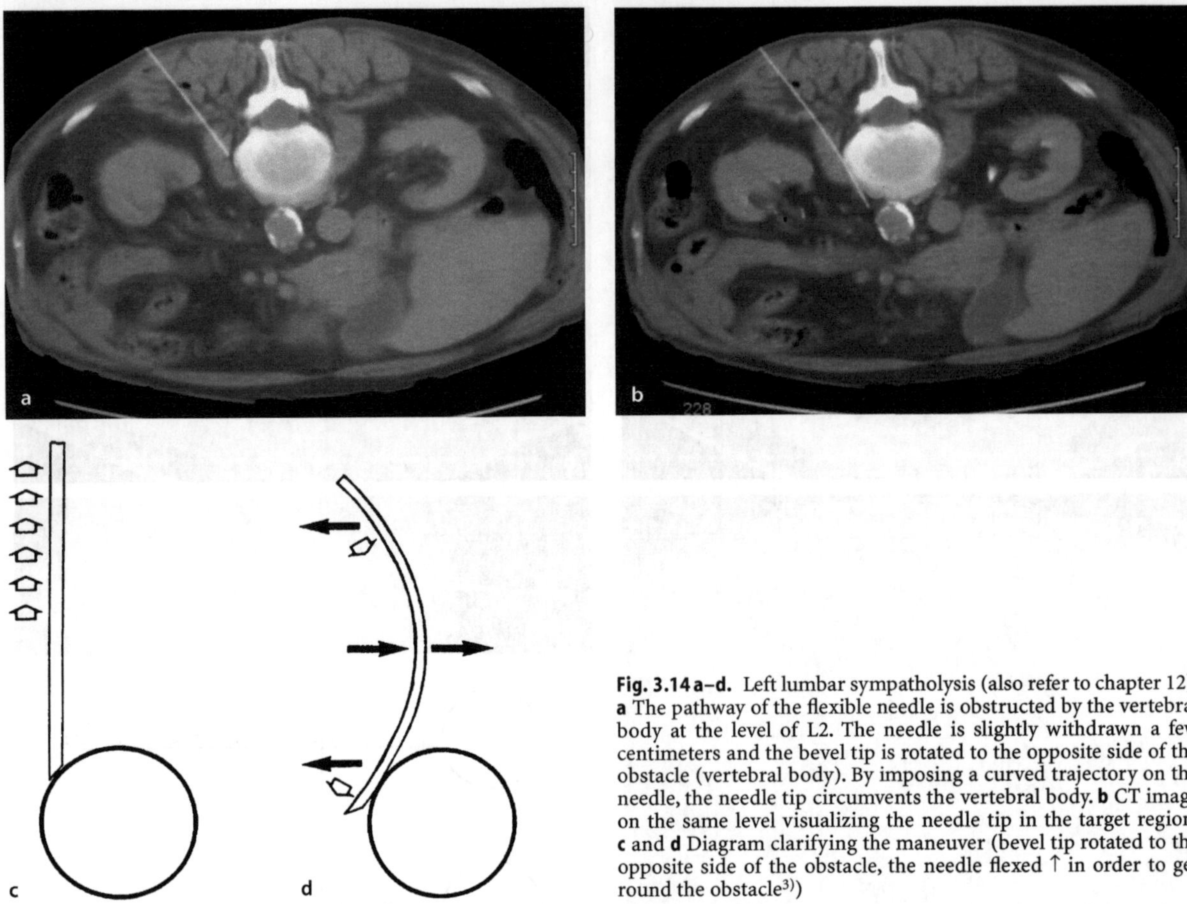

Fig. 3.14 a–d. Left lumbar sympatholysis (also refer to chapter 12). **a** The pathway of the flexible needle is obstructed by the vertebral body at the level of L2. The needle is slightly withdrawn a few centimeters and the bevel tip is rotated to the opposite side of the obstacle (vertebral body). By imposing a curved trajectory on the needle, the needle tip circumvents the vertebral body. **b** CT image on the same level visualizing the needle tip in the target region. **c** and **d** Diagram clarifying the maneuver (bevel tip rotated to the opposite side of the obstacle, the needle flexed ↑ in order to get round the obstacle[3)])

Rigid needles (inferior to 22 Gauge) always adhere to a rectilinear track in soft tissues. Changes of direction and reorientation in deeper levels can only be achieved by moving the whole needle together with the surrounding tissue at the skin level, or by withdrawing and penetrating again in an altered direction (Fig. 3.15). In solid tissue such as bone (for biopsy or vertebroplasty) a rigid needle tends to deviate to the side of the bevel tip. A zigzag course is necessary in order to keep a rectilinear trajectory; and multiple obstacles can be circumvented by a zigzag course of the needle. This can be achieved with a 180° needle tip rotation at each step to adapt the orientation of the bevel tip. Needle tips with a diamond-shaped bevel (symmetrical) do not require this type of zigzag maneuver.

An epidural infiltration of the left fifth lumbar nerve root was performed in a patient presenting with persistent pain originating in this region. CT images were obtained with increased inclination of the gantry initially in order to achieve a more convenient approach. The needle tip (a flexible needle of 22 gauge) was placed at the level of the origin of the nerve root by carrying out a double rotation technique during placement (Fig. 3.16). A first rotation positioned the tip of the needle bevel opposite to the spine, then followed a second 180° rotation in the opposite direction (Fig. 3.16a). Thus, we avoid the obstacle, which would have been impossible by using a strictly linear trajectory. The correct positioning of the needle tip was assessed by injecting contrast medium that diffused at the expected location around the nerve root (Fig. 3.16b).

3) like a ski ...

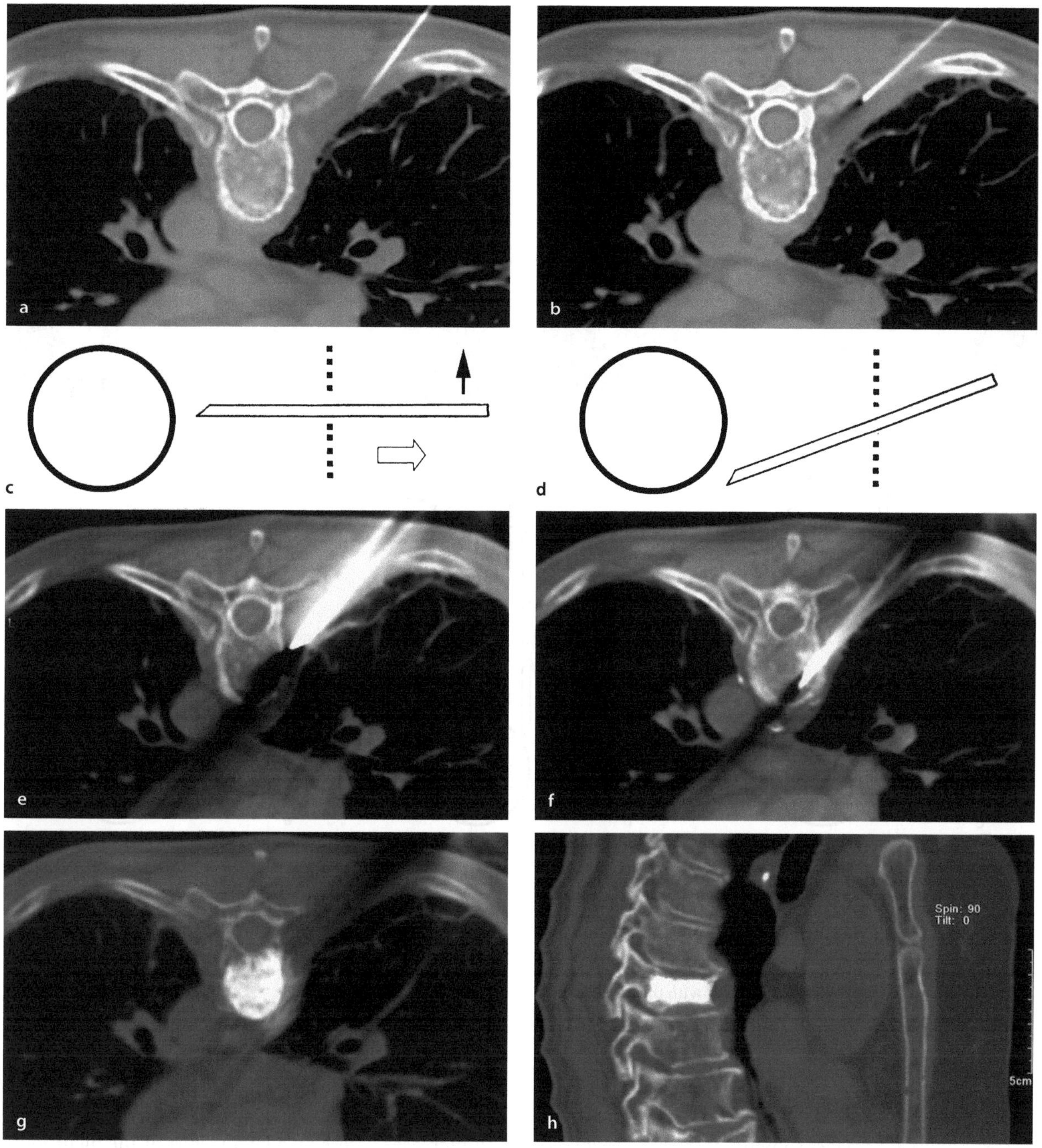

Fig. 3.15 a–h. Vertebroplasty in a patient with multiple myeloma (also refer to chapter 15). **a** CT image showing the therapy needle (needle tip not seen) wrongly aimed at penetration of the lung parenchyma. **b** CT image showing the reoriented therapy needle. **c** and **d** Diagrams clarifying the maneuver. In contrast to the flexible needle, the unbending needle changes its path by withdrawal and directional reorientation of the needle on an upper level. **e** CT image showing the therapy needle penetrating the cortex of the vertebral body. **f** The needle tip is located in the vertebral body. **g** and **h**). CT images following the intervention. The hyperdense signal indicates the injected acrylic cement

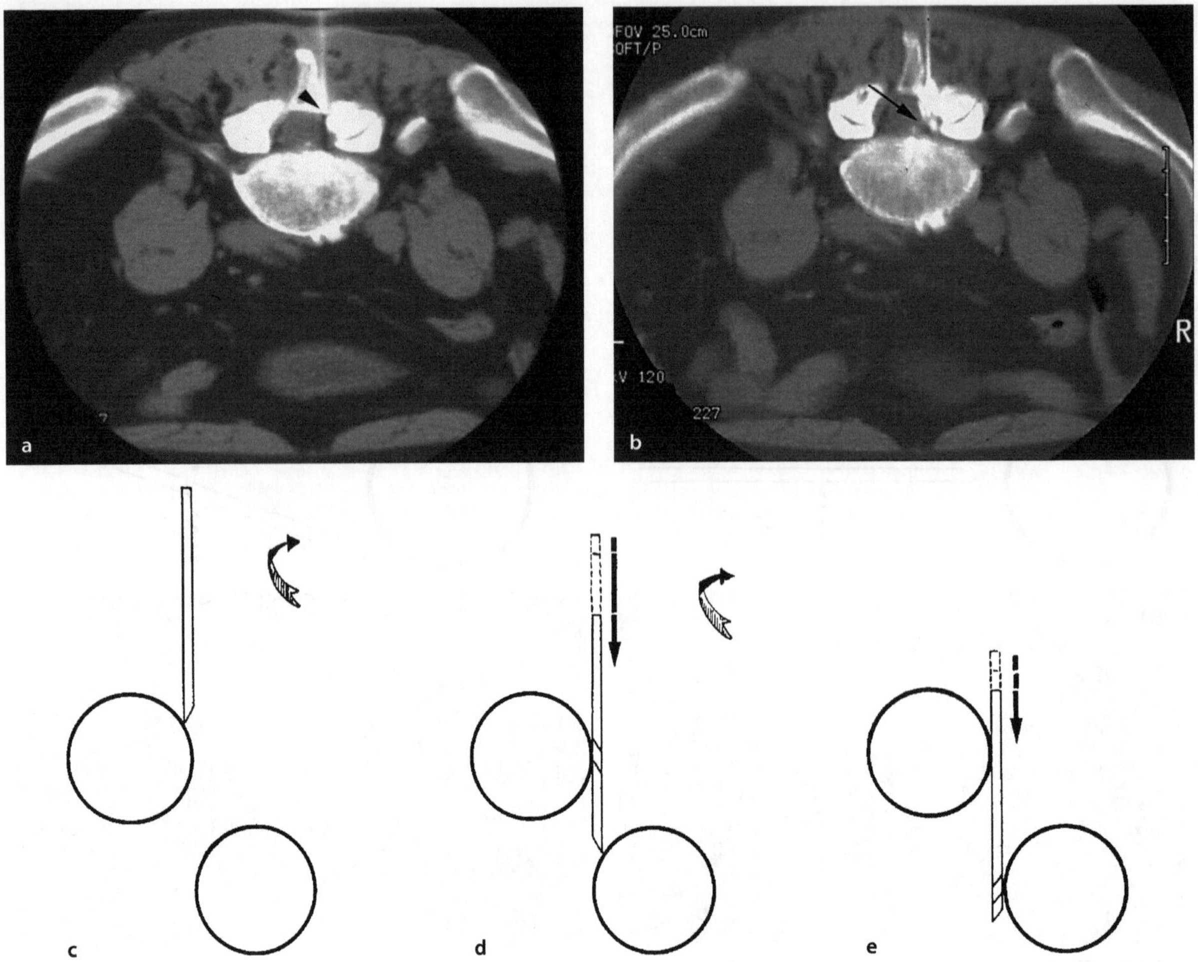

Fig. 3.16 a–e. Infiltration of the left L5 root (also refer to chapter 5). Needle placement using a technique (180°) of double rotation of the needle. **a** CT image showing the needle tip (needle tip artifact, *arrowhead* on image **a**. at the right lateral base of the spinous process. To circumvent the base the bevel tip is directed to the right, opposite the base while introducing the needle. To skirt the articular process the procedure is continued with the bevel tip now oriented to the left. **b** Verification of the correct position of the needle tip by injecting a small volume of contrast medium (*arrow* on image **b**) around the emergence of the nerve root. **c–e** Diagrams clarifying the maneuver. **c** Rotation and reorientation of the bevel tip to pass the first obstacle **d**. Opposite rotation by 180° to pass the second obstacle. **e** The needle tip comes finally to lie behind the obstacles

Pathway Enlargement

Preprocedural CT images sometime reveal narrowing of the potential needle pathway. Soft tissue narrowing can be counteracted during needle approach by injecting physiological saline solution or lidocaine via the therapy needle. This technique often leads to a wider path and enables progress of the needle without complications (Figs. 3.4c, 3.17, 3.18, 3.19).

In the dorsal approach for a right-sided thoracic sympathicolysis (here at the level of the third thoracic vertebra) the space between the vertebral body and the pleuropulmonary parenchyma often is narrowed (see Fig. 3.17). A needle approach is encumbered with a certain amount of risk of perforating the pleura. The injection of physiological saline solution widens the passage and increases access by a lateral shift of the pleuropulmonary parenchyma (see Fig. 3.17a and c). The needle passes in this widened space without problems.

In another patient, a neurolysis of the right lumbar sympathetic chain at the level of the second nerve root was performed (Fig. 3.18). The needle pathway was narrowed by the right renal vein. The injection of physiological saline solution during the approach of the needle shifted the vein anteriorly and avoided damaging it (see Fig. 3.18b). Additional safety can be achieved by rotating the needle tip so that the bevel tip is opposite the vessel.

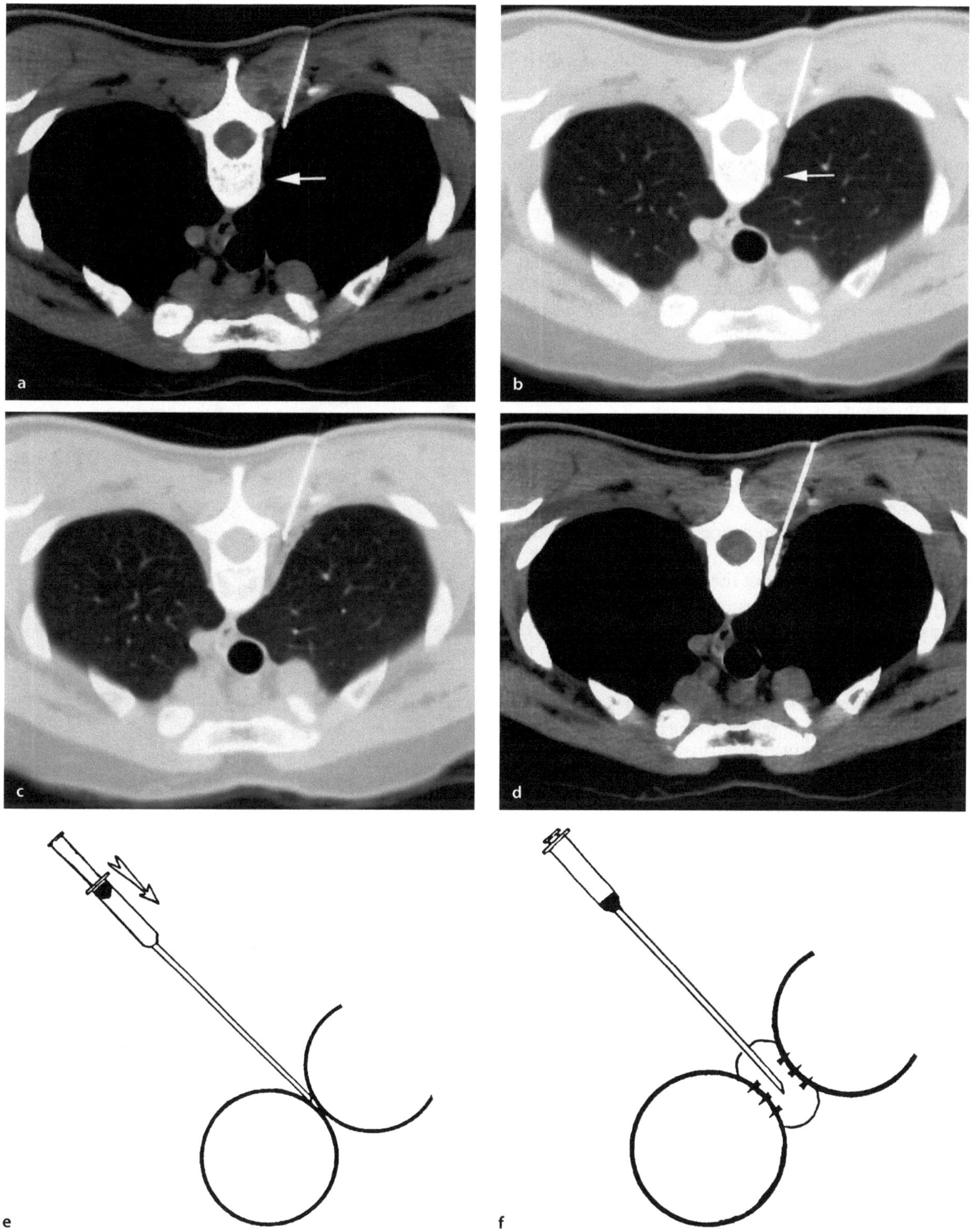

Fig. 3.17 a–f. Right thoracic sympatholysis (also refer to chapter 12): narrowing of the intervertebropleural channel. **a** and **b** CT images demonstrate a narrowed channel between the vertebral body and the lungs. **c** The injection of physiological saline solution results in widening of the channel thus inducing in a lateral pleuropulmonary shift. Needle positioning can be continued without risk of (**d**) perforation of the pleura or the lung. **e** and **f** Diagram clarifying the principle of the maneuver. The injection of physiological saline creates a channel by pushing tissue aside

Fluid Diffusion Assessment

Following the successful positioning of the needle tip, any of several therapeutic agents may be administered: local anesthetics for temporary blocks, anti-inflammatory drugs in combination with steroids for a prolonged anti-inflammatory effect. Finally, dehydrated (absolute) alcohol can be delivered for permanent blocks and neurolysis or radiofrequency ablation, which is often preceded by a temporary diagnostic block.

In the application of anesthetics or anti-inflammatory drugs a relatively large volume of several milliliters is injected. Apart from a possible inadvertent intravascular injection, to be avoided by an aspiration test maintained for 5 to 10 seconds prior to injection to make sure of no blood reflux, the procedure is relatively safe – as are the agents used.

In neurolysis, the situation is quite different. Complications can occur by diffusion of the alcohol to surrounding structures such as nerve roots. These serious events can be reduced:

- By injecting a small predefined but sufficient volume of alcohol
- By precise positioning of the needle tip
- By anticipating the diffusion of alcohol with a previous injection of a precise quantity (according to the procedure) of a lidocaine–contrast mixture (5:1). The preliminary injection of a lidocaine–contrast mixture further serves as a therapeutic test block, but also to reduce pain[4] related to the neurolysis (alcohol injection) (Fig. 3.18 and 3.19). Furthermore, it can identify an intravascular puncture (large perivertebral vascular plexus) by the absence of contrast medium at the needle tip following the test injection. In the estimation of the diffusion of alcohol it must be remembered that alcohol is simultaneously hydrosoluble and liposoluble. The diffusion of absolute alcohol thus cannot be completely controlled, nor will its diffusion be strictly consistent with that of the preliminarily injected mixture, which is of an exclusively hydrosoluble character.

In addition, to realize an adequate neurolytic effect a final alcohol concentration of 66% to 75% is required. The calculation for the concentration thus follows a simple rule: the injected total quantity of absolute (close to 100%) alcohol A, which follows the injection of lidocaine–contrast mixture X must be at least twice or better three time the quantity of X (A=2 X or = 3 X) to obtain a sufficient alcohol concentration C = 66% to 75% (C = A/A+X). With the injection of high concentrated alcohol smaller total volumes can be achieved! At the end of the procedure, the injection of one-fourth of a milliliter of physiologic serum or lidocaine (to rinse away the alcohol), just off the main site provides relief from pain as the needle is removed.

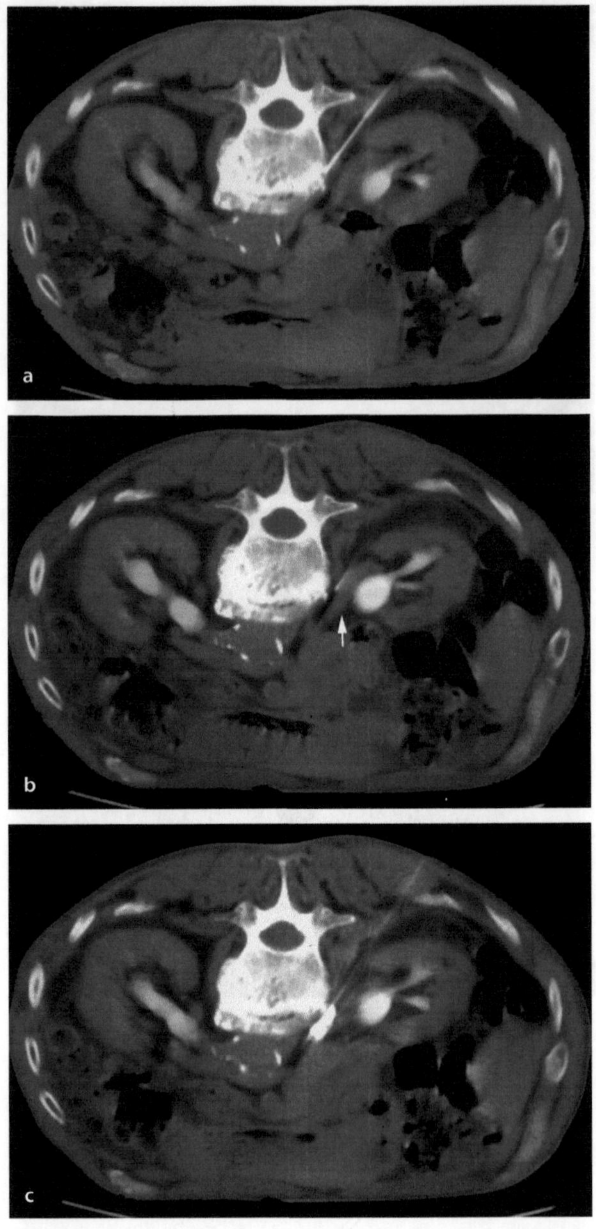

Fig. 3.18 a–c. Neurolysis of the right lumbar sympathetic chain at the level of L2 (also refer to chapter 12). **a** and **b** The needle passes the vertebral body by the rotation maneuver of the bevel. The injection of physiological saline solution during the approach of the needle shifts the right renal vein (*arrow*, **b**) anteriorly and avoids trauma to the right renal vein (on image **b** only the needle tip is visualized). To be on the safe side the tip of the needle bevel is still rotated (180°) to the opposite of the vessel. **c** The injection of an anesthetic-contrast mixture ensures the correct extravascular location of the needle tip. The fluid distributes around the lumbar sympathetic chain

4) In the event of intolerable pain, it is generally helpful to distract the patient with inspiratory and expiratory maneuvers. The pain should ease in less than one minute by which time the nervous fibers should be destroyed.

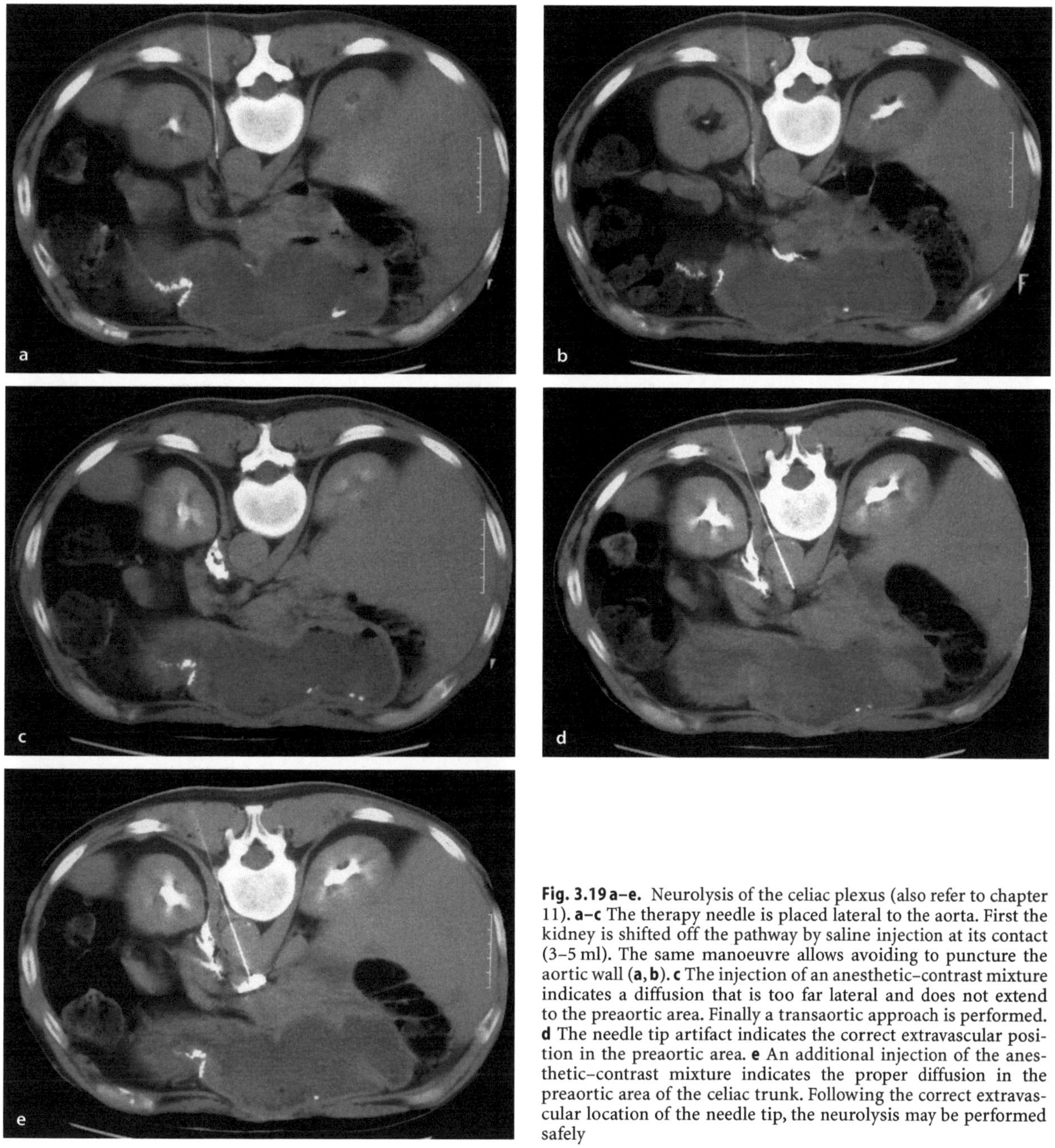

Fig. 3.19 a–e. Neurolysis of the celiac plexus (also refer to chapter 11). **a–c** The therapy needle is placed lateral to the aorta. First the kidney is shifted off the pathway by saline injection at its contact (3–5 ml). The same manoeuvre allows avoiding to puncture the aortic wall (**a**, **b**). **c** The injection of an anesthetic-contrast mixture indicates a diffusion that is too far lateral and does not extend to the preaortic area. Finally a transaortic approach is performed. **d** The needle tip artifact indicates the correct extravascular position in the preaortic area. **e** An additional injection of the anesthetic-contrast mixture indicates the proper diffusion in the preaortic area of the celiac trunk. Following the correct extravascular location of the needle tip, the neurolysis may be performed safely

References

1. Kastler B, Gangi A, Allal R, Litzler JF, Sohm O, Abbes A (1995) Optimizing interventional procedures under CT guidances: tips and hints. Scientific exhibit. Radiological Society of North America, 81st scientific assembly and annual meeting, Chicago, 26 Nov – 1 Dec 1995. Radiology [Suppl] 197:516
2. Kastler B, Couvreur M, Clair C, Litzler JF, Perreira P, Allal R et al (1999) Tomodensitométrie interventionnelle: suivez le guide. Feuillets Radiol 39:421–432
3. Schmutz G, Kastler B, Fournier L, Leproux F, Provost N, Delassus P (1999) Tomodensitométrie interventionnelle : techniques, indications, résultats. EMC Radiodiagnostic, appareil digestif 33-680, A10, 13 pp
4. Clair C, Kastler B, Couvreur M, Boulahdour Z, Litzler JF, Fergane B (2000) Interventional procedures under CT guidance in pain management. Scientific exhibit. Radiological Society of North America, 86th scientific assembly and annual meeting, Chicago, 26 Nov – 1 Dec 2000. Radiology [Suppl] 217:671
5. Kastler B, Clair C, Fergane B (2001) Radiologie interventionnelle sous contrôle tomodensitométrique dans le traitement de la douleur. EPU JFR

6. Kastler B, Clair C, Michalakis D, Boulahdour Z, Brunelle S, Fergane B (2002) Interventional procedures under CT guidance in 756 patients, incidents, side effects and how to reduce their incidence. Scientific exhibit. Radiological Society of North America, 88th scientific assembly and annual meeting, Chicago, November, 2002. Radiology [Suppl] 225:724
7. Gangi A, Kastler BA, Dietemann JL (1994) Percutaneous vertebroplasty guided by a combination of CT and fluoroscopy. AJNR Am J Neuroradiol 15:83–86

Complications and Patient Management

Type of Agents Infiltrated

Pierre Delassus, George Hadjidekov, Bruno Kastler

4

Analgesic nerve blocks have a number of indications outside of the operating theatre. These are specific forms of anesthesia that consequently require precise knowledge of the regional anatomy concerned and the techniques used. Under these circumstances, they are effective, safe, and relatively nontoxic provided that the pharmacology of the products used is observed – in other words that the doses, concentrations, and volumes are respected. Contraindications should always be borne in mind. Accidents cannot be excluded, whatever the precautions taken.

Type of Agents Infiltrated

Local Anesthetics

Indications

Local anesthetics infiltrated at appropriate concentrations on contact with any nerve structure, reversibly block the propagation of action potentials [5]. Blockage of the nerve conduction involves not only the sensory and motor fibers, but also the sympathetic fibers. Their use in pain of neurological origin may serve different purposes:

- Diagnostic: a diagnostic block may enable the origin of the pain to be determined: for example, a crural nerve block may confirm neuralgia in this region. It may also distinguish visceral or parietal pain from neurogenic pain.
- Prognostic: the block may enable the effects of a neurolytic block or a surgical procedure for nerve destruction to be evaluated. For example, a celiac block with an injection of lidocaine can, if the result is positive, establish the pancreatic and celiac origin of abdominal pain in a patient suffering from chronic pancreatitis, and may help determine the indication for celiac neurolysis or surgical splanchnic ablation.
- Therapeutic: the technique of local anesthetic infiltration may be of therapeutic value in the relief of certain chronic pain syndromes, either through administration of one or more repeated blocks, or of a continuous anesthetic block.

Products Used

A pair of references meriting consultation on this topic are: [2, 4]

Please see Table 4.1. The choice of a local anesthetic is based on its clinical effects: potency, onset and duration of action, and potential toxicity. The most widely used products are lidocaine , bupivacaine, and ropivacaine.

- Lidocaine possesses the best therapeutic index, but also the shortest duration of action: its efficacy generally does not exceed 3 hours following infiltration. Conversely, the possibility of using large volumes

Table 4.1. Local anesthetics

	Maximum doses		Onset of action	Duration of action
	Without adrenaline	With adrenaline		
Lidocaine 5 mg/mL 10 mg/mL	5 mg/kg	7 mg/kg	Rapid 5 to 10 min	2 h
Bupivacaine 2.5 mg/mL 5 mg/mL	1.5 mg/kg	2 mg/kg	Delayed 20 to 30 min	4 to 6 h
Ropivacaine 7.5 mg/mL	3 mg/kg	–	Delayed 15 to 25 min	3 to 4 h

without any risk of systemic toxicity is of benefit in some cases.

- Bupivacaine is more toxic with a more potent and more prolonged action (4 to 6 hours). It is best to avoid its use in heart diseases with disorders of excitability or conduction and in treatments with beta-blockers or calcium inhibitors. In these patients, lidocaine is always preferable.
- Ropivacaine, a new local anesthetic (available in France since 1998) appearing to have the same efficacy and the same duration of action as bupivacaine with lower cardiovascular toxicity, although greater than that of lidocaine.

Adrenaline, possibly combined with local anesthesia, reduces blood absorption, prolongs the duration of action and improves the quality of the block. However, sympathomimetic effect may lead to tachycardia and/or blood pressure instability ranging from hypo- to hypertension, thus constituting risk, particularly in elderly subjects.

Maximum Doses

From the combined comparative pharmacological properties of local anesthetics it is possible to establish the maximum doses that must not be exceeded in a single injection: 300 mg for lidocaine and ropivacaine, 150 mg for bupivacaine.

Incidents and Events

Allergic reactions to local anesthetics with an amide bond (lidocaine, bupivacaine, ropivacaine) are exceptional [7]. They must be considered upon the appearance of an urticarial rash, angioneurotic edema, bronchospasm, or anaphylactic shock. Treatment is not specific to the causative agent and combines epinephrine (adrenaline), ventilation, and volume replacement with crystalloids. Allergy testing should be performed following an episode of this nature.

Side effects and events reported as being related to an allergy are in fact usually due to overdoses or technical errors, such as the intravenous injection of normally harmless doses, but administered too rapidly.

Local anesthetics absorbed from injection areas or injected directly into the circulation, cross the blood-brain barrier and are likely to cause central neurological manifestations, of major concern the onset of generalized convulsive seizures. The most common preconvulsive manifestations, to be taken as alarm signals, are somnolence, headache, a metallic taste in the mouth, and perioral paresthesia.

Convulsions usually occur at plasma concentrations greater than 8 mcg/mL of lidocaine. A rapid increase in the cerebral concentration of local anesthetic signals danger. Treatment requires maintenance or restoration of good ventilatory conditions, administration of oxygen, and injection of a benzodiazepine: diazepam 0.20 mg/kg or midazolam (Hypnovel; Roche, Basel) 0.10 mg/kg.

Cardiac problems associated with local anesthetics come predominantly from the more potent ones, such as bupivacaine, and are dose-dependent. Delayed conduction rates responsible for extreme bradycardia, atrioventricular blocks or tachycardia, and even ventricular fibrillation can be observed. This cardiotoxicity also reduces myocardial contractility, making resuscitation of a disastrous event particularly difficult. In the case of bradycardia, acceleration of the heart rate with adrenaline is not recommended; a parasympathetic agent such as atropine is, however, appropriate. In the case of depression of contractility, dobutamine (Dobutrex; Lilly, Strasbourg) is recommended, and. upon the appearance of ventricular rhythm disorders, electric shock should be applied. In the event of cardiac arrest, adrenaline remains the drug of choice, combined with external heart massage (CPR) and oxygen therapy.

Rules of Use

The use of a neurostimulator for nerve trunk localization block allows greater precision for the injection during truck block. This does not guarantee the absence of problems, but it can prevent excessive administration of solution to offset the lack of precision in the needle positioning. The local anesthetic is injected slowly after checking aspiration. During the injection, the doctor must maintain verbal contact with the patient to immediately detect the premonitory signs of an untoward event, particularly of a neurological variety. Close monitoring must be continued for one hour following this injection; this is independent of the monitoring required as a result of the nerve block itself.

If the solution contains adrenaline, a trial injection of 0.5 to 1 ml must be given 1 minute before the total dose is injected in order to detect any heart disorders. Irrespective of the local anesthetic used, any regional anesthesia requires that an intravenous line be placed, and blood pressure and an electrocardiographic tracing be monitored. Full respiratory and circulatory resuscitation facilities must be available at hand along with personnel trained in their use [3].

Neurolytic Substances

The destruction of nerve tissue by injection of neurolytic agents is a very old practice. The two neurolytic agents most widely used in the treatment of chronic pain are phenol and alcohol [6]. They act by selectively destroying the small and large nerve fibers and have an effect on all aspects of nerve function. The size of the lesions varies according to the concentration. In addition, they cause sequelae in the axonal membrane, which might explain cases of painful paresthesia observed several months following a neurolytic block.

In all cases, it is essential to obtain the patient's informed consent before undertaking a procedure with normally permanent consequences.

Phenol

This comes in two forms: a 1/15 aqueous solution and a 5% solution in glycerol (the latter is hyperbaric and used only intraspinally). Aqueous phenol is easy to use and does not cause violent pain on injection. Its mode of action is primarily the denaturation of proteins. Axons of all sizes are affected non-selectively by phenol at concentrations greater than 2%. Phenol is responsible for a transient local anesthetic effect. The duration of action of the analgesia following phenolization varies between 5 and 20 weeks.

It should be noted that many serious complications observed during blocks with phenol are due to vascular lesions, hence the need to constantly monitor neurolytic injections in order to prevent the risk of intravascular injection. Phenol toxicity appears at doses greater than 8 g. In practice, the use of phenol is therefore considered to be risk free only when the total amount used is less than or equal to 600 mg, i.e., 10 ml of 1/15 solution.

Alcohol

The neurolytic effects of ethyl alcohol at a concentration greater than 50% are well-known, but absolute alcohol (95% to 100%) is required for nerve destruction to be permanent. Alcohol acts on the neurons through the extraction of cholesterol and phospholipids. It causes the precipitation of lipo- and mucoproteins. The use of lower concentrations (80 and even 65%) causes partial or incomplete nerve destruction.

Alcohol is extremely irritating to neighboring tissues, causing pain, burns, and local hypersensitivity. It is therefore essential to use the smallest effective quantity and to place it as close as possible to its target. Alcohol must be injected slowly, and it can thus be appreciated that neurolytic blocks must always be given under visual control – after prior administration of local anesthetic and carrying out an aspiration test before the injection.

The use of a preliminary test dose (1 to 2 ml) of local anesthetic is desirable, particularly if there is any doubt about the nerve concerned and if the efficacy of the block in suppressing pain is to be assessed. After the injection of alcohol or phenol, it is advisable to rinse the needle with a small quantity of local anesthetic or physiological saline to prevent pain from occurring along the path of the needle.

Corticosteroids for Local Infiltration

Indications

Corticosteroids are used for their anti-inflammatory and/or analgesic action. They can be used in peripheral, peri-articular, or intra-articular nerve infiltrations [7].

Products Used

Suspensions have lower systemic diffusion and prolonged action, but an appreciable local atrophic effect; conversely, solutions, which are rarely used, have a brief effect with rapid diffusion, comparable to that of an intramuscular injection. (See Table 4.2)

Complications

The major problem in using these infiltrations is dominated by the risk of infection. Most significant is septic arthritis which has a usual latency period of 24 to 72 hours. This risk can and should be greatly minimized by meticulous aseptic technique. More benign incidents can occur following an infiltration: an immediate and generally transient painful reaction is common. A later inflammatory reaction, occurring after a few hours, may reflect microcrystalline peri- or intra-articular precipitation. This acute microcrystalline arthritis generally regresses in 24 to 48 hours (although microcrystalline suspensions have been used).

Corticosteroid infiltrations may have an atrophic effect on the skin and subcutaneous and musculotendinous tissues with a risk of tendon rupture in the case of injection into the tendons. It is predominantly fluorinated corticosteroids such as triamcinolone that occasion this sort of risk, and these must therefore be reserved strictly for intra-articular infiltrations. Allergic reactions can be seen and are usually due to sulphites in the excipients of certain products.

Precautions

As stated, the potential septic risk requires strict surgical asepsis. The use of prefilled sterile syringes reduces the risk of inadequate asepsis. Infiltration of any inflammatory joint for which no diagnosis has been made should be prohibited. Prior joint puncture for examination of the joint fluid represents an essential diagnostic tool.

Table 4.2. Corticosteroids for local infiltration used for their anti-inflammatory and analgesic action

Generic name	Commercial name	Presentation – Composition	Administered Dose	Duration of action	Indications
Cortivazol	Altim; Sanofi Aventis, Paris	Aqueous suspension Prefilled syringe 1.5 ml – 3.75 mg	0.25 to 1.5 ml	Intermediate	Deep peri-articular or intra-articular disease (not intraspinal)
Methylprednisolone	Depo-Medrol; Pfizer, New York	Aqueous suspension 1 ml – 40 mg 2 ml – 80 mg	0.1 to 2 ml	Intermediate	Idem
Dexamethasone	Dectancyl; Sanofi Aventis, Paris	Aqueous suspension 3 ml – 15 mg	0.25 to 2 ml	Intermediate	Idem
	Soludecadron; MSD International, Wadeville, South Africa	Hydrosoluble suspension 1 ml – 4 mg	NB: Sulphites 0.25 to 2 ml	Intermediate	Idem
Triamcinolone	Kenacort Retard; BMS -UPSA, Waterloo, Belgium	Aqueous suspension 1 ml – 40 mg 2 ml – 80 mg	0.25 to 2 ml	Prolonged	Idem (intra-articular route exclusively)
	Hexatron (long-acting); Wyeth Lederle, Paris	Microcrystalline suspension 2 ml – 40 mg	0.5 to 2 ml	Prolonged	Idem
Betamethasone	Diprostene; Schering-Plough, Kenilworth, NJ, USA	Microcrystalline suspension 1 ml – 7 mg Prefilled syringe	0.25 to 2 ml	Prolonged	Deep peri-articular or intra-articular disease
Hydrocortisone	Hydrocortisone Roussel; Sanofi Aventis, Paris	Aqueous suspension 25 mg/mL 125 mg/5 ml	0.25 to 3 ml	Short	Superficial or small joint disease
Prednisolone	Hydrocortancyl suspension; Laboratoires, Roussel, France	1 ml – 25 mg	0.1 to 2 ml	Short	Idem

For any superficial infiltration or infiltration of small joints, suspensions of hydrocortisone or hydrocortancyl should be preferred to other suspensions, most any of which have an excessive atrophic effect. The forms containing polyethylene glycol as well as highly microcrystalline forms should not be injected intrathecally because of the danger of arachnoiditis and epiduritis. The number of corticosteroid infiltrations should be limited: a minimum interval of one week should be allowed between infiltrations, not to exceed three successive infiltrations at the same site.

Patient Management

Useful references: [1, 8].

Before undertaking any invasive procedure, it is essential to obtain the patient's informed consent. The doctor must provide the patient with all relevant details regarding the proposed procedure and any risks of complications.

Data from the clinical examination and particularly from the neurological examination must be recorded in the patient's medical records. Likewise, evaluation of the different components of pain – somatic, affective and cognitive – and of its behavioral and social repercussions is compulsory. In 1999, the French National Agency for Accreditation and Evaluation in Healthcare (ANAES) proposed recommendations and references prepared for a working party based on an analysis of literature and professional opinions concerning the evaluation and monitoring of chronic pain in adult outpatients.

In case there is a neurological deficit present at the time the treatment procedure is begun, it is essential to carefully observe the signs and symptoms presented, to record them, and to draw the patient's attention to them before performing the procedure. The duration of postoperative monitoring and the measures to be applied should also be included in the patient care record. Finally, the patient should be given instructions necessary for monitoring after discharge from the treatment facility, and given the telephone number of the doctor and/or institution, where someone should be available in the event of problems.

Conclusion

Although a number of publications report lasting and even permanent improvement of chronic pain following analgesic infiltration, their relative and sometimes all too temporary efficacy would suggest that these procedures be incorporated into global, multidisciplinary management. They should only be offered after weighing the analgesic and functional benefits against the complications that these blocks can occasion in patients with chronic pain.

References

1. Anaes (1999) Évaluation et suivi de la douleur Chronique chez l'adulte en médecine ambulatoire. ANAES/service des recommandations et references professionnelles, février 1999
2. Brasseur L, Chauvin M, Guilbaud G (1997) Douleurs. Maloine, Paris
3. Bruce Scott D (1989) Techniques illustrées d'anesthésie loco-régionale. Arnette, Paris
4. Bruxelle J (1998) Techniquesd'anesthésie locorégionale en douleur chronique: du concept à la pratique. Évaluation et traitement de la douleur, 40e congres national d'anesthesie et de reanimation. Lab Elsevier et SFAR, pp 87–96
5. Charlton JE (1997) Les blocs nerveux: place des blocs thérapeutiques, pronostiques et diagnostiques. In: Brasseur L, Chauvin M, Guilbaud G (eds) Douleurs, bases fondamentales, pharmacologie, douleurs aiguës, douleurs chroniques, thérapeutiques. Maloine, Paris, pp 766–774
6. Devoghel JC (1988) Les blocs: phénolisation, alcoolisation. In: Scherpereel P (ed) La douleur et son traitement. Arnette, Paris, pp 359–371
7. Morel D, Duvauferrier R (1996) Les infiltrations nerveuses sous contrôle dans le traitement de la douleur. In: Gauthier-Lafaye P, Muller A (eds) Anesthésie loco-régionale et traitement de la douleur, 3rd edn. Masson, Paris
8. Scherpereel P (1998) Complications et implications médico-légales des blocs dans la douleur chronique. Évaluation et traitement de la douleur, 40e congres national d'anesthesie et de reanimation. Lab Elsevier et SFAR, pp 121–127

Foraminal Injections of Corticosteroids Under Tomodensitometric Control

5

Olivia Delmer, Vincent Dousset

Introduction

Corticosteroid injections represent a symptomatic treatment for radicular pain of spinal origin (cervicobrachial neuralgia, intercostal neuralgia, cruralgia, and sciatica) where resistance is shown to appropriately given medical treatment. Several methods of local injection are possible, e.g., epidural, intrathecal, and periradicular with fluoroscopic guidance. Monitoring exact position and progression of the needle, and injection of the corticosteroids all under tomodensitometric guidance appears to be the most reliable technique, readily reproducible for the treatment of radiculalgias caused by foraminal stenosis. Furthermore, the method does not involve irradiation of the person performing the procedure.

Anatomical Review

Among worthwhile references are these: [2,12,13,16]
The intervertebral foramen connects with the end of the radicular groove containing the nerve root in its subpedicular segment. The first foramen connects with the occipitoatlantoid space while the last is located between the fifth lumbar and the first sacral vertebra. In the sacrum, the intervertebral foramina are called sacral openings.

Each foramen links two vertebrae and is bounded (Fig. 5.1) [16]:

- In front by the posterolateral aspects of the vertebrae immediately above and below and by the posterolateral aspect of the disc, covered by the posterior common vertebral ligament
- Above by the pedicle of the overlying vertebra
- Below by the upper edge of the underlying vertebral pedicle
- Behind by the anterior aspects of the articular apophyses of the overlying and underlying vertebrae lined with the ligamentum flavum

The foramen contains (Fig. 5.2) [13]:

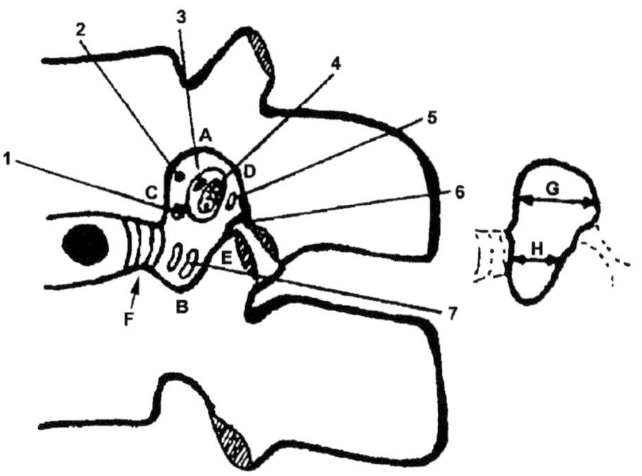

Fig. 5.1. Sagittal section of intervertebral foramen (Vital; [16]). Boundaries: *A*: superior pedicle; *B*: inferior pedicle; *C*: body of vertebra; *D*: isthmus; *E*: upper articulation of underlying vertebra; *F*: intervertebral disc; *G*: fixed part of foramen; *H*: mobile part of foramen. Contents: *1*: radicular artery; *2*: sinuvertebral nerve of Luschka; *3*: anterior root; *4*: posterior root; *3+4*: spinal ganglion; *5*: radicular vein; *6*: articular capsule; *7*: foraminal venous plexus

- The spinal nerve is formed from the anterior (motor) and posterior (sensory) roots and carries the spinal ganglion containing the cell bodies of the sensory neurons. This is the largest element in the foramen.
- Lushka's sinuvertebral nerve is a collateral stemming from the spinal nerve which, via proprioceptive pathways to the CNS, transmits the variations in tension to which the ligaments are subjected, thus facilitating postural adaptation.
- Meningeal envelopes accompany the ventral and dorsal nerve roots as far as the foramen, merging thereafter with the envelopes of the spinal nerve.
- The foraminal spinal nerve is accompanied by a vascular pedicle comprising a radicular artery, a large venous plexus, and lymphatic vessels.
- Foraminal fat plays a natural role in lubricating and physiologically cushioning the nerve roots.

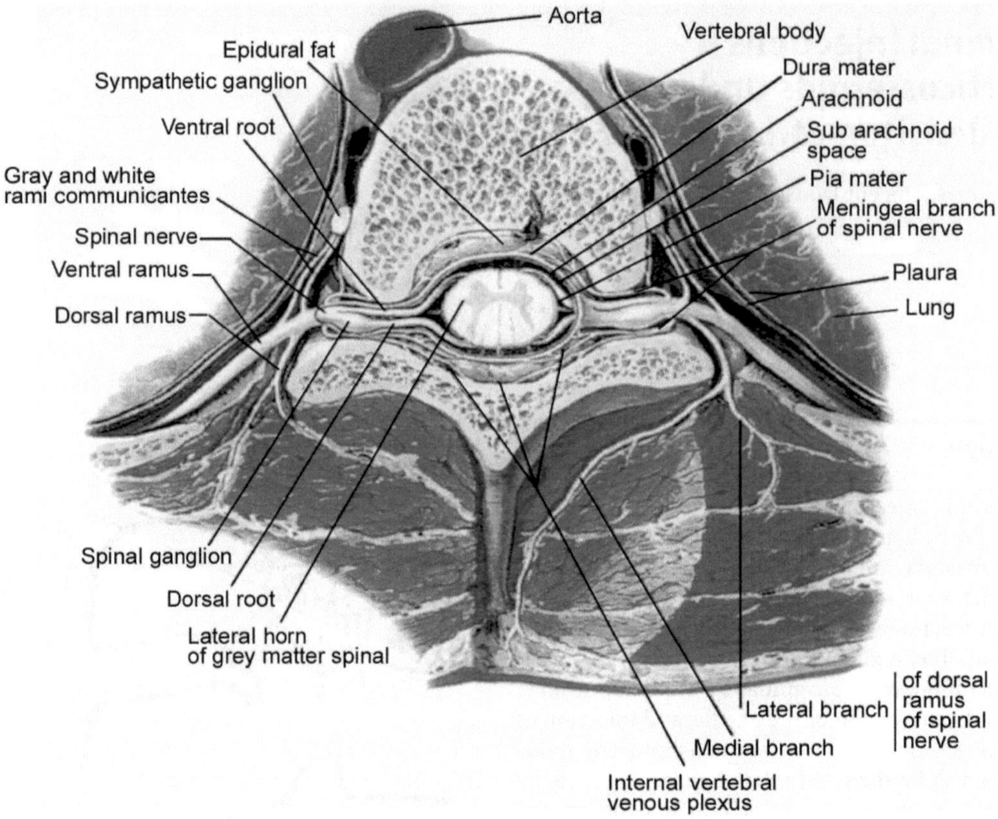

Fig. 5.2. Spinal nerve and meninges [13]. Aorta; Body of vertebra; Dura mater; Arachnoid; Subarachnoidal space; Pia mater; Recurrent meningeal rami of spinal nerve; Pleura; Lung.; Lateral branch, median branch of dorsal ramus of spinal nerve; Internal vertebral venous plexus; Lateral horn of gray matter of spinal cord; Dorsal root; Sensory spinal ganglion; Dorsal ramus; Ventral ramus (intercostal nerve); Spinal nerve; White and gray communicating rami; Ventral root; Sympathetic ganglion; Fatty tissue in the epidural space

Etiology of Foraminal Radicular Constrictions

The size and morphology of the foramina vary with the position of the subject (standing, load-bearing) and with the flexion–extension movements of the spine. When upright and/or in extension, there is a reduction in the anteroposterior diameter and a decrease in the height of the foramen. In addition to these dynamic changes, there may be morphological changes associated with stenoses originating essentially in the discs or in osseous degeneration (Fig. 5.3) [11].

Static images may underestimate foraminal constriction.

Stenosis of Discal Origin

Herniated discs tend to regress spontaneously in a few weeks. Posterolateral herniated discs with foraminal and strictly foraminal herniated discs, as well as extraforaminal or excluded herniated discs are all indications for CT-guided foraminal injections (Fig. 5.4) [7, 14].

Stenosis of Osseous Origin

In general, degenerative pathology occurs in older patients and develops chronically. It involves posterior articular deterioration, erosion of the disc, and hypertrophy of the ligamentum flavum, causing compression of the foramen, which may increase with active movements such as extension(Fig. 5.5) [5].

Spondylolisthesis, caused by isthmic lysis or degeneration associated with discal and posterior articular degeneration producing instability of the spine, is responsible for shrinkage of the intervertebral foramina (Fig. 5.6) [8].

Fibrosis

In patients who have undergone spinal surgery, corticosteroids may reduce residual pain if there is persisting periradicular inflammation.

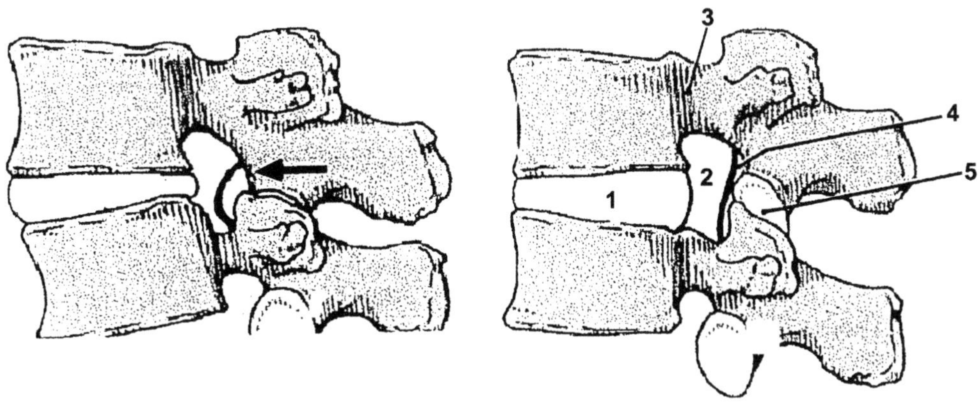

Fig. 5.3. Variation in size of foramen when flexion-extension movement occurs [11]. *1*: disc; *2*: intervertebral foramen; *3*: pedicle; *4*: yellow ligament; *5*: zygapophysal articulation. Left (extension): narrowing of the distal part of the intervertebral foramen caused by the forward bulging of the disc, and particularly by the bulging of the yellow ligament (ligamentum flavum) and the articular capsule being forced back by the anterior projection of the lower articulation. Right (flexion): normal inverted pyriform, almost oval, view of foramen

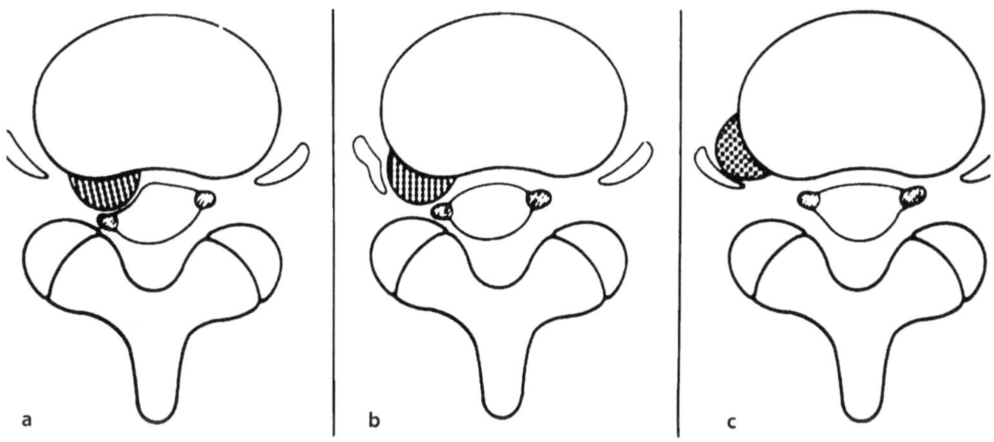

Fig. 5.4. **a** Foraminal extension; **b** foraminal, and **c** lateral posterolateral herniated discs [8]

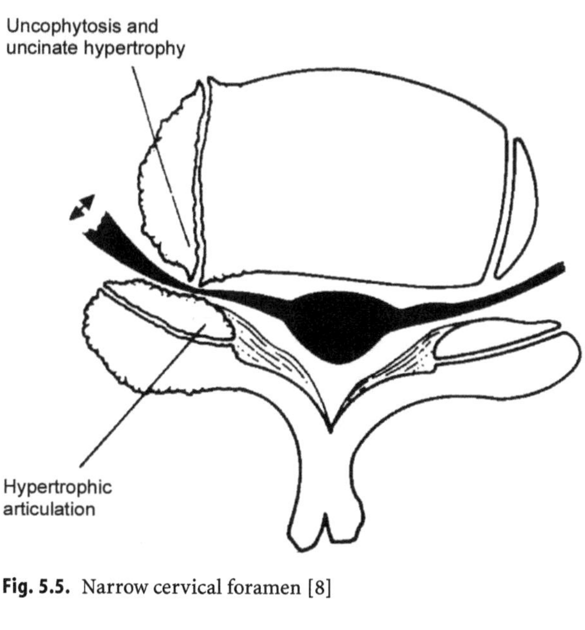

Fig. 5.5. Narrow cervical foramen [8]

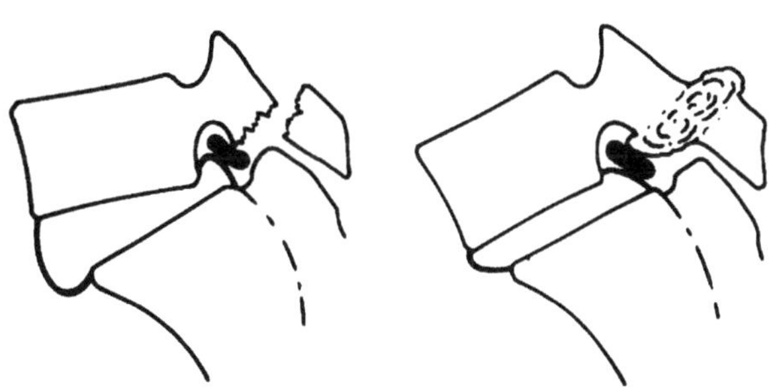

Fig. 5.6. Foraminal stenosis attributable to isthmic lysis [8]

The rare etiologies of foraminal stenosis, notably those involving tumors, are not covered here because the related patient care is entirely different.

Hypertrophic articulation.

Mechanisms Governing Pain in Radiculalgias

Radicular pain caused by compression in the foramen is multifactorial [18]. Mechanical compression of the spinal nerve and ganglion in the foramen produces:

- Chemical phenomena: the degeneration of the nucleus pulposus releases substances (histamine, prostaglandins) that irritate the nerve and the ganglion, causing chemical radiculitis.
- Edematous phenomena: compression of the nerve causes increased permeability of the intraneural vessels, leading to intraneural edema, and consequently a nervous dysfunction causing pain.
- Vascular phenomena: compression of the venous plexuses leads to dilatation and then foraminal venous congestion, disturbing the local circulation and producing ischemia, edema and demyelinating lesions.
- Local inflammation: an autoimmune reaction with respect to discal material causes an inflammatory reaction with secondary development of perineural fibrosis.

The spinal ganglion is the vulnerable part of the spinal complex and its mechanical compression can produce neuronal hyperactivity in the nociceptive transmission system. It plays an important role in expressing radicular pain.

Indications

Spontaneous resolution of radiculalgia occurs in more than 50 % of cases. The main objective in treating the remainder is to improve quality of life through long-term pain control.

The initial symptomatic treatment is medical, combining systemic anti-inflammatories and/or corticosteroids with restriction if necessary. In the event of failure, guided injections under tomodensitometry allow the steroid anti-inflammatory drug to be administered locally and thus make it possible to greatly increase the dose delivered to the site of pain compared to doses given via oral or parenteral routes.

These techniques can benefit patients with radiculalgia in the absence of neurological deficit, in cases where this pain resists appropriate medical treatment and is maintained for more than 3 to 4 weeks, and when foraminal stenosis is shown using modern imaging of the spine, i.e., CT and/or MRI. Local injections of corticosteroids have a limited effect on radicular pain and are not aimed at the treatment of lumbar pain.

In a few cases where symptomatic treatment fails and/or severe neurological effects occur, etiological treatment is employed, which in the event of true disc herniation involves surgery or nucleolysis.

Contraindications

- Absolute: allergy to corticosteroids
- Contingent: blood dyscrasias, severe chronic respiratory insufficiency (for the posterior approach), pregnancy.

Technique

Care of the Patient

The simple procedure can be used with ambulatory patients. The indication is confirmed by means of different imaging methods (CT and/or MRI). The patient should be asked about hemostatic problems and allergies. Patients with atopy receive an antiallergic preparation; in patients with a real allergy to iodine the examination is performed without the injection of a contrast medium. The patient is informed beforehand about the conditions of the examination and about the benefits and risks involved. A venous route is systematically employed. Written consent must be obtained as required by regulations.

Placing the Patient

The position of the patient depends on the injection level; for the cervical level the patient is supine; for injections at the dorsal and lumbar levels the patient is prone.

Cardiac function, arterial blood pressure and oxygen saturation are monitored in frail patients.

Materials

The usual consumable items are: an iodized contrast medium, 1 % lidocaine, and prednisolone acetate. The examination is conducted under strictly aseptic conditions: sterile disposable compresses, syringes, needle for local anesthesia, and needle for injection (PL 22 G). Asepsis requires the use of sterile drapes, clothing, and gloves, and scrupulous disinfection of the surface of the skin.

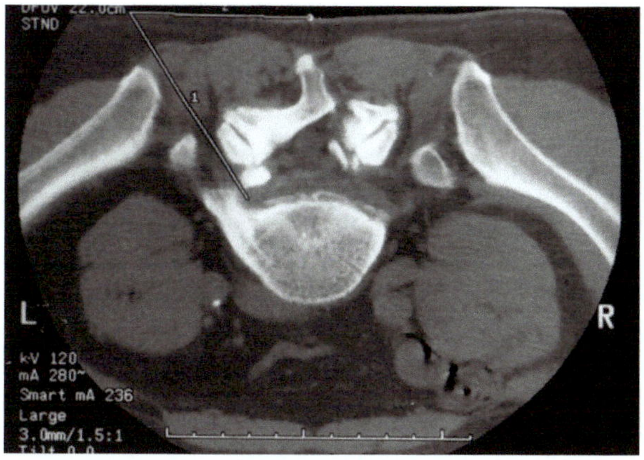

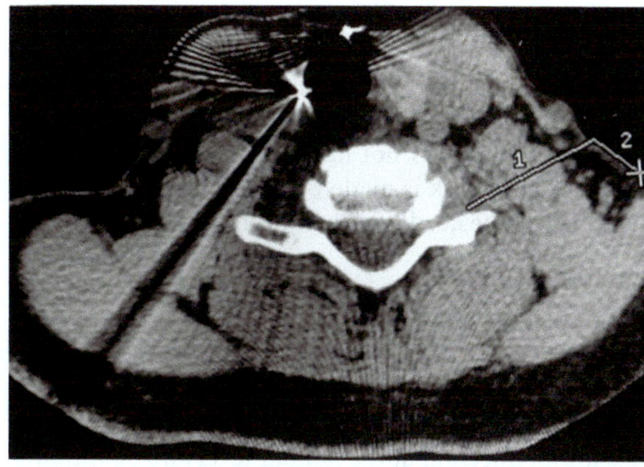

Fig. 5.7., Fig. 5.8. Determination of puncture courses at the lumbar (Fig. 5.7) and cervical (Fig. 5.8) levels

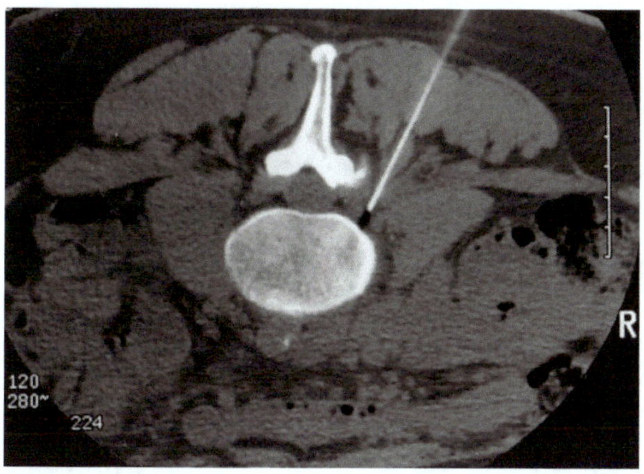

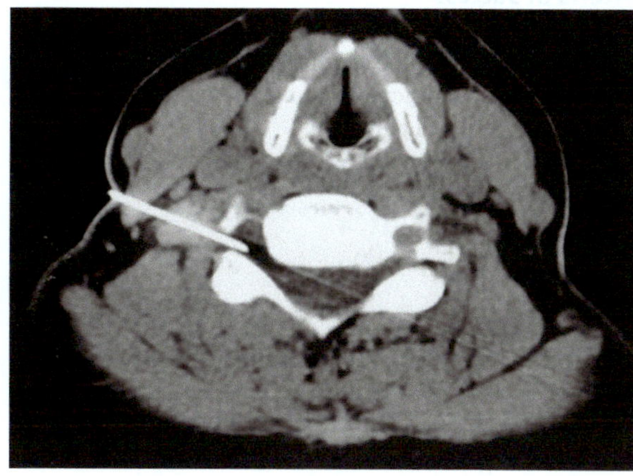

Fig. 5.9., Fig. 5.10 Monitoring the position of the needle

Method

After location by means of a frontal and lateral topogram, contiguous 3-mm axial sections centered on the affected spinal segment are made in double fenestration, during apnea and without inclination of the stand in order to locate the spinal ganglion in its intervertebral foramen. A reference incision is then selected. The cutaneous point of entry should allow a posterolateral approach to the ganglion in the upper part of the foramen at the dorsal and lumbar levels such that the needle passes close to the posterior articular mass.

At the cervical level the entry point is lateral, behind the sternocleidomastoid muscle, avoiding the vascular structures. The puncture course is determined on the console by tracing a virtual line between the cutaneous point of entry and the foramen. The cutaneous entry point is marked on the patient's skin by means of the luminous center-finder projecting the selected incision plane, the distance determined on the console being measured in relation to a metallic marker positioned laterally on the patient's neck, as a lateral approach does not enable location of a palpable structure (Fig. 5.8).

At the dorsolumbar level the entry point is marked on the patient's skin by means of the luminous center-finder projecting the selected incision plane; the distance determined on the console is measured in relation to the median line (Fig. 5.7).

After local anesthesia of the cutaneous and muscular planes on the predetermined course, a 22 G lumbar puncture needle is introduced as far as the point of contact with the spinal ganglion, the position of the needle being monitored by iterative scanographic sections, the number of which depends on the experience of the operator and the anatomical situation (Figs. 5.9, 5.10).

The correct positioning of the needle tip is assessed on the basis of imaging (seeing the needle tip artifact in contact with the ganglion) and the patient's reporting (usually reproduction of the pain). The injected solution is a mixture of 75 mg prednisolone with approximately 1 ml lidocaine and 1 ml iodized contrast medium.

A tomodensitometric check is made at half-syringe in order to verify proper diffusion of the mixture and, in the event that this is not happening, to reposition the needle. A last check is made when the injection is complete, before the needle is finally withdrawn.

Duration of the Procedure

This depends on the operator's experience.

After the learning stage, it is considered to be 15 minutes for an injection at the lumbar level and 30 minutes for an injection at the cervical level.

Criteria of Success

Success of the procedure includes these elements:

- Recurrence of radicular pain usually felt
- Molding of spinal ganglion
- Periradicular entry
- Foraminal entry
- Epidural entry
  (See Fig. 5.11, Fig. 5.12)

Refining Technique; Variations for Different Levels

- Injection must be performed slowly in order to avoid reflux along the needle.
- The shortest possible needle must always be used for maneuvering purposes (4 cm for the cervical level, 9 cm if possible for the lumbar level).
- For the dorsolumbar levels, preference must be given to the most lateral approach possible, in order to maximize the obliqueness of the needle, thereby enabling intraforaminal diffusion of the solution and epidural entry. For pathway S1 radiculalgias, the injections go into the first sacral cavity.
- At the cervical level it is rarely possible to position the needle very far forward in the foramen because of the closeness of the vertebral artery and because hyperalgia is much more of a problem than at the lumbar level. Lidocaine should not be included in the injection mixture without previously checking that the tip of the needle is in a strictly extradural position by injecting iodized contrast medium on its own.

It is not always possible to reach the lowest cervical levels because of a short neck and an elevated position of the shoulders.

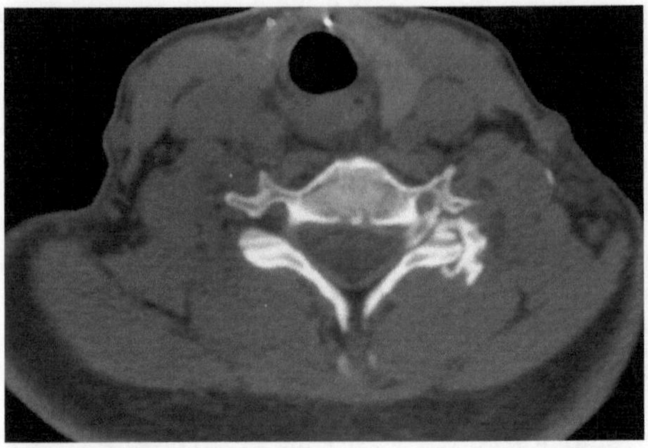

Fig. 5.11. Monitoring after injection at the cervical level (C6–C7 Left: molding of spinal ganglion, periradicular and foraminal entry

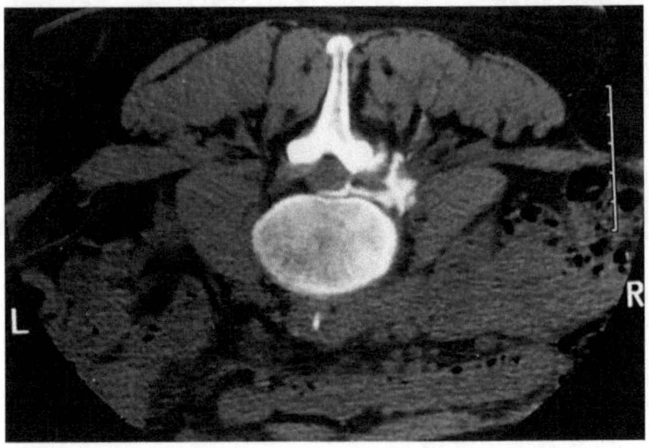

Fig. 5.12. Monitoring after injection at the lumbar level (L3–L4 G): the same criteria are used as in Fig. 5.11 plus epidural entry.

Complications, Side Effects, Monitoring

References to consult include these: [3, 6, 15, 17].

Complications

These are exceptional: we have observed some rare allergic skin reactions, nausea, vomiting, and other vagal disturbances that cleared up spontaneously. Complications reported in the literature should be avoidable by strict adherence to the rules for asepsis and by monitoring the needle position with CT. There have been reports of hyperadrenocorticism, hematomyelia, epidural abscess, meningitis or severe headaches, pleural puncture, dural puncture, and damage to the vertebral artery. Punctures of the foraminal venous plexus occur frequently and have no consequences.

Side Effects

Rapid transitory anesthesia may occur in the dermatome concerned, and prudence should be exercised in consequence. The patient should be accompanied by someone since the he or she should not drive immediately after the procedure. Exacerbation of pain in the first 48 hours is commonly observed: it is therefore important to advise the patient about this beforehand and to prescribe antalgics if necessary.

Monitoring

The patient is systematically monitored for half an hour after completion of the procedure. No special convalescent measures are necessary.

Results

The effectiveness of the procedure is assessed on the basis of the decline in pain measured on a visual analogue scale before and one and three weeks after injection, and on the reduction or cessation of the use of antalgics. Various studies [1, 19] have demonstrated that 65% of patients experience lasting improvement (mean duration: 15 months) and that on average an improvement is evident after 13 days. In 90% of the patients showing lasting improvement, the intensity of radiculalgias declined by at least 50%. Eighty percent of the patients with lasting improvement stopped taking medication after the injections were given.

These injections are effective without difference among the spinal levels involved (cervicobrachial neuralgia, intercostal pain, cruralgia and sciatica) and also without difference with respect to the radiological anomaly in question (degenerative phenomena, herniated disc, post-operative fibrosis). Long-term improvement is probably attributable to the corticosteroids. We have observed that the mechanisms controlling pain are multifactorial and that the "neuralgic center" is the spinal ganglion. Two hypotheses concerning effectiveness can be put forward:

- A direct anti-inflammatory effect
- An action on the C fibers

The latter is based on the fact that the mechanosensitivity of the ganglion induced by a mechanical stimulus is partly mediated by the amyelinated C fibers. It has been shown that the local application of corticosteroids decreases both the hyperactivity of the nerve fibers and the conduction in the afferent amyelinated C fibers.

Some patients experience only a temporary reduction in pain. This is attributable to the lidocaine and its rapid-action mechanism.

Specific Advantages of Injection Under CT

The advantages of this technique over other local injections of corticosteroids are that the exact position of the needle tip is identified and that the correct diffusion of the solution is monitored. In fact observations have shown that needles are in poor positions in 30% to 40% of periradicular injections performed under fluoroscopy [4, 9, 10]. The complete absence of irradiation for the operator is an additional reason for preferring this technique to those involving fluoroscopy.

Future development of fluoroscopy-CT techniques should reduce the time taken for the procedure, still without irradiating the doctor (the technique allowing the operator to be at least 1 m from the source of radiation).

Lastly, we recommend giving a maximum of three injections at intervals of at least 3 weeks. Surgery should be considered if there is no improvement after three procedures.

Conclusion

The tomodensitometry-controlled technique of periradicular injections of corticosteroids in contact with the spinal ganglion is simple and easily reproducible and can be performed on ambulatory patients. It should be included among the therapeutic procedures for dealing with radicular pain of discal or degenerative origin. The purpose is to achieve a rapid decline in symptoms, thereby improving a patient's quality of life.

References

1. Berger O, Dousset V, Delmer O et al (1999) Évaluation de l'efficacité des infiltrations foraminales de corticoïdes guidées sous tomodensitométrie, dans le traitement des radiculalgies par conflit foraminal. J Radiol 80:917–925
2. Bouchet A, Cuilleret J (1985) Anatomie topographique, descriptive et fonctionelle, in Le système nerveux central. SIMEP
3. Chan ST, Leung S (1989) Spinal epidural abscess following steroid injection for sciatica. Spine 14:106–108
4. Dreyfuss P (1993) Epidural steroid injections. A procedure ideally performed with fluoroscopic control and contrast media. Int Spinal Infect Soc Newslett 1:34–40
5. Giles L, Kaveri M (1990) Some osseous and soft tissue causes of human intervertebral canal stenosis. J Rheumatol 17:1474–1481
6. Gutknechi DR (1987) Chemical meningitis following epidural injections of corticosteroids. Am J Med 82:570
7. Kunnert JE, Vautravers P, Martin JC et al (1982) Les hernies discales lombaires foraminales: particularités cliniques, électrologiques et thérapeutiques. Masson, Paris
8. Manelfe C (1989) Imagerie du rachis et de la moëlle. Vigot, Paris
9. Rapp SE, Haselkorn JK, Elamm JK et al (1994) Epidural steroid injection in the treatment of low back pain: a meta-analysis. Anesthesiology 81:923

10. Renfrew DL, Moore TE, Kathol MH et al (1991) Correct placement of epidural steroid injections: fluoroscopic guidance and contrast administration. AJNR 12:1003–1007
11. Revel M, Mayoux-Benhamou MA, Aaron C, Amor B (1988) Variations morphologiques des trous de conjugaison lombaires lors de la flexion-extension et de l'affaissement discal. Rev Rhumat 55:361–366
12. Rouvière H, Delmas A (2002) Anatomie humaine. Masson, Paris
13. Sobotta. Atlas d'anatomie humaine, vols I and II, 3rd French edn. Éditions Médicales Internationales
14. Stephens M, Evans J, O'Brien J (1991) Lumbar intervertbral foramens: An in vitro study of their shape in relation to intervertebral disc pathology. Spine 16:525–529
15. Tuel SM, Meythaler JM, Cross LL (1990) Cushing's syndrome from epidural methylprednisolone. Pain 40:81–84
16. Vital JM (2000) Foramen intervertébral lombaire: anatomie, exploration et pathologie. Cahier d'Enseignment de la SOFCOT. Expansion Scientifique Publications, Conférences d'Enseignement
17. Williams KN, Jackowski A, Evans PJD (1990) Epidural haematoma requiring surgical decompression following repeated cervical epidural steroid injections for chronic pain. Pain 42:197–199
18. Zennaro H (1996) Les infiltrations foraminales péri-ganglionnaires de corticoïdes. Thèse Médecine Bordeaux II
19. Zennaro H, Dousset V, Viaud B et al (1998) Periganglionic foraminal steroid injections performed under CT control. AJNR 19:349–352

Spinal Infiltrations: Technical Difficulties and Potential Complications

6

Philippe Brunner, Patrick Chevallier,
Nicolas Amoretti, Jack Sedat,
Elodie Cazaux, Françoise Fuerxer,
Jean-Michel Cucchi, Michel-Yves Mourou

Periradicular infiltrations are effective for treating radicular pains at the cervical, dorsal, lumbar, and sacral levels [1].

Physicians in varied specialties perform these infiltrations, e.g., general practitioners, physical therapists, rheumatologists, orthopedic surgeons, and radiologists. They use very different localization means : from simple anatomic reference to a most sophisticated imaging technique, namely, scanography.

In last few years, these treatments have been too widely and/or too easily prescribed and performed. More or less serious complications have therefore occurred.

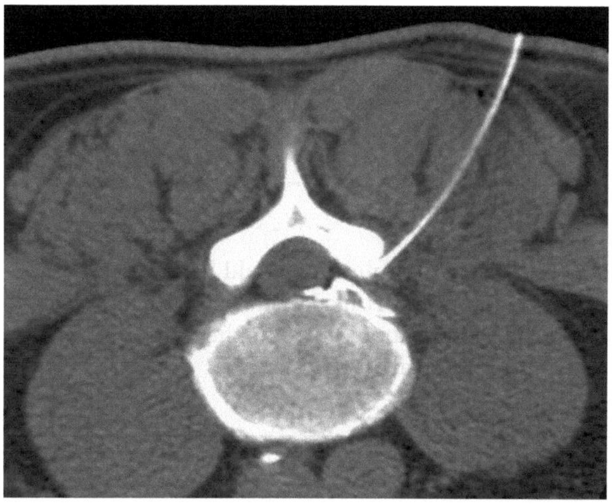

Fig. 6.1. Periradicular diffusion of the radiopaque contrast

What Are the Potential Complications of Periradicular Infiltrations?

Inefficacy

Of course, inefficacy is not a complication beyond having imposed an unnecessary risk, even if minimal. Of course, the results of each infiltration are not guaranteed and depend on different factors (e.g., type of problem addressed, age, anatomic factors, psychological profile), but the result is disappointing if, for instance, the injected product does not diffuse into the planned location.

- If the product (corticosteroid) is injected too far from a target, it will be less efficient. Clinical localization during the infiltration in such cases is illusory.
  - Radiologic localization also has its failings; it is often difficult to obtain a casting of the nerve root targeted by a radiopaque contrast as needed for good periradicular diffusion [2]. On the other hand, periradicular diffusion is not afflicted with targeting problems when scanographic control is used. (Fig. 6.1).
- If the medication is injected in a vascular network, more exactly in the epidural venous plexus, failure is possible. The injected corticosteroids simply enter systemic circulation. In this case, radiologic control is again inadequate while scanographic control highlights this risk.
  - The infiltration needles employed here are 22 gauge small caliber (external diameter 0.7 mm).
  - It should be noted that blood reflux, even with withdrawal, occasionally will not occur when the needle is inside an intravascular network. It is therefore important to first inject contrast medium in order to inspect its diffusion into the target area. If the contrast medium is not visible in the slices under scanographic control, it means the end of the needle is in an intravascular space and it has to be adjusted.
- If the end of the needle is in the posterior epidural space, the contrast medium often diffuses into a lateral epidural space only, and consequently it cannot be of help at the expected site. The needle has to be repositioned before injecting the medication [3, 4].

Hematoma

When the hemostatic conditions are respected (normal coagulation values, no platelets given within 8 days before the procedure), epidural hematoma is an exceptional complication during an epidural infiltration within the spinal canal.

Infection

Strict asepsis is necessary.

Every infiltration must be made in an adapted room, respecting aseptic conditions which are almost surgical.

Personnel involved must wear sterile clothes (mask, head cap, gloves).

Vagal Reaction

The rate of this complication could be lowered by having a previous comforting patient visit with one or more of the radiology team performing the procedure, and by an appropriate local anesthesia.

Hypersensitivity

Iodinated contrast medium may be contraindicated because of prior reactions.

In some cases, infiltrations can be performed using sterile air (Fig. 6.2).

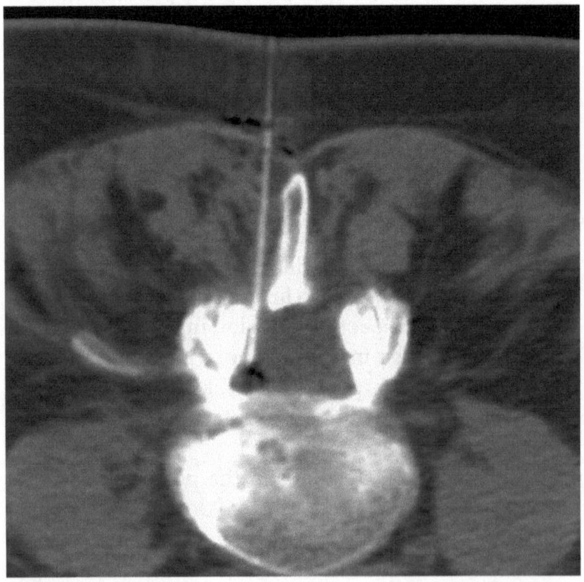

Fig. 6.2. Negative contrast: sterile air

At the cervical and dorsal levels air injection is forbidden as air in a vertebral or anterior spinal artery could induces very serious ischemic consequences.

Puncture of Important Organs

Spinal Cord Puncture

This is a very exceptional case.

Scanographic control can avoid this problem during the needle's progression in the cervical peridural infiltrations.

Absolute immobility of the patient is necessary.

Arterial Puncture

This is a complication with a variety of possible serious consequences.
As stated above, such a puncture could be innocuous but major-risk vessels are:

- Vertebral artery
- Carotid artery(most exceptional)
- Anterior spinal artery.

The serious problems that may ensue from such a perforation include:

- Dissection
- Thrombus
- False aneurysm
- Perivascular hematoma
- Air embolism
- Embolism by particular elements from corticosteroids (more exactly those with big crystals).

The potential risk is an ischemic (cerebral) stroke or medullar ischemia [6].

Epidural Venous Puncture

This is a frequent procedure, normally without great consequence except in the possible inefficacy of the infiltration.

Such a puncture has to be detected by a previous contrast injection and must be surgically corrected if considered necessary.

Nerve Root Puncture

This mishap might occur during a rushed act when the needle is too rapidly advanced.

The immediate pain felt by the patient is ordinarily sufficient to induce repositioning.

Residual paresthesia could occur. If spontaneous resolution does not occur as is usual, B vitamin therapy may give relief.

Intrathecal Puncture

Such a puncture may of course be intended in certain situations, but can also be accidental.

Its detection is easy under scanographic control, bringing into prominence the intrathecal contrast.

Spinal fluid reflux is not always obvious for the same reason that blood reflux sometimes doesn't occur through the fine needles used.

These problems can occur:

- Leakage of spinal fluid
- Meningeal irritation syndrome

Subdural Puncture

This is a very rare occurrence; it can be detected on scanography slices when the virtual subdural space fills with contrast fluid. (Fig. 6.3, 6.4, 6.5).

Besides yielding no benefit, such mistakes can lead to back pain [5].

Radicular Sheath Puncture

This puncture is easily seen on the scanner (Fig. 6.6).

The techniques and problems here are the same as with intrathecal punctures, though at the dural sheath level.

Injection of corticosteroid is likewise disallowed here if contraindicated intrathecally [7].

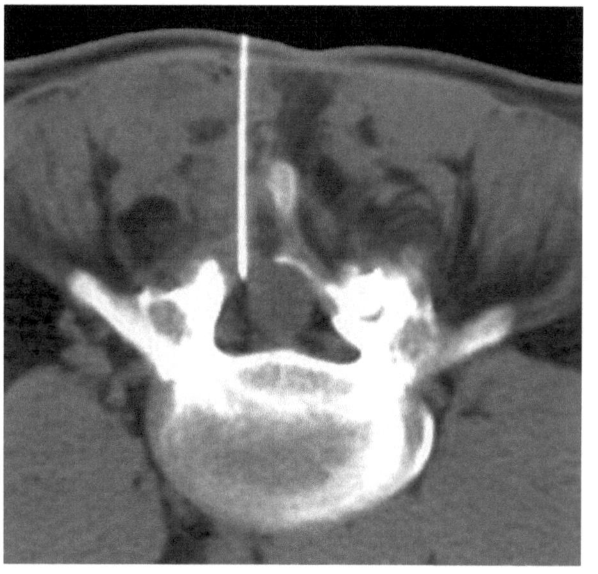

Fig. 6.3. Intracanalar infiltration

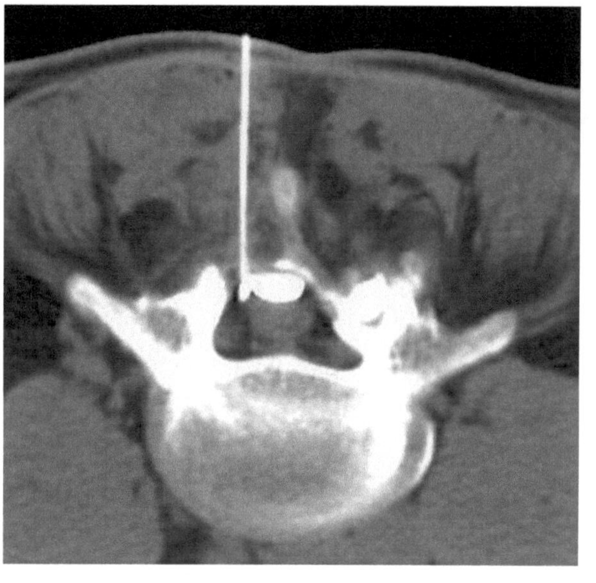

Fig. 6.4. Subdural puncture

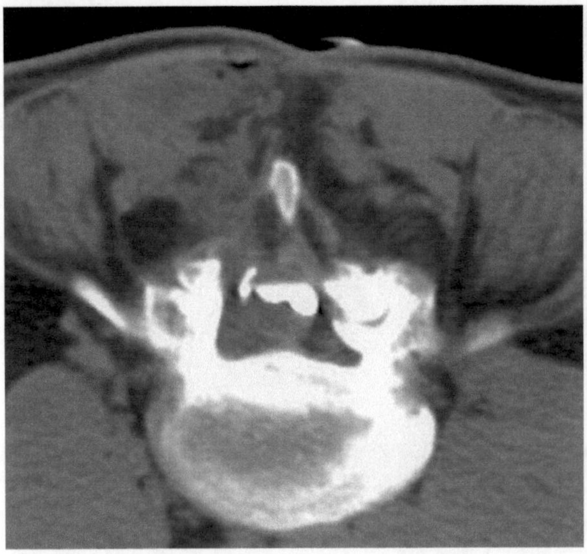

Fig. 6.5. Subdural contrast difusion

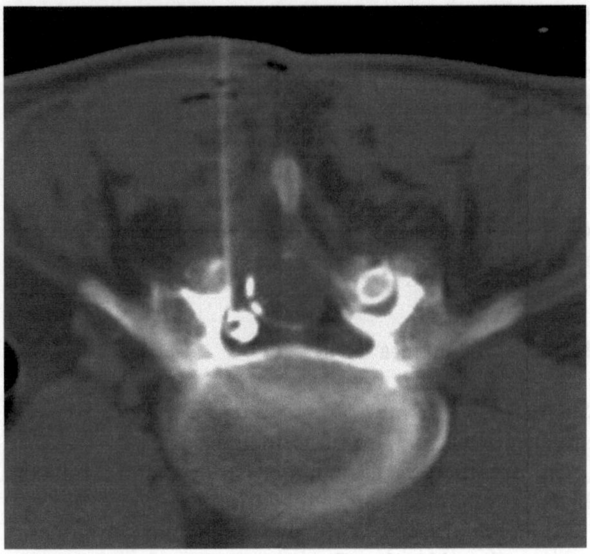

Fig. 6.6. Radicular sheath puncture

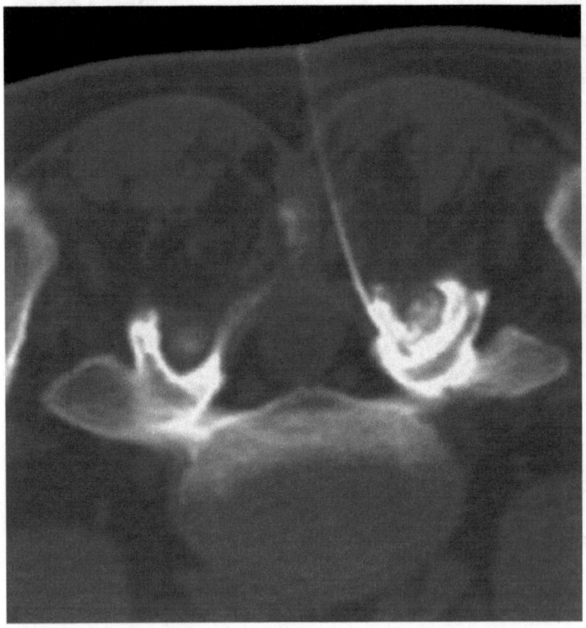

Fig. 6.7. Posterior intraarticular puncture

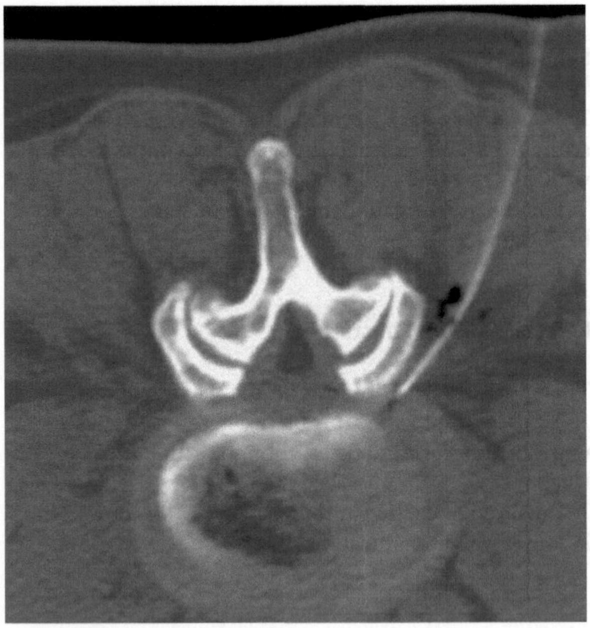

Fig. 6.8. Intradiscal puncture

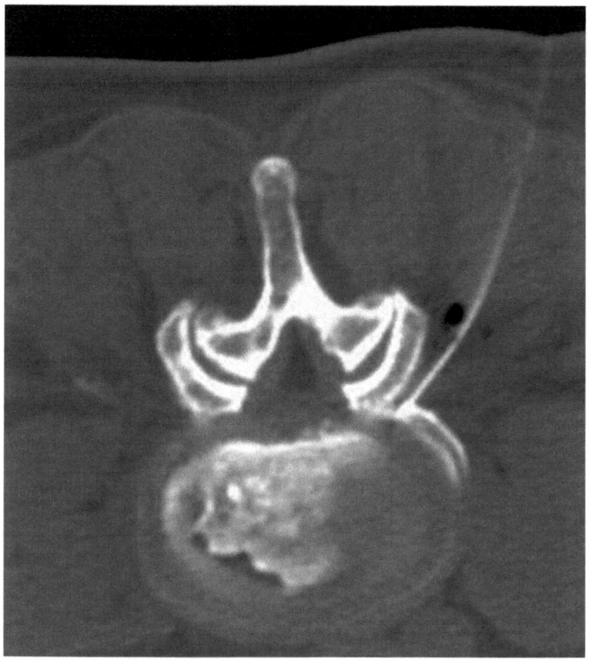

Fig. 6.9. Discography

Intra-articular Posterior Puncture

This situation can lead to inefficacy problems. It cannot be detected by anatomic means or simple radioscopic measure (Fig. 6.7).

As articular puncture occurs, a "loss of resistance" of the syringe pump is felt similar to that in an accidental < epidural entrance.

Intra-annular or Intranuclear Discal Puncture

This puncture happens most often during a foraminal infiltration.

It unfortunately remains unsuspected during scope operation (Fig. 6.8, 6,9).

Except the inefficacy problem, consequences are not particularly significant.

How to Avoid These Problems

- Scanography provides the best control for the monitoring of all infiltrations procedures. This control is most important for all infiltrations at the cervical level.
- While the use of non-iodine contrast may be necessary for safety, the procedure is of great importance in that it allows one to detect an incorrect position of the needle tip, not otherwise seen.
- Pre-curved 22 gauge needles permit an optimum approach to the target while avoiding important intervening structures and other obstacles.
  - These needles are used as landmark keys for avoiding the obstacles [5].
  - For iodine-hypersensitive patients, sterile air for contrast is a potential solution at the lumbar level.
- Scan can be undertaken with different tilts of the gantry (cranial, caudal).
  - A variety of needles and their approaches can likewise be used (cranial or caudal, medial or lateral routes).
- For local anesthesia, lidocaine 0.5% is recommended. This relatively small dose allows a nerve puncture still to be felt, and does not induce a peri-dural anesthesia, which could be problematic for an ambulatory, or " day surgery" patient.
- The safest route must be chosen. At the cervical level, safety indicates a posterolateral approach. This technique allows one to avoid articular structures.
  - In order to stay away from an anterior spinal artery, entry of the spinal foramina must be avoided.
- Finally, it should be kept in mind that the operator is an essential part of the scenario. She/he is the person who defines the indication and performs the infiltration.

It is essential to examine every patient at the beginning of the process, correlating the physical exam and clinical history with the procedure to be undertaken.

Infiltrations are not harmless; they require the experience acquired only through the performance of a large number of procedures.

Conclusion

Indications for infiltrations have expanded in recent years.

Most of them are performed under simple scope control.

Scanography is used to visualize as clearly as possible the sites of interest, avoiding vital organs and controlling the diffusion of contrast.

Procedures can thus be efficient and fully effective while maintaining the highest of safety standards.

References

1. Gangi A, Dietemann JL (1996) Tomodensitométrie interventionnelle en anesthésie locorégionale. In: Muller A (ed) Anesthésie loco-régionale et traitement de la douleur. Masson, Paris, pp 555–564
2. Siebel RM, Grönemeyer DH (1990) Periradicular therapy. In: Seibel RM (ed) Interventional computer tomography. Blackwell, Boston, pp 100–115
3. Brunner P, Chanalet S, Sedat J et al (2002) Percutaneous infiltrations of cervical, thoracic and lumbar spine. Semin Intervent Radiol 19:219–228
4. Windsor RE, Falco FJE (2001) Paraplegia following selective nerve root blocks. Int Spinal Inject Soc Sci Newslett 4:53
5. Gangi A, Dietemann JL (1994) Tomodensitométrie Interventionnelle. Vigot (Paris) 24:213–225
6. Krause D, Cognet F, Dranssart M et al (2002) Syllabus FMC. Soc Franç Radiol (Paris) 157–161

7 Trigeminal Neuralgia

Alain Czorny, Romain Billon-Grand

Facial, or trigeminal, neuralgia was identified as a clinical entity at the end of the 17th century. The well-known term "tic douloureux" (Nicolas André, 1756), is often wrongly attributed to Trousseau (1864) who did, however, quite rightly describe the condition as "epileptiform neuralgia." It is one of the most intense pains found in humans.

Anatomical Review, Secondary Neuralgias

The anatomy of the trigeminal system must be firmly in mind when undertaking radiological examination. Such examination should focus on the whole route taken by the nerve (Fig. 7.1):

- Pons cerebellum (from which the nerve emerges)
- Nerve trunk (1) in the pontocerebellar cistern and relationship with vessels (arteries and veins, sometimes with vascular loops, an ectatic basilar artery, or aneurysms)
- Gasser's ganglion (2) in Meckel's cavity on the roof of the apex of the petrous bone
- Cavernous sinus
- Nerve root outlets across the cranium
- Foramen ovale (3) in the horizontal part of the large sphenoid wing (V_3 and motor root);
- Foramen rotundum (4) in the coronal plane in the pterygomaxillary fossa (V_2);
- Superior orbital fissure (V_1; 5).

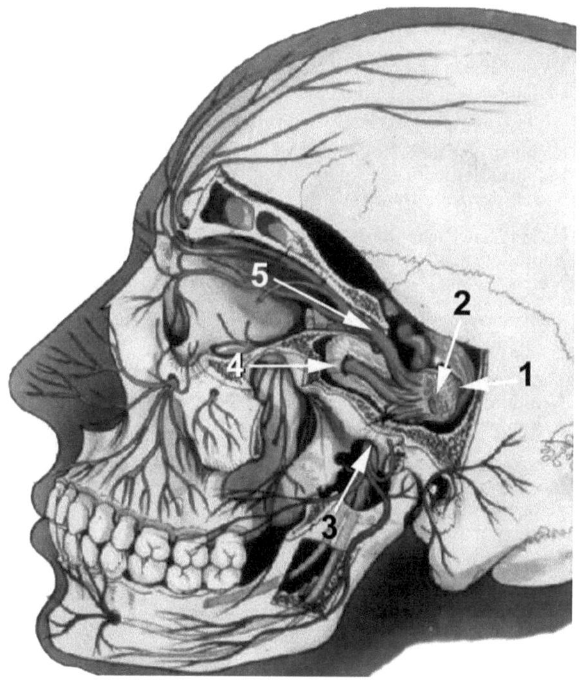

Fig. 7.1. Anatomy of the trigeminal system

The trigeminal nerve is the main facial sensory nerve. Roughly, the skin areas are: V_1 spread above a line between the outer corner of the eye and the tragus, plus the nasal bridge, V_2 below the previous line and above a line from the labial commissure to the tragus, and V_3 below this line (Fig. 7.2).

Trigeminal neuralgia, in its so-called essential form, can be compared item by item with cluster headaches, which is the main differential diagnosis for other facial pains (Table 7.1). Its particularity lies in the fact that it responds only to specific treatment, both medically and surgically. A deafferentation type pain, it resists peripheral analgesics and even opiates. The cornerstone of diagnosis is the clinical description of pain. Clinical examination only aims at ruling out trigeminal neuropathies, i.e., trigeminal neuropathic pains secondary to any neurological disease.

The etiologies of secondary neuralgias of cranial nerve V must be investigated when clinical examination reveals that a sensory or motor branch is affected or that there is a change in the type of pain. Clinical features of such a secondary neuralgia include:

- Young adult, man or woman
- Nocturnal pain and/or a permanent background pain
- Pain involving more than one branch of the trigeminal nerve
- Corneal or cutaneous hypoesthesia or anesthesia
- No distinct trigger zone

Table 7.1. Clinical comparison of trigeminal neuralgia with vascular facial algia. Of the so-called essential orofacial pains, two can be compared schematically point by point from a symptomatological perspective

Facial or trigeminal neuralgia	Vascular facial algia
Known as "Trousseau's tic douloureux," it is characterized by intense, stabbing, short-lived pain in the area of the trigeminal nerve (V). 5/100,000 inhab.	Known as "cluster headache," it is characterized by repeated pain which is highly characteristic. With respect to its symptomatology and its medical treatment, it is closely resembles a migraine. 80/100,000 inhab.
Women aged over 65; 60 % women	Young men aged under 40; 80 % men
Intense, very short bursts of pain (several seconds to 2 minutes)	Continuous pain (not pulsating)
Unbearable, stabbing, burning.	30 minutes to 3 hours Burning, crushing, tearing
Patient tense, fixed features.	Agitated "could jump out of the window"
Trigger zone	Alcohol triggers attacks
Topography: 1 or 2 roots of cranial nerve V Unilateral	Periorbital Retro-ocular Unilateral
No particular time. Not at night No periodicity 5 to 10/day, subintrant	Stereotyped timing: daytime 1 to 8/day Same time (clock symptom) Seasonal periodicity: 3 to 10 weeks duration
No associated symptoms Neurological examination normal	Positive symptoms associated: vegetative symptoms, lacrimation, Horner's syndrome, conjunctival and hemifacial redness
Carbamazepine (and gabapentin):	Initial treatment: oxygen therapy + triptans. Basic chronic and/or episodic treatment:
Therapeutic and diagnostic test Imipraminic baclofen, clonazepam, morphine ineffective	Verapamil (1200×3), beta-blockers (AVC 40×2), indomethacin, lithium (300×2)
Surgical treatment: percutaneous thermocoagulation, microvascular decompression, percutaneous compression, glycerol, premotor cortex stimulation	No surgical treatment Treatment of attacks Basic treatment

If a secondary affection is suggested, an MRI should be performed systematically

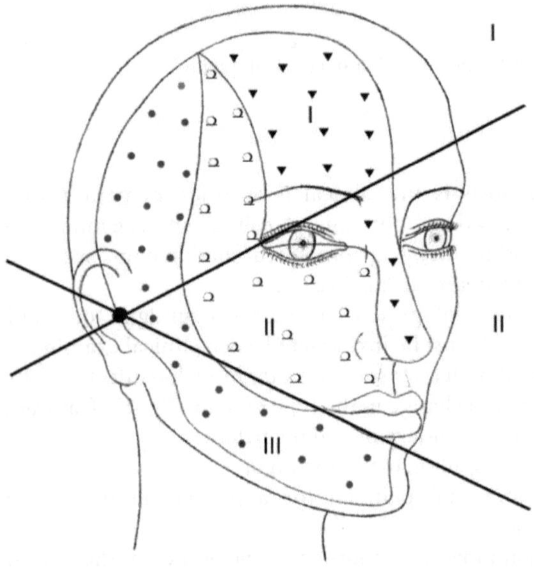

Fig. 7.2. Sketch of the skin areas affected by the trigeminal nerve (Drawn by Andia Hashemizadeh)

- Poor reactivity to treatment with carbamazepine: this molecule remains the reference medical treatment, other treatments playing only a secondary role.

The main etiologies of trigeminal neuropathies, as opposed to trigeminal neuralgias are:

- Affection of bulboprotuberantial and medullar nuclei of the fifth cranial nerve
- Wallenberg's syndrome
- Syringobulbia
- Occipitocervical junction malformation
- Multiple sclerosis in a young adult (which is one of the major differential diagnoses)
- Peripheral affections:
  - Petromastoid lesion with epidermoid cyst in the pontocerebellar angle, post-otitic osteitis, neoplastic metastases
  - Cranial nerve V lesion in the outer wall due to meningioma of the cavernous compartment (Fig. 7.3) or clivus chordoma

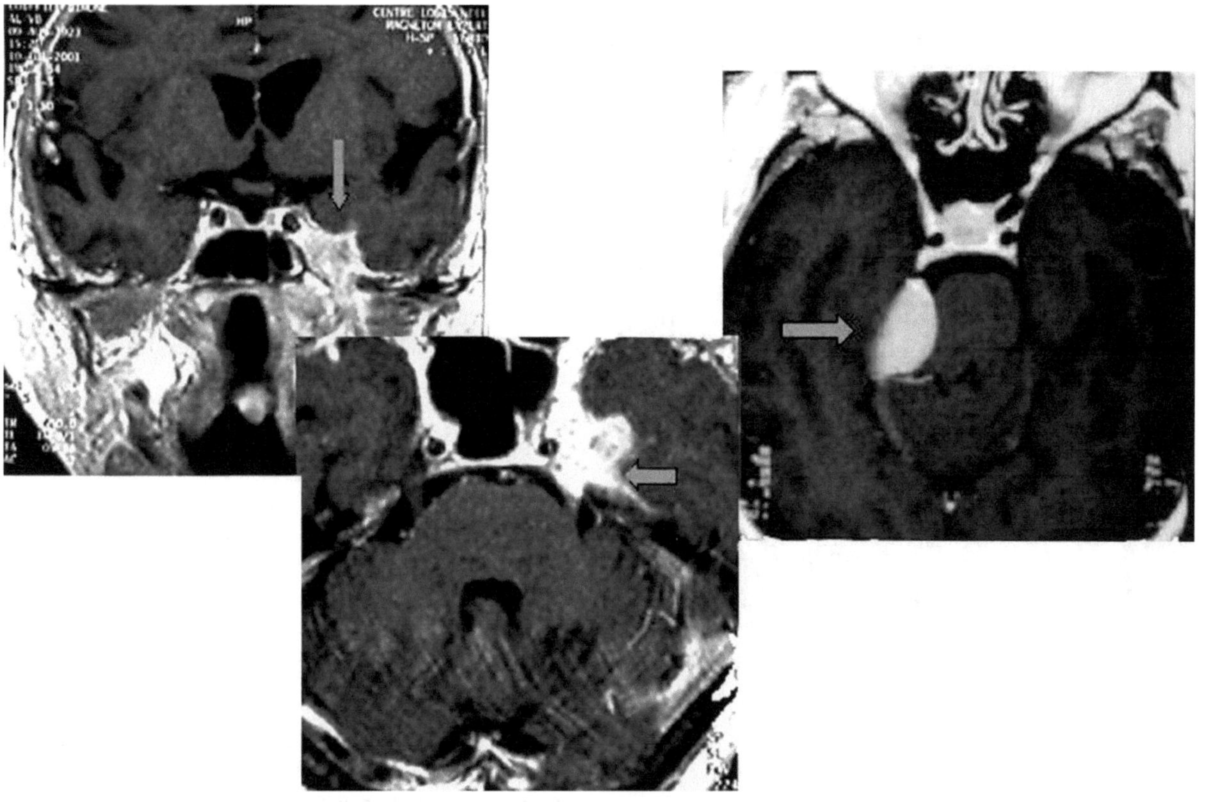

Fig. 7.3. Meningiomas of the cavernous sinus and tentorial notch responsible for trigeminal neuralgia

- Vestibular Schwannomas, in which trigeminal pain can occur before facial paralysis, but usually after cochleovestibular signs (loss of hearing and vertigo).

CT scan with coronal and axial sections in bone resolution and three-dimensional reconstruction is informative (Paget, petromastoid malformation).

MRI on 3D weighed sequences can show either contact of the fifth nerve and vascular loops, or neurovascular compression between them. Once each structure are differentiated reliably, MRI can also specify the nerve's relationships with its environment in Meckel's cavity and perhaps disclose a rare cranial nerve V Schwannoma. It is very difficult to confirm neurovascular compression through imaging. On occasion, however, operative findings disclose compressing not seen on MRI (Fig. 7.4).

Surgical Treatment

Percutaneous or open, retromastoid micro-vascular decompressions are the most performed procedures in these patients.

Percutaneous Approach

Percutaneous techniques aim to destroy some of the C fibers to reduce the pattern of nociceptive influx reaching the thalamus, given that the deep sensory filter is deficient, this being a deafferentation pain. For all these approaches the cheek is penetrated between 1.5 and 2.5 cm laterally to the labial commissure with a needle that is led through the foramen ovale (Fig. 7.5) at the base of the large sphenoid wing, to reach Gasser's ganglion (under brief general anesthesia using propofol).

X-ray verification can take place in three ways:

- Lateral view, wherein the needle in retroclival projection is in the angle intercepted by the roof of the petromastoid and the dorsum sellae (Fig. 7.6)
- Plain X-rays of the skull using Hirtz incidence are useful for viewing the foramen ovale, but difficult to perform in elderly patients suffering from cervical arthritis
- A special view projecting the foramen ovale in the angle of the vertical and horizontal branches of the mandible.

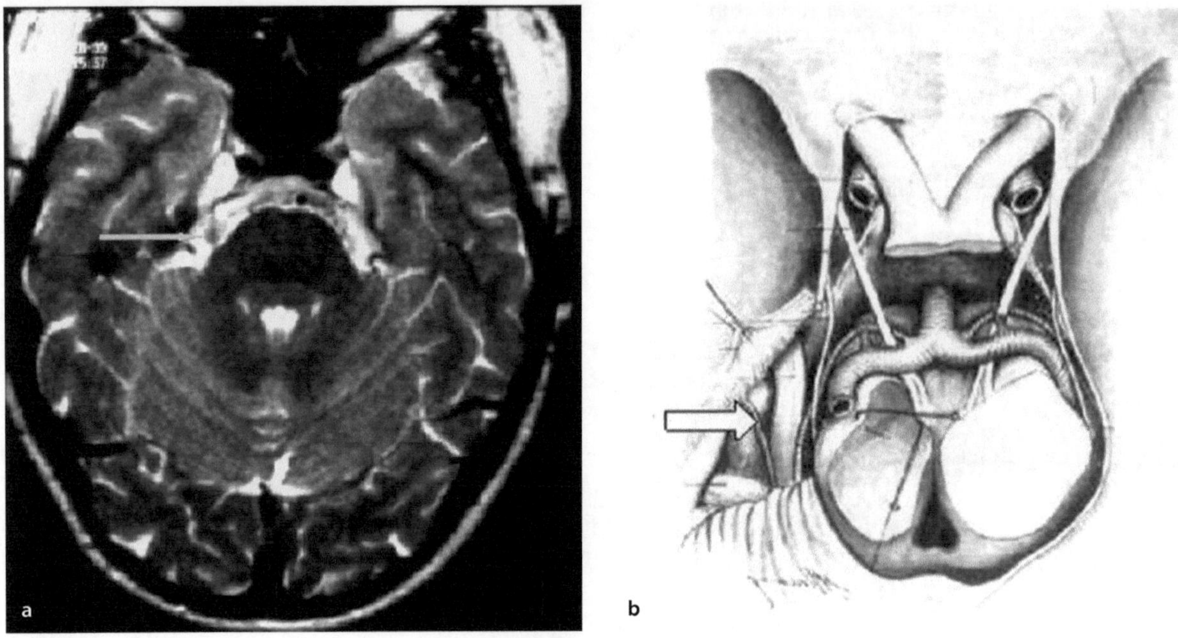

Fig. 7.4. **a** MRI: axial section in T2 showing the route of the nerve (*arrow*) in the pontocerebellar cisterna. **b** Anatomical sketch

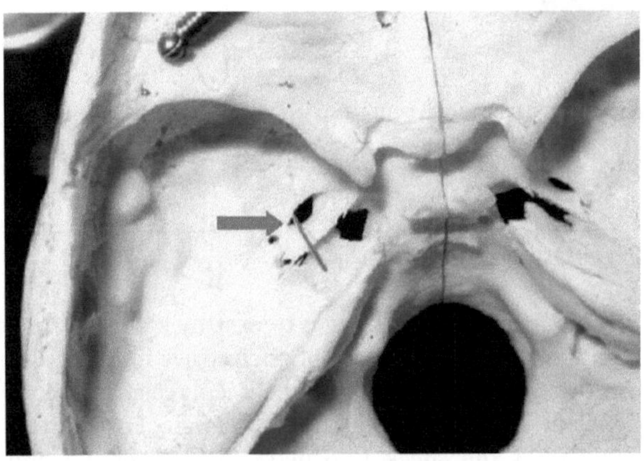

Fig. 7.5. Base of the cranium with penetration of a needle into the foramen ovale in the direction of Meckel's cavity

The needle can be used to provide:

- Chemical neurolysis using glycerol, which affects the stability of the lipoprotein-containing membranes of the nerve fibers. After performing a reference cisternography in seated position using an opaque product, in order to check the position of the needle, 0.2 to 0.4 ml of glycerol are injected into Meckel's cavity.
- Mechanical neurolysis by inserting a Fogarty probe and inflating it with several ml of X-ray-opaque liquid for 10 minutes to compress the ganglion in the inextensible dural foramen, which is Meckel's cavity (introduced in 1979; see Fig. 7.3). Verification is carried out by lateral-view fluoroscopy (Fig. 7.7).
- Thermal neurolysis by inserting a thermistor into the ganglion. Intensity is adjusted in order to reach a temperature between 60 and 75 °C, to inactivate the small nociceptive amyelinic C and A delta fibers. The less fragile large myelinized A beta and gamma fibers are preserved (1969).

Once the anesthesia protecting the patient against the very painful penetration of the foramen ovale has dissipated, the patient is tested to reproduce the pain in the area concerned (highly precise somatotopia in Gasser's ganglion) and obtain very low stimulation thresholds (the lower they are the closer the electrode is to the target zone).

After adjusting the position of the needle to reach the chosen stimulation zone, the patient is anesthetized once more and heat is provided by thermal frequency for 1 to 2 minutes. As soon as the patient awakens (3 to 5 minutes later), the stimulation test is performed once again and much higher thresholds should be obtained. The greater the heat the higher the control thresholds, but also the greater the risk of complication. These complications include:

- Disturbing paresthesia, hypoesthesia or, in the worst cases, cutaneous and particularly corneal anesthesia with risk of neuroparalytic keratitis
- Paralysis of the masseter muscle with chronic disturbance of temporomandibular articulation, the symptoms mimicking an intra-articular foreign body.

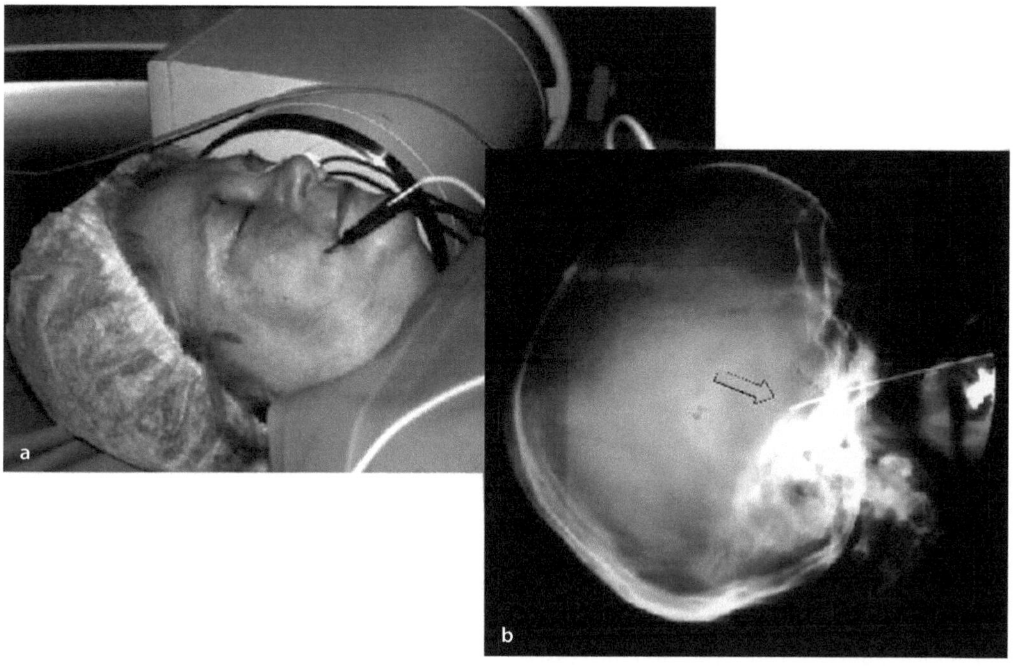

Fig. 7.6. **a** Percutaneous puncture and control of the needle in the cranium. **b** X-ray of cranium in profile, with needle in place (*arrow*)

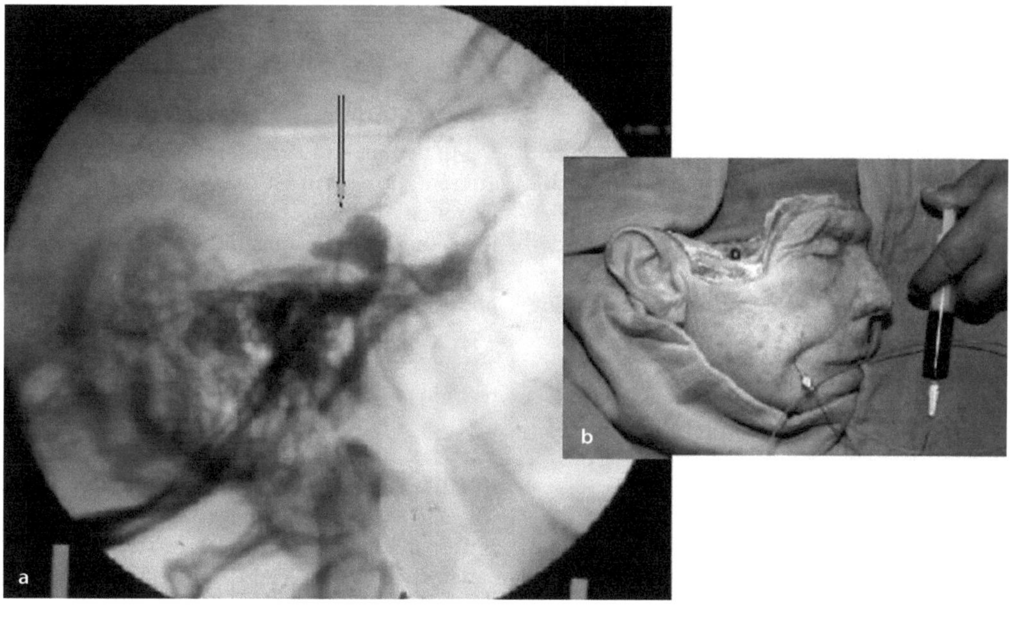

Fig. 7.7. **a** X-ray control and **b** anatomical specimen of a percutaneous compression

Contraindications are anticoagulant treatment, Wernicke's aphasia, evolved dementia, and tumor at the base of the cranium. An interpreter should be present as needed.

Surgical Approach

The intention is to alleviate a vascular compression affecting the nerve due to hardening of the arteries with age (most such patients are of advanced age) in non-acute soft contact with cranial nerve V.

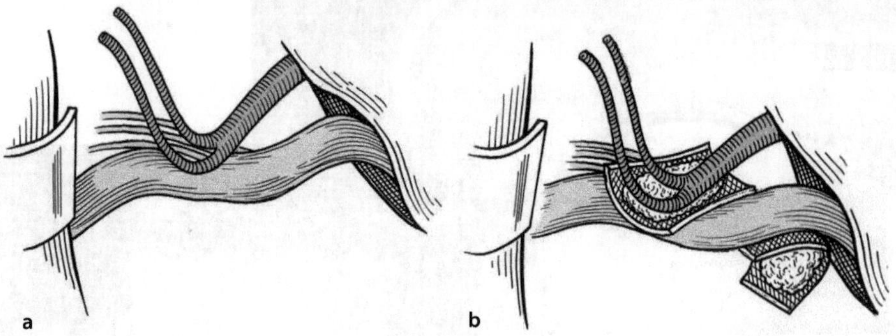

Fig. 7.8. **a** Drawing of microvascular decompression. From Marc Sindou. **b** Surgical view after treatment

Microsurgical Decompression (1959)

An arciform retro-auricular incision is used to approach the mastoid, which is trepanned below the asterion and cerebellum and reclined downwards. The high, deep nerve is approached. The arachnoid environment, which is more or less adhesive, is released and the vessel responsible for the compression can quite easily be identified. It is carefully dissected away from the nerve. These elements must be manipulated with great care. After careful exploration to eliminate any other cause of compression (e.g., vein, bone anomaly) a Gore-Tex, polyurethane, or muscle graft is inserted between nerve and artery, forming a harmonious loop with the latter. The field is then flooded with biological adhesive. The dura mater is carefully closed with an artificial patch or temporal aponeurosis to prevent cerebrospinal fluid from leaking (Fig. 7.8).

The cerebellum must be handled very gently in order to avoid tearing the petrous veins, and it must not be reclined too far because there is a risk of thus damaging the acousticovestibular and facial nerves and causing a cerebellar contusion.

Juxta-protuberantial Radiculotomy (1929)

This measure consists in cutting the sensory root in the pontocerebellar angle. It is rarely used, mostly when no neurovascular compression is found..

Additional surgical techniques are much less frequently used, some falling into disuse, others seemingly headed for an interesting future. A few of these are now described.

Bulbar Trigeminal Tractotomy (1939)

This intervention interrupts the tractus descending from the trigeminal on its way to the spinal core; retrogasserian neurotomy, using the subtemporal approach (1901), cuts the fibers immediately behind Gasser's ganglion, these procedures, along with the alcoholization of Gasser's ganglion, are no longer used.

Radiosurgery by Stereotaxy

Also known as *Gamma Unit*, this procedure disrupts the nerve blood supply, thereby modifying function of the cranal nerve V by itself.

Extradural Stimulation of the Premotor Cortex

This technique plays a retrograde inhibiting role on the thalamus and can therefore be used to control deafferentation pain. It is mainly indicated for post-ischemic thalamic pain. Under neuronavigation and local, then general anesthesia, we can identify the facial premotor zone and stimulate it by placing an electrode opposite the chosen area. It is secondarily connected to a generator placed under the clavicle.

We do not have a long-term history for these last two techniques.

Results

Both percutaneous and open procedures have had very satisfactory results. In the often frustrating attempts to find adequate pain relief by increasing doses of carbamazepine and/or combining this drug with clomazepan, surgery should be considered. Similarly, when treatment is effective but not well tolerated (somnolence, gastralgia, dizziness), surgery should also be considered.

Designed for a population of patients aged over 60, thermocoagulation should be proposed first. When typical essential neuralgia is involved, immediate results are close to 90% successful, with disappearance of the pain. This result is proportional to the degree of heating; the higher the temperature the better the results in terms of analgesia and the lack of recurrence. Complications (8% recurrence; 10 to 12% relatively disturbing paresthesia, usually disappearing in less than two months; hypoesthesia or corneal anesthesia with keratitis type complications) are avoidable if care is taken not to exceed certain temperatures (<60 °C for V_1, <65 °C for V_2, <70 °C for V_3). However, recurrence of pain is more likely when lower temperatures are used. When there is no cutaneous or corneal anesthesia, the same procedure can be repeated in the event of recurrence.

If these effects do occur, the procedure must not be repeated as it would aggravate the problem: persistent pain (painful dysesthesia) with anesthesia observed in a similar area. While oculomotor paralysis is a very rare complication, paralysis of the motor branch of V with masseter paralysis (injury to the nerve on its way through the foramen ovale or possibly from heating) is common. This is reflected in temporomandibular joint discomfort.

Meningitis is an exceptional complication as are intracranial hematomas; hematoma of the cheek is more common but not serious.

Secondary neuralgia (MS and shingles) obtain slightly less satisfactory results from this treatment. Patients find it harder to identify the target zone and thresholds are less clear.

Microdecompression using the direct approach must be performed by trained surgeons to insure precise graft installation, atraumatic handling of the cerebellum and acousticofacial ganglion, and finally careful detection of any cause of disturbance of the nerve. Results approach 80% cure with 10% failure, recurrence, and very rare complications.

Other techniques such as chemical neurolysis or percutaneous compression are easier to perform (they do not require patient cooperation) but also less specific (persistent paresthesia) and less effective in the long run (recurrence within a year is not uncommon).

Conclusion

Trigeminal neuralgia is an interesting pathological entity for clinicians, because formal diagnosis can be made exclusively by questioning, radiologic tools being used only to try and detect secondary causes, and in the specific medical and surgical treatment.

The results of treatment are excellent if careful diagnosis is made based on trigeminal unilateral radicular topography and the neuralgic nature of the pain. Carbamazepine is used as a therapeutic and diagnostic test. Poor response to this medication raises doubts over the diagnosis of trigeminal neuralgia and of course contraindicates percutaneous treatment as well as microvascular decompression. At times, however, tailored procedures can be offered for those specific cases.

References

1. Keravel Y, Sindou M, Ollat H, Laurent B (1988) La névralgie du trijumeau. Monogr ANPP 2, 108 pp

Arnold's Neuralgia

8

Bruno Kastler, Zakia Boulahdour, Sebastien Aubry, Bernard Fergane, Zoltan Patay

Clinically Relevant Anatomy

The greater occipital nerve (GON) or nerve of Arnold (Fig. 8.1, Fig. 8.2), which corresponds to the posterior ramus (sensory) of the second cervical nerve, has a complex winding course comprised of three segments (S1, S2, S3) and having two bends (b1, b2). During its curving route the GON comes into relationship with anatomical structures that have been well described in classic works [9, 11, 20–23].

The GON nerve originates between the posterior arch of the atlas (C1) and the lamina of the axis (C2) and courses in its first segment (S1) obliquely downward, posteriorly, and laterally. The origin of the GON ("or" Fig. 8.1) is in a space bounded in front by the C1–C2 joint capsule (which it innervates), behind by the lateral margin of the atlanto-axial membrane (Fig. 8.2b). The vertebral artery lies 6 to 12 mm lateral and posterior to it. This landmark is important because the artery (which should be off the needle pathway) is well visualized after an iodated contrast bolus injection (Fig. 8.2). The GON then courses behind the inferior obliquus capitis muscle, reaching its inferior border, there to curve more or less transversely around the muscle in the nerve's "first bend" (b1; Fig. 8.1), giving off a few muscular branches as it does so.

In the second segment (S2) the GON ascends obliquely upwards and inwards, between two muscular layers, a deep layer where the nerve crosses successively the dorsal aspect of the inferior obliquus capitis m. and rectus capitis posterior m. and a superficial layer represented by the semispinalis capitis m.

The GON then passes through the muscular fibers of the semispinalis capitis m., where the second bend (b2) is located proximal to the midline, thence to enter its third segment (S3), traveling laterally and upward. In this muscular channel, which is actually between the dorsal aspect of the semispinalis capitis m. and the deep aspect of the trapezius m., the GON is rarely cramped. The GON finally pierces the trapezius m. through an aperture in its tendinous portion, which is always narrow and rigid and is a source of potential entrapment. The GON emerges from it medial to the occipital artery at 2.5 to 3 cm from the midline, in line with the nuchal ridge (see em Fig. 8.1 and Fig. 8.6b, c).

The GON gains the posterior part of the scalp, communicates with the 3rd cervical nerve (and occasionally the 1st cervical nerve), and divides into terminal cutaneous branches that supply half of the scalp over the vertex and top of the head.

Areas of Vulnerability on Nerve Pathway

The winding pathway, comprising a series of segments and angles, exposes the nerve to possible compression and/or stretching, particularly with [8, 18], movement of the head [23]. Two zones where the nerve is anatomically vulnerable and where infiltrations can be of benefit can be outlined [1–5, 8, 16,23]:

- Proximally: at its origin ("or," "first site") and at its first bend (b1, "second site") where the GON curves around the inferior obliquus capitis muscle (see Fig. 8.1): compression of the C2 ganglion during extension of the head combined with contralateral rotation [23] or direct pressure on the C1–C2 joint; stretching of the nerve exacerbated during contralateral rotation and flexion of the head [23]; extension does not affect any portion of the nerve, only the C2 ganglion.
- Distally: at its emergence at the narrow and rigid aperture when perforating the tendinous area of the trapezius m. [23] (em, "third site"; see Figs. 8.1 and Fig. 8.6 b, c): pain induced by palpation at the emergence point (trigger zone).

Between the first bend (b1) and the emergence (em) the nerve is rarely a source of direct, anatomically well-defined trouble, but it can be stretched by forced flexion of the head [23].

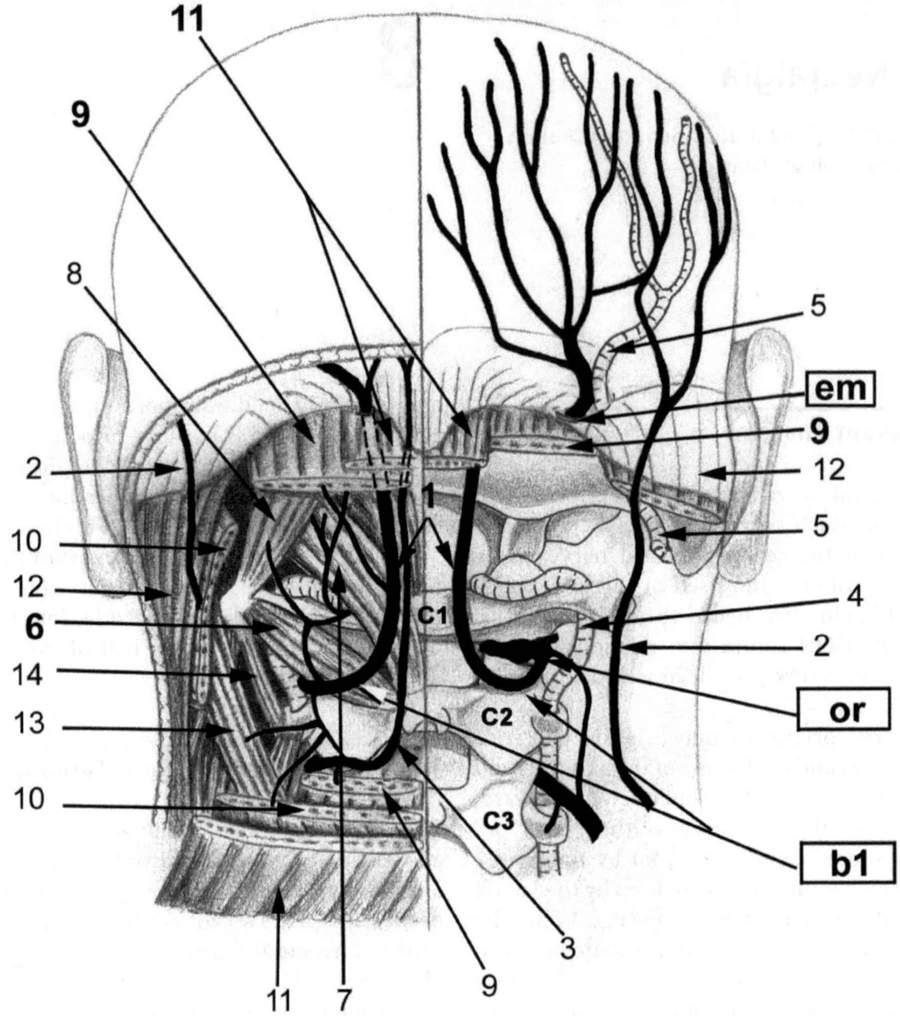

Fig. 8.1. Anatomical view of the origin, course, and emergence of the great occipital nerve (GON) or nerve of Arnold (see text for further explanation). (Drawing by Andia Hashemizadeh). Proximal infiltration sites: 1. at the origin "*or*" posterior to the C1–C2 joint; 2. at the first bend (b1) where the GON curves around the inferior obliquus capitis muscle (*6*). Distal infiltration site: at the GON emergence (*em*) through an aperture in the tendinous portion of the trapezius muscle (11). Also note: lesser occipital nerve (*2*), dorsal ramus of the 3rd cervical nerve (*3*), vertebral artery (*4*), occipital artery (*5*), rectus capitis posterior m. (*7*), superior obliquus capitis m. (*8*), semispinalis capitis m. (*9*), splenius capitis m. (*10*), sternocleidomastoid m. (*12*), longissimus m. (*13*), intertransversalis m. (*14*)

Etiopathogenesis

Most cases of Arnold's (or occipital) neuralgia have no apparent etiology. But besides this idiopathic form, structural pathology that can harm the proximal portion of the GON, ("or" to bend b1) has multiple known causes: trauma of the neck (most frequently),nervous and osseous tumors, Arnold-Chiari type 1 malformation, osteoarthritis of the spine, particularly C1–C2 degenerative joint disease [8], inflammatory rheumatism. We have also found several cases of elongation and buckling of suppress and of the vertebral artery on the side of the neuropathy (see Fig. 8.5 a).

Anesthetic blockades of the GON resulting in complete transitory pain freedom can be quite useful to rule out other headaches involving the occipital region, e.g., cervical headache, muscle tension headache or migraine,[1, 2] with possible overlapping features with these latter two.

1) A large number of patient suffer from muscle tension headaches with occipital distribution, but few experience concomitant true neuralgia.

2) It is not always possible to distinguish formally neuralgic and vascular pain: some patients can have migraine-like symptoms with at least hints of the autonomic features as found in cluster headaches.

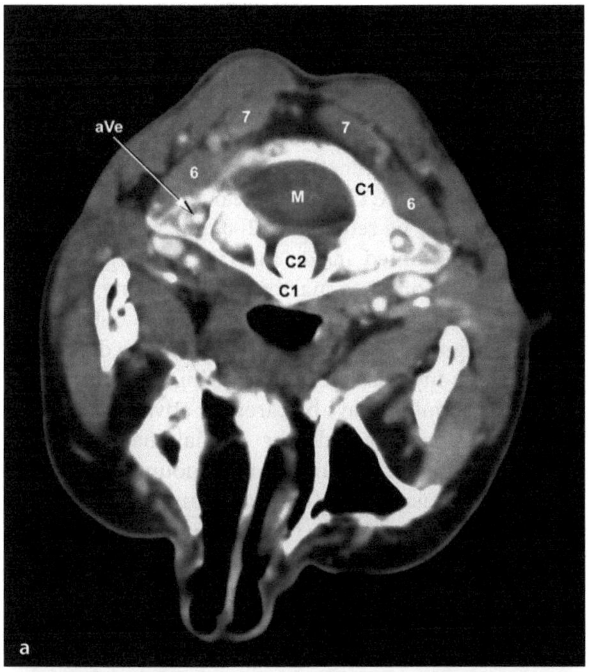

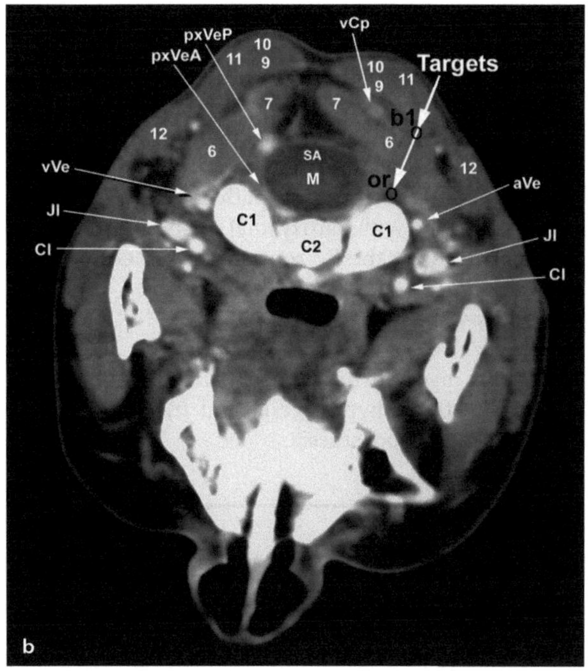

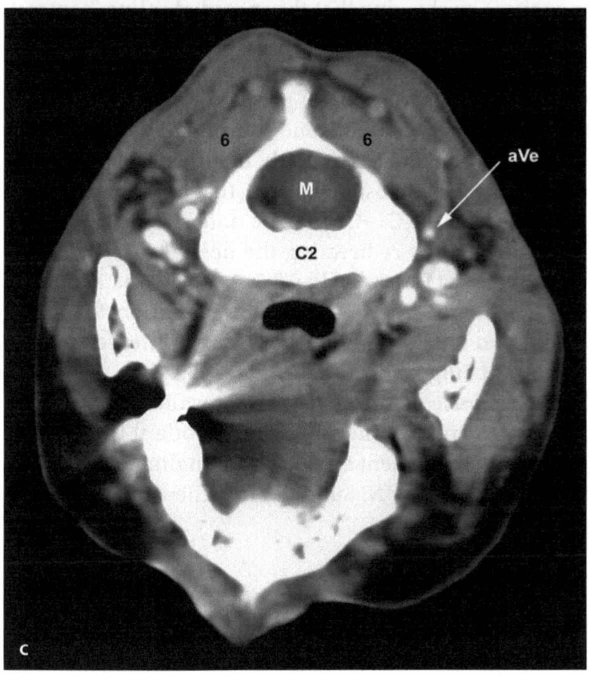

Fig. 8.2 a–c. Anatomical axial CT slices (3 mm) from C1 to C2. **a** Axial slice at the level of the posterior arch of C1, **c** at the posterior arch of C2, and **b** at an intermediate level between these two slices where the targets (see circles) for the proximal GON infiltration are best displayed: 1. at the origin ("or") posterior to the C1–C2 joint; 2. at the first bend ("b1") where the GON curves around the inferior obliquus capitis muscle (*6*). Note also: rectus capitis posterior m. (*7*), superior obliquus capitis m. (*8*), semispinalis capitis m. (*9*), splenius capitis m. (*10*), trapezius m. (*11*), sternocleidomastoideus m. (*12*), vertebral artery (aVe), vertebral vein (vVe), plexus vertebralis internalis anterior (pxVeA), plexus internalis posterior (pxVeP), cervicalis profundis vein (vCp), spinal cord (*M*), subarachnoid space (*SA*)

Pain originating in the occipital region caused by a pathological derangement at the emergence ("third site") of the GON or of the terminal branches (where tenderness or trigger zones are found), can also be due to a myofascial syndrome. This can be caused by trauma, muscular tension, neck positional problems, or tendonitis of the insertion of the trapezius muscle.

Clinical Considerations

The symptoms have been well described [8, 18]; two forms have been described:

- A paroxysmal form: these patients, predominantly women, experience unilateral (rarely bilateral) intermittent aching and throbbing pain, non clustering, variable in duration, on which shock-like jabs can be superimposed. The pain starts in the suboccipital region and radiates over the posterior scalp and top of the head. Retro-orbital pain may be present in severe attacks. The pain is induced by sneezing or turning of the head (limiting movement), and can be exacerbated by pressure over the GON.

- A continuous form: these patients experience unremitting pain with paroxysmal episodes. Here again tenderness over the C2 root and at the GON emergence can be found, as well as restricted voluntary head movement due to pain.

The patient may note mild sensory changes in the territory of the GON: hyperalgesia and hyperesthesia or hypalgesia and hypoesthesia.

Contraindications

Uncorrected coagulopathies or seriously altered coagulation profiles are contraindications for proximal infiltrations (see Chap. 3). For distal infiltration the risk-to-benefit ratio should discussed with the patient; using a 25–27-gauge needle can minimize the risk of bleeding. The patient must be informed about the procedure and its sequence of events and give consent. Written consent must be obtained as required by regulations.

Technique

Besides the usual specific medication, particularly in the case of a patient not responding well, or as diagnostic test, steroid and/or anesthetic GON blocks can be performed at the two proximal main sites at "or," or "b1", and/or distally at emergence "em."

Infiltration of the Greater Occipital Nerve at Its Origin Under CT Guidance

(Please also see Fig. 3.9, Chap. 3.) The approach is posterior or posterolateral and the patient is placed in a comfortable prone position with a pillow under his or her chest (Figs. 8.3–8.5). The patient's head is turned opposite to the puncture site for a unilateral infiltration and face down on a padded surgical ring for a bilateral infiltration. After bolus contrast injection, an initial series of axial 5 mm slices covering the occipital bone to C3 is obtained in order to visualize vascular structures particularly the vertebral artery and insure that it lies off the chosen pathway)

The posterior arches of C1 and C2 are the bony landmarks (Fig. 8.2). The target "or" is at an intermediate level between the two arches, slightly below the posterior margin of the posterior arch of C1, directly behind the C1–C2 joint capsule. The progression of the needle (check for the tip artifact) can be followed step by step using the iterative CT control. Near the target the slice thickness has to be reduced to 2–3 mm, and the needle tip should be aimed inside the lateral margin of the C1–C2 joint, in order to make sure of avoiding inadvertent puncture of the vertebral artery, and outside the medial margin in order to avoid piercing the dura matter. To avoid any possibility of injuring the spinal cord the needle should always be carefully advanced with its aim being, again, outside the medial margin of the C1–C2 joint. Before the injection the mounted syringe is maintained in aspiration (under vacuum) for 5 seconds in order to detect blood (vascular puncture) or cerebrospinal fluid.

First a mixture 1 ml of saline and contrast media (90%/10%)[3)] confirms that the needle tip is safely positioned (outside of a vascular structure and the foramen magnum) by showing that the spread of saline–contrast mixture molds the dura matter (and ideally the spinal C2 ganglion). The steroid is then administered: slow depot steroid instillation of prednisolone 2 ml or cortivazol 1 ml (50 mg prednisone equivalent).

We recommend, particularly in an elderly patient or one suffering from osteoarthritis, that a complementary infiltration of the C1–C2 joint be undertaken, which can be performed by redirecting the needle so that the tip faces the joint capsule (Fig. 8.3 e). Again the mounted syringe should be maintained in aspiration for a few seconds to insure no blood return, the intervertebralis vein now being its likely source (see Fig. 8.2).

If a radiofrequency generator is available, initially a test is performed in the stimulation mode at the C1 ganglion level; the patient should feel a tingling effect in the territory of the GON. Subsequently thermolysis can be performed [6, 10].

3) Saline instead of a local anesthetic in case inadvertent subarachnoid administration occurs, which can result, if a significant amount of the latter should be given, in an immediate total spinal anesthesia and/or possible cardiorespiratory arrest. It should be verified that the hyperdense mixture spreads strictly outside the dura matter (see Fig. 8.3 d, 8.4 a, 8.5 d and 8.6 e).

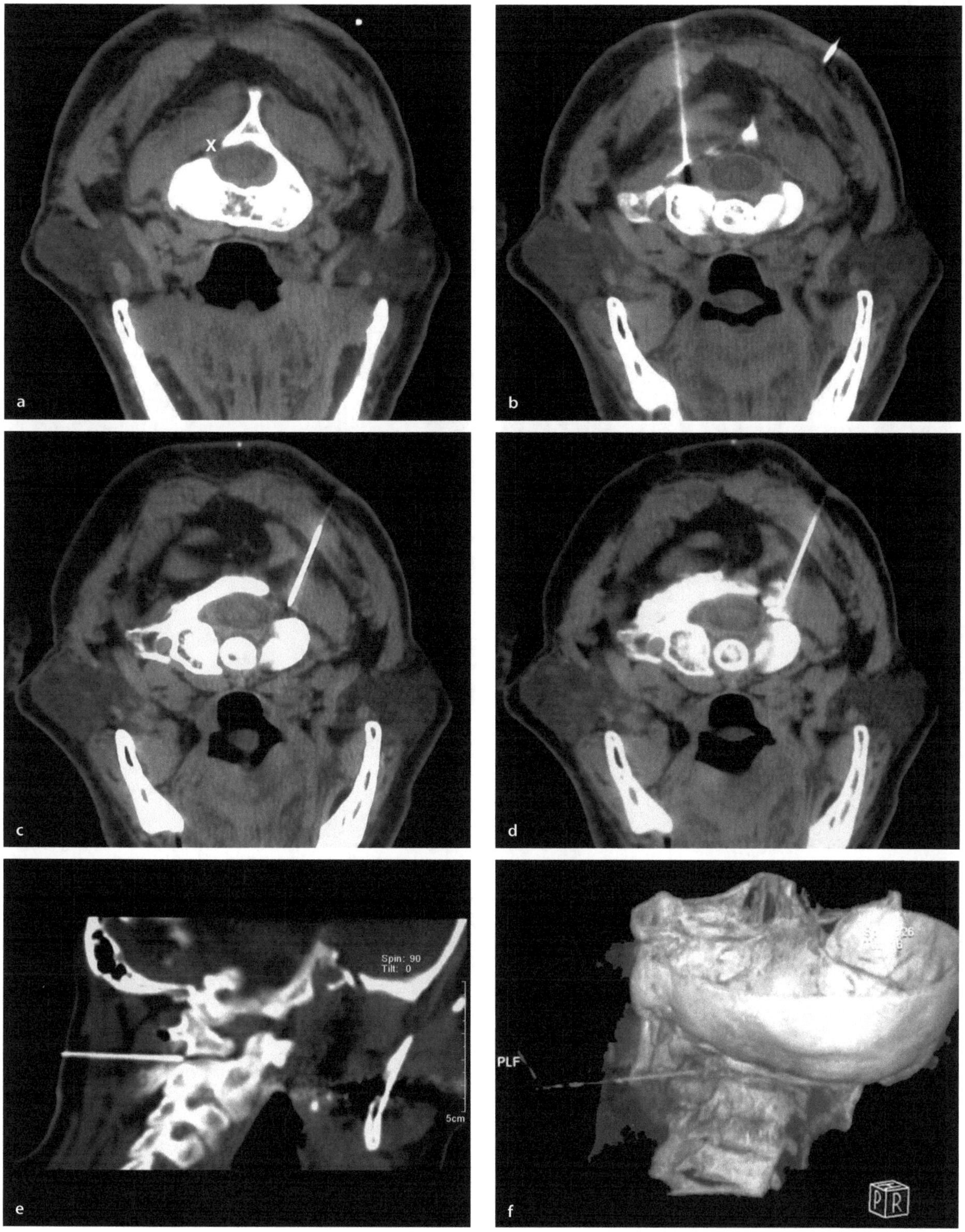

Fig. 8.3 a–f. Bilateral infiltration of the greater occipital nerve at its origin ("or"). Metallic landmarks are placed on the skin for optimal entry point location here in a bilateral approach. **a** the "*X*" pinpoints the left target at a level slightly above the axis lamina. **b** Left needle and **c** right needle are on target slightly under the posterior arch of the atlas directly behind the C1–C2 joints (close to the nerve origin). **c, d** Proper spread of saline-contrast mixture molding the dura matter (from outside), before the depot steroid injection is made. **e** A complementary infiltration of the C1–C2 joint can be performed, by repositioning the needle tip to face the C1–C2 joint capsule, as can be verified on reformatted coronal oblique slices. **f** Three-dimensional reconstruction. (See also Chap. 3, Fig. 3.9)

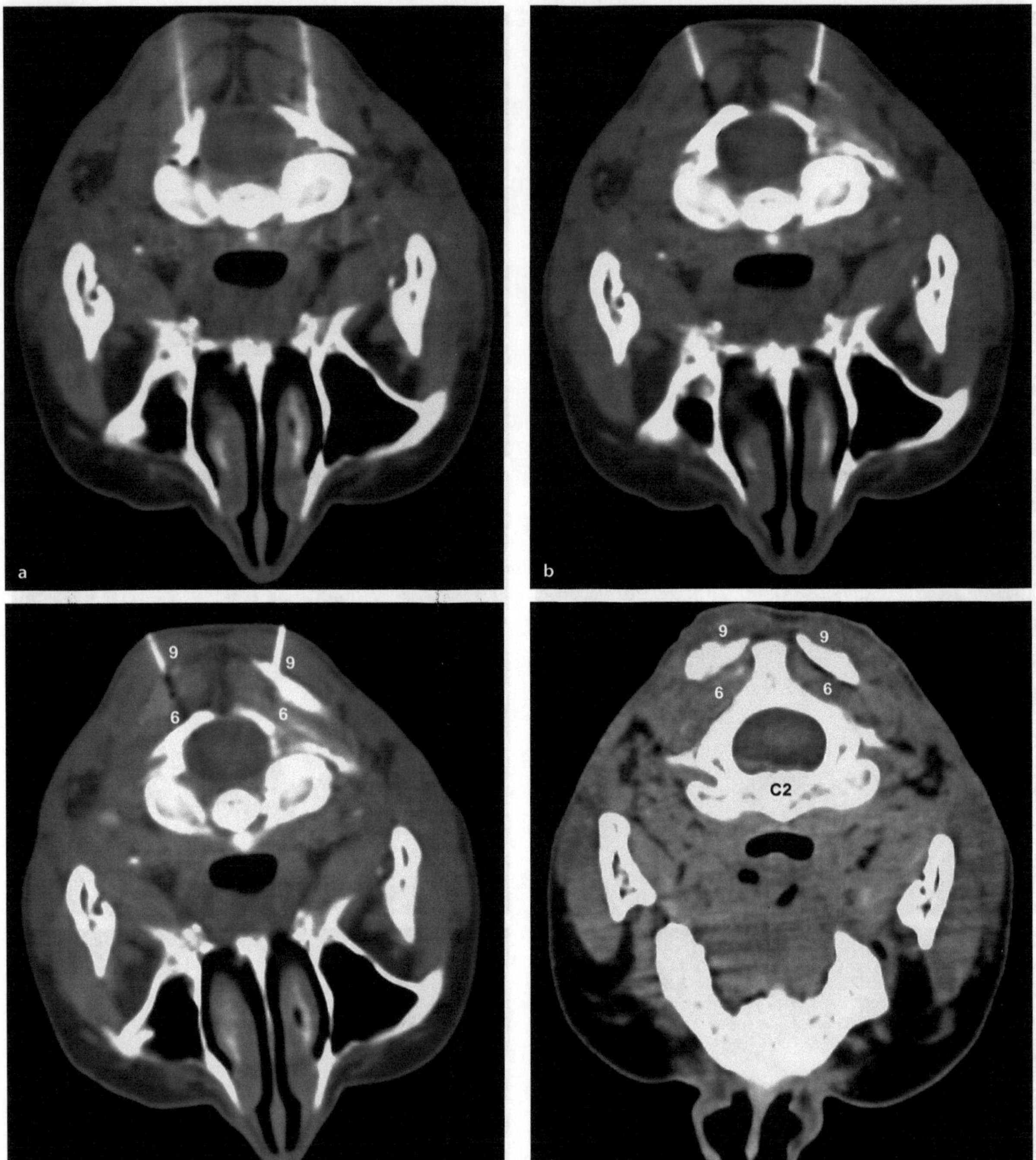

Fig. 8.4 a–d. Infiltration of the greater occipital nerve on the second proximal site, first bend (b1). **a, b** An infiltration has been accomplished at the first site at the origin "or" (posterior to the C1–C2 joint). See the hyper dense mixture molding the dura matter (from outside). **c** A second infiltration is performed by pulling back on the needles to arrive at the first bend: b1 (around the inferior obliquus capitis muscle, *6*); the needle tips recognized by the *needle tip artifacts* are located in the fatty compartment located between the dorsal aspect of the inferior obliquus capitis m. (*6*) and the deep aspect of the semispinalis capitis m. (*9*). This infiltration on the second site can also be performed when initially advancing the needle(s). The infiltration constitutes a block with a mixture of anesthetic and contrast media followed by a depot steroid. **d** The proper spread of this hyperdense mixture between the two muscles (especially towards the b1 bend) can be verified on control CT slices. The depot steroid injections may appear as lowering the density of the hyperdense contrast mixture (see "b1" left site on **c**, and "or" right site on **b** and **c**)

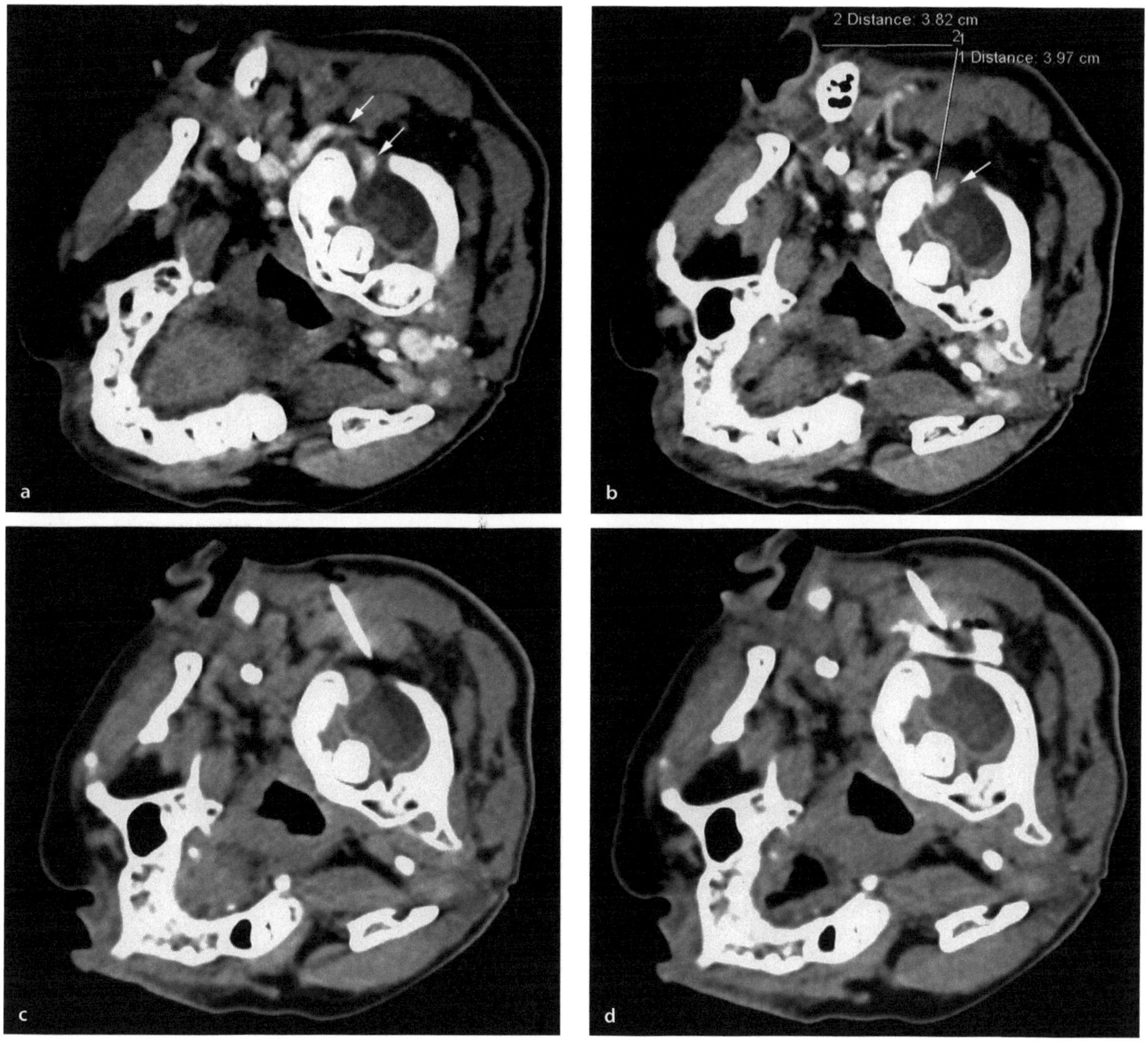

Fig. 8.5 a–d. Infiltration of the greater occipital nerve at its origin ("or"). **a, b** The vertebral artery (*arrows*) describes a large buckle (possibly the cause of neuralgia). **b** Optimal entry point of pathway is determined with respect to the ear and marked on the skin. **c** The *needle tip* at the target is at a safe distance from the vertebral artery. **d** Proper spread of saline–contrast mixture molding the dura matter (from outside); the depot steroid injection appears as a hypodensity at the *needle tip* within the hyperdense saline–contrast mixture. (See also Chap. 3, Fig. 3.9)

Infiltration of the Greater Occipital Nerve at the Second Proximal Site (b1)

We advocate when retrieving the needle (or, alternatively, when aiming at the target), that a second infiltration be given behind the inferior obliquus capitis muscle around which the GON describes its first bend b1 (a possible symptomatic site). The needle tip visualized by the tip artifact should be located in the fatty compartment between the dorsal aspect of the inferior obliquus capitis m. and the deep aspect of the semispinalis capitis m. The infiltration starts with a block comprising a 3 ml mixture of short and long acting anesthetics (lidocaine 1/3 and ropivacaine 2/3) and contrast media 10%. The proper diffusion of this hyperdense mixture between the two muscles confirms that the needle tip is safely positioned (Fig. 8.4). It is also necessary to verify that the mixture spreads caudally ideally reaching the inferior border of the inferior obliquus capitis muscle, i.e., to b1. The steroid injection of prednisolone 1 ml or cortivazol 1 ml (50 mg prednisolone equivalent) can then by performed.

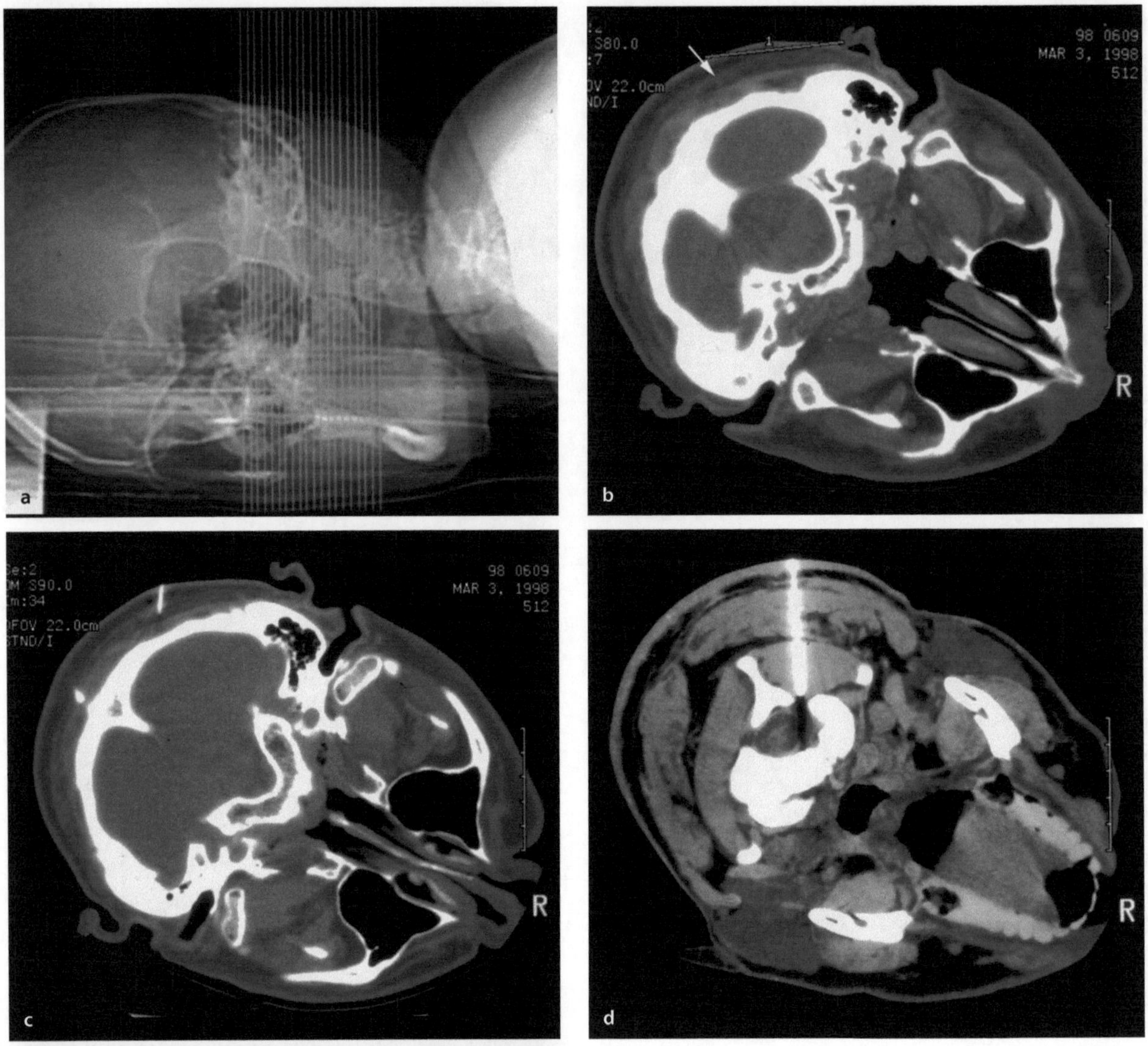

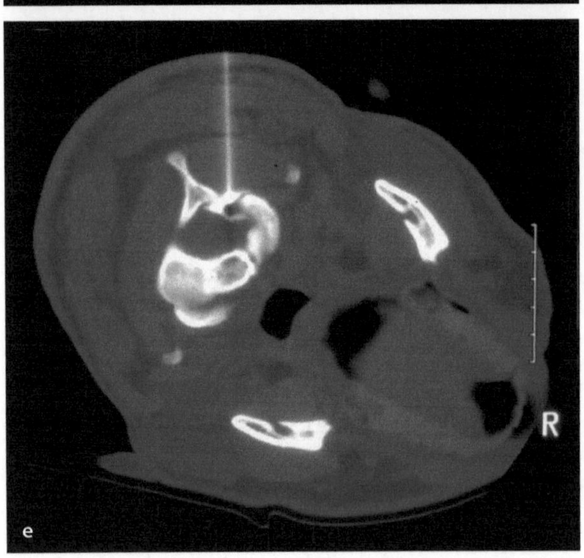

Fig. 8.6 a–e. Infiltration of the greater occipital nerve a its emergence (em). **a** Scout view displaying the 5 mm slices from the occipital bone to C3. **b** Optimal entry point (facing the occipital artery) is determined on line with the nuchal ridge. **c** The *needle tip* is placed in proximity and medial to the artery. The infiltration consists of a block with local anesthetic and depot steroid. **d, e** An infiltration at the origin is also accomplished. Needle tip artifact is clearly visualized on **d**, and the depot steroid injection appears as a hypodensity at the *needle tip* within the hyperdense saline–contrast mixture **e** (molding the dura matter from inside)

Infiltration of the Greater Occipital Nerve at its Emergence

The infiltration can be conducted using bony and palpable landmarks (Fig. 8.6b, c). The GON is usually blocked just above the superior nuchal line, about 2.5 to 3 cm lateral from the external occipital protuberance, just medial to the occipital artery, which can be palpated (tenderness or pain trigger zone). The needle is placed and advanced perpendicularly until it comes in contact with the periosteum, then pulled back 1 or 2 mm before injecting 3 to 4 ml of a local anesthetic (lidocaine 1/3 and ropivacaine 2/3) followed by a long acting steroid prednisolone 1 ml or cortivazol 1 ml (50 mg prednisolone equivalent). Other authors use a different landmark for a thermolysis: 2 cm lateral to and 3 cm above the external occipital protuberance [10].

The infiltration can also be performed under CT guidance (see Fig. 8.6b, c) by finding the occipital artery on the slice where the occipital artery becomes subcutaneous (accompanying the GON), usually close to the superior nuchal line (pain trigger zone). This distal site is infiltrated before or after an infiltration of the proximal sites. To optimize the localization of the emergence of the nerve a test is performed in the stimulation mode of a radio frequency (RF) generator; a thermolysis may follow.

Pain originating in the occipital region caused by restriction at the emergence (em) of the GON or on the terminal branches (where tenderness or trigger zones are found), can also be due to a myofascial syndrome, as aforementioned.

Whenever a myofascial syndrome is suspected, tenderness zones and/or trigger points (located by palpation) can by inactivated by the instillation of a few milliliters of local anesthetic (e.g., ropivacaine). When the needle tip (25–27 gauge) hits trigger points the pain is exacerbated, but it however disappears after the injection and cannot be evoked again even by strong palpation on the trigger point. When appropriate, we perform this instillation as a complement to the infiltration of the GON under CT guidance.

Complications

At the origin of the nerve, the most frequent complication is the inadvertent puncture of the vertebral artery. This is avoided by CT guidance, which is far more precise than fluoroscopic guidance [12–14]. The same applies for piercing the dura matter or infiltration of the neck muscle on the pathway. Pain at the puncture site, transitory torticollis, nausea, and dizziness are rare adverse reactions.

As the scalp is highly vascular and the occipital artery is in close proximity to the emergence of the GON there is a risk of arterial puncture and hematoma formation, particularly when only a sole palpable cutaneous landmark is used to locate the GON at its emergence. Expansion of such a hematoma can be prevented by immediate manual pressure on the site of the infiltration. No other side effects have been noted at this peripheral site of injection.

Results

The results are diverse, and ours in a series of 34 patients infiltrated at the origin of the GON [3–14] compare favorably with those published in the literature [6, 7]: Forty-two percent of our patients responded well and on a prolonged basis. In some patients the infiltration had to be repeated once or twice a year. In 10 to 20% of our patients the effect was more transitory, lasting for but a few weeks. With a complementary infiltration at the second site (bend b1) the results were significantly better, 84.5% in our series of 24 individuals thus treated now experiencing prolonged relief.

Thermolysis seems to give satisfactory long-term results [6, 10]; we have only limited experience with this form of treatment. Surgical decompression has also been advocated. [1, 10, 15, 17].

References

1. Arnold G (1969) Die örtliche Injecktiosbehandlung okzipitaler und subokzipitaler Schmerzzustände. Munch Med Wochenschr 138–141
2. Baret J (1983) Techniques des infiltrations locales dans les torticolis. Rhumatologie 64:57–59
3. Biehr V (2004) Infiltration du nerf d'Arnold en deux site sous guidage scanographique. Thèse de médecine Besançon
4. Bogduk N (1980) The anatomy of occipital neuralgia. Clin Exp Neurol 17:167–184
5. Bogduk N (1981) Local anesthetic blocks of the second cervical ganglion: a technique with application in occipital headache. Cephalgia 1:41–50
6. Bovim G, Fredriksen T, Stolt-Nielsen A, Sjaastad O (1992) Neurolysis of the greater occipital nerve in cervicogenic headache. A follow up study. Headache 32:175–179
7. Bovim G, Sand T (1992) Cervicogenic headache, migraine without aura and tension-type headache. Diagnostic blockade of greater occipital and supra-orbital nerves. Pain 51:43–48
8. Ehni G, Benner B (1984) Occipital neuralgia and CI C2 arthrosis. N Engl J Med 310:127
9. Guerrier Y, Colin R (1954) Le deuxième nerf cervical (valeur topographique de ses racines et de son segment tronculaire). CR Assoc Anat 813–816
10. Horst G (1975) Radio frequency denaturation for the treatment of the occipital nerve? Radionics
11. Hovelacque A (1927) Anatomie des nerfs crâniens et rachidiens et du système grand sympathique. Doin, Paris
12. Kastler B, Couvreur M, Clair C et al (1999) Tomodensitométrie interventionnelle: suivez le guide. Feuillets Radiol 39:421–432
13. Kastler B, Gangi A, Allal R et al (1995) Optimizing interventional procedures under CT guidances: Tips and hints. Scientific exhibit. Radiological Society of North America, 81st scientific assembly and annual meeting, Chicago, 26 Nov – 1 Dec 1995. Radiology [Suppl] 197:516

14. Kastler B (2004) Greater occipital nerve infiltration under CT Guidance: an anatomical and Radiological study for aiming at two possible sites. Scientific exhibit. Radiological Society of North America, 90th scientific assembly and annual meeting, Chicago, 28 Nov – 3 Dec 2004. Radiology [Suppl]
15. Lang G (1977) Quelle est la place du traitement chirurgical de la névralgie d'Arnold? J Med Strasbourg 8:541–544
16. Lazorthe G, Gaubert J, Chancholle AR (1962) Les rapports de la branche postérieure des nerfs cervicaux avec les articulations interapophysaires vertébrales. Assoc Anat Toulouse 887–895
17. Ody (1934) Traitement chirurgical de la névralgie essentielle et paroxystique du grand nerf d'Arnold (résection ganglionnaire du grand nerf d'Arnold par trépanation atlanto-occipitale). Rev Neurol 6:774–782
18. Pobeau D (1979) Névralgie occipitale d'Arnold. Thèse Marseille, no 467
19. Pougnard-Bellec F, Rolland Y, Morel D et al (2002) Efficacité de l'infiltration de C1-C2 par voie parasagittale postérieure dans le traitement de la névralgie d'Arnold de 24 patients. J Radiol 83:133–139
20. De Ribet RM (1953) Les nerfs rachidiens, vol 1. Doin, Paris
21. Tillaux P (1897) Traité d'Anatomie topographique, 9th edn. Asselin et Harzeau, Paris
22. Villemin F (1928) Précis d'Anatomie topographique. Ballière, Paris
23. Vital JM, Grenier F, Dautheribes M et al (1989) An anatomic and dynamic study of the greater occipital nerve (n. of Arnold). Applications to the treatment of Arnold's neuralgia. Surg Radiol Anat 11:205–210

Pterygopalatine Ganglion Neurolysis Under CT Guidance

Christophe Clair, Bruno Kastler, Gilles Cadel, Bernard Fergane

9

Introduction

Neurolysis or blockade of the pterygopalatine ganglion (PPG) is an efficient method in the management of pain for patients suffering from cluster headaches, PPG neuritis, postherapeutic neuralgia, atypical facial headache, trigeminal neuralgia, and severe intractable cancer-related pain. We will first describe the anatomy of the pterygopalatine fossa to better understand the surrounding structures which determine a possible percutaneous pathway. Secondly, we will describe our technique under CT guidance [4, 5, 9, 12, 14].

Anatomy of the Pterygopalatine Fossa

The following references merit consultation: [6, 8, 9, 10, 11, 13, 15–18].

A topographical division of the fossa infratemporalis is suggested on the basis of CT images. Three distinct regions are discernable (Fig. 9.1):

1) The retromaxillozygomatic region (RMZR), anterior and lateral, contains the fat pad of the cheek.
2) The pterygoid muscle region (PMR), posterior and medial, is crossed horizontally by the internal maxillary artery.
3) The pterygopalatine fossa (PPF), medial and superior, is the deepest part of the fossa infratemporalis.

The pterygopalatine fossa is located directly posterior to the maxillary sinus (Fig. 9.2).

- Posteriorly it is bordered by the fused medial and lateral pterygoid plates of the sphenoid bone. It communicates with the middle cranial fossa through the sphenoid bone via the pterygoid canal and the foramen rotundum.
- Inferiorly the fossa narrows and becomes the pterygopalatine canal, which communicates with the oral cavity.
- Superiorly it is in continuity with the inferior orbital fissure.

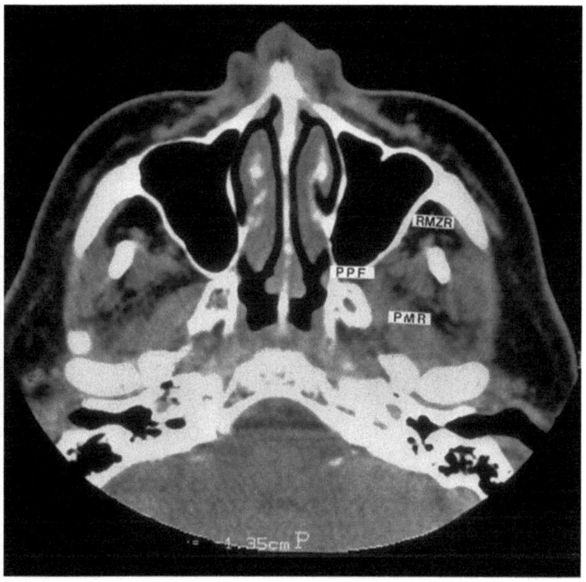

Fig. 9.1. Axial CT scan at the lower level of the PPF shows the three regions of the fossa infratemporalis (see text for further explanations)

- Laterally there is direct communication with the infratemporal fossa through the pterygomaxillary fissure.
- Medially it is bound by the perpendicular plate of the palatine bone except at its upper limit where the sphenopalatine foramen accesses the nasal cavity.

The pterygopalatine fossa houses the internal maxillary artery, the pterygopalatine ganglion, and the maxillary nerve. In general, the arterial component of the fossa lies anteriorly and the neural component posteriorly.

- The internal maxillary artery, arising from the external carotid artery, enters through the pterygopalatine fissure taking generally an anterior, medial, superior and horizontal direction (see Fig. 9.3). In its course, it classically forms fourteen branches before entering the sphenopalatine foramen.

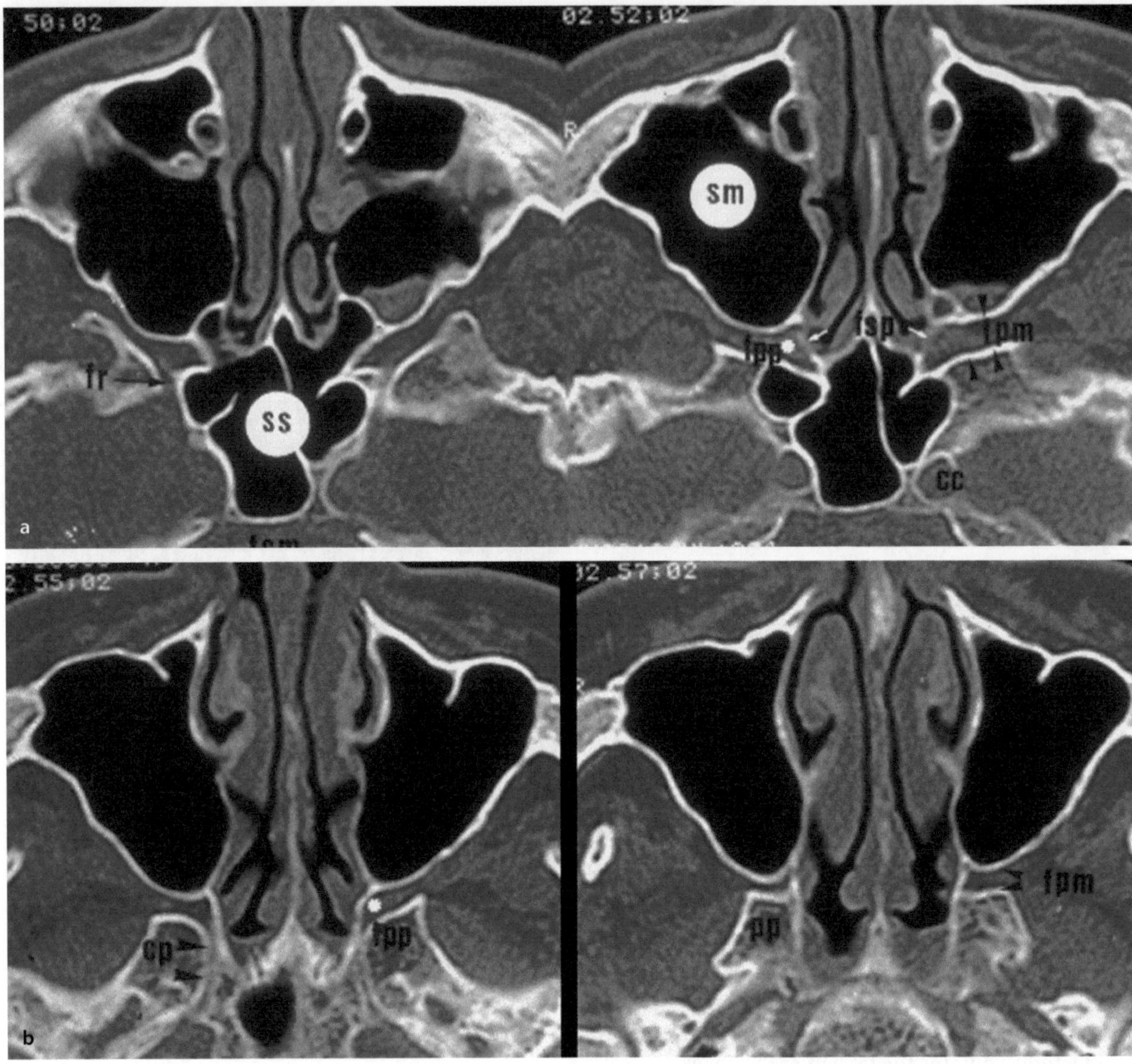

Fig. 9.2 a, b. Axial CT scans from the upper (**a**) to the lower (**b**) part of the pterygopalatine fossa. Key anatomic structures: *Cc* internal carotid canal, *Cp* pterygoid canal, *Fcm* middle cranial fossa, *Fpm* pterygomaxillary fissure, *Fpp* pterygopalatine fossa, *Fr* foramen rotundum, *Fsp* sphenopalatine foramen, *Pp* pterygoid process of the sphenoid bone, *Sm* maxillary sinus, *Ss* sphenoid sinus

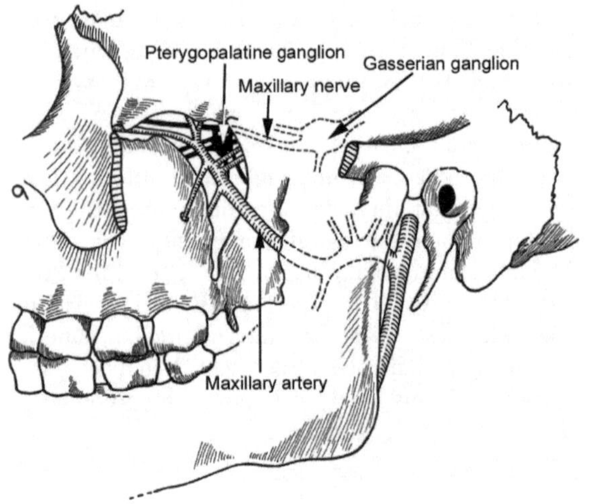

Fig. 9.3. Anatomical lateral view of the pterygopalatine fossa, which houses the internal maxillary artery, the pterygopalatine ganglion, and the maxillary nerve. The pterygopalatine ganglion lies deeply in the fossa (see text for further explanation; drawing by Jean-Louis Vannson)

- The maxillary nerve (second division of the trigeminal nerve) enters the fossa via the foramen rotundum and continues its course through the infra orbital canal where it supplies sensory innervation to the skin of the cheek, side of the nose, and upper lip. Branches of the maxillary nerve cross the pterygopalatine ganglion, leading to the palate (greater and lesser palatine nerves), the nose (pterygopalatine nerve), the upper jaw (superior posterior alveolar branches) and the orbit (zygomatic nerve).
- The pterygopalatine ganglion lies deep in the fossa under the maxillary nerve, laterally near the sphenopalatine foramen, and posteriorly near the pterygoid canal. The PPG is a relay station for the autonomic innervation of the nasal mucosa, soft palate, and lachrymal gland.
- The remainder of the pterygopalatine fossa is filled with fatty tissue in continuity with the infratemporal fat pad.

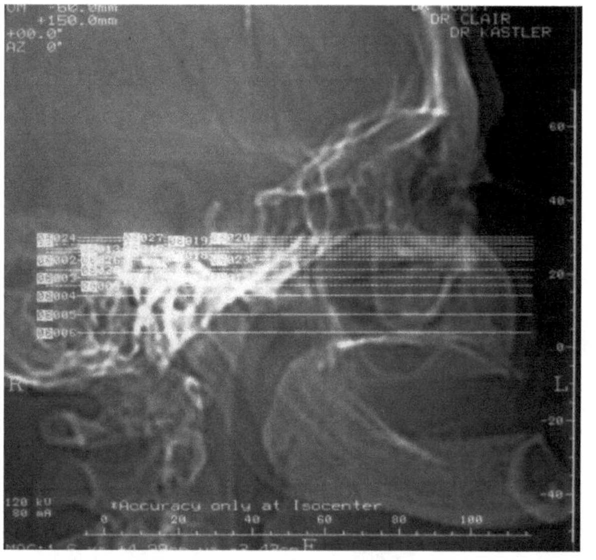

Fig. 9.4. Scout view displaying the acquired slices

Neurolysis Technique

These references may be consulted: [2, 7].

- After verifying the patient's coagulation rates are normal, the patient is informed about the procedure to be carried out, its expected benefits and risks, and permission is obtained, if possible during a previous consultation. Written consent must be obtained as required by law.
- The patient is placed in a supine position on the CT table with the head turned opposite to the side of puncture and fixed with a strip of adhesive tape.
- Axial CT contiguous slices of 5 mm in thickness are made from the upper part of the zygomatic arch to the lower part of the maxillary bone (see scout view Fig. 9.4).
- The pterygopalatine fossa is seen posterior to the maxillary sinus and anterior to the lateral pterygopalatine plate. The pterygopalatine ganglion is located at the slice level of the sphenopalatine foramen.
- In order to avoid intervening structures (zygomatic arch in particular) and obtain a direct pathway to the target, it may be useful to tilt the gantry 10° caudally.
- The optimal entry point is located just below the sigmoid notch of the zygomatic arch between the condylar and the coronoid process of the mandible (Fig. 9.5). It should be marked on the skin with a felt tip pen.
- The patient is draped in a sterile fashion, the skin scrubbed and sterilized, and local anesthetic instilled at the entry point and on presumed initial pathway. The procedure is performed under local anesthesia.
- The correct needle/target orientation should be determined with respect to the orientation and skin entry point of the anesthetic needle left in place (either parallel to that orientation or at a slight angle thereto, see chapter 3).

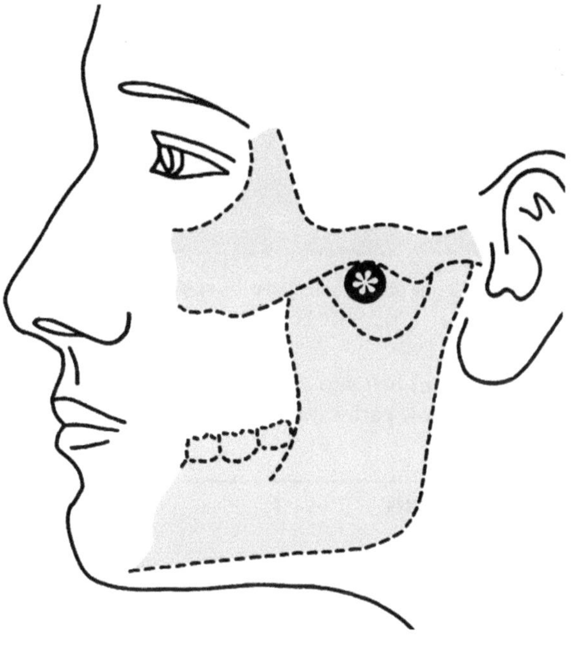

Fig. 9.5. Lateral view of the face showing the entry point (*asterisk*)

- A safe pathway is chosen in order to avoid damage to the internal maxillary artery, which runs in a horizontal line across the fat of the infratemporal fossa. Bolus contrast injection can be useful to display the artery.
- The needle is slowly and carefully advanced under step-by-step CT guidance until the needle (check for the needle tip artifact) tip is within the pterygopalatine fossa (Fig. 9.6). Saline injection combined with needle tip lateral displacement and rotation (bevel-

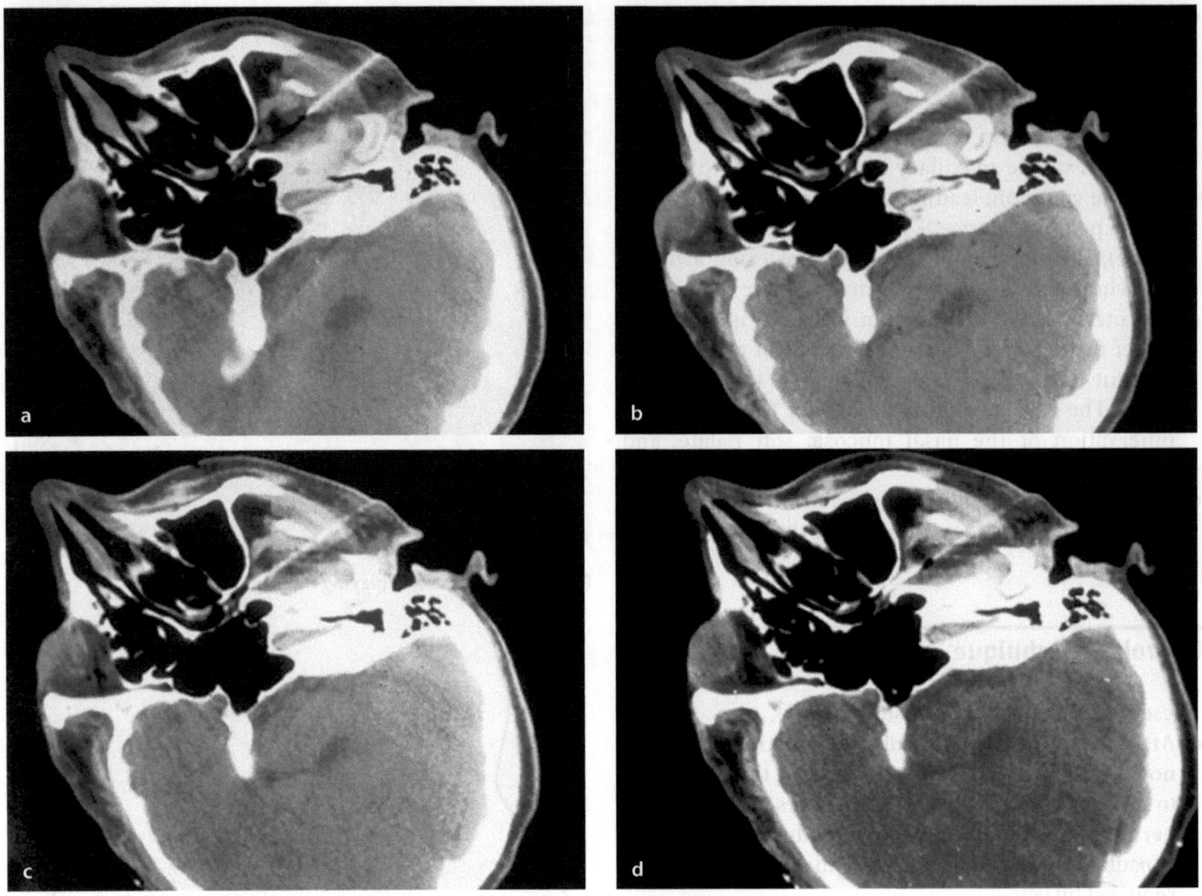

Fig. 9.6 a–d. Needle placed under step-by-step CT guidance

edge rotation) helps to avert intervening organs and enlarge narrow pathways (see Chap. 3).

Ethanol Neurolysis

- The needle used is a disposable 22 gauge, 7 cm spinal needle.
- The correct position of the needle tip at target is determined by an injection of contrast media diluted with local anesthetic (1:5, a total of 0.5 ml in a 2 ml syringe) which makes it possible to anticipate possible diffusion of the alcohol (checked by CT) and also perform a test block (see Fig. 9.7). Prior to injection the syringe is maintained in aspiration (under vaccum) for 5 s to ensure against vascular puncture.
- The patient may observe a decrease in symptoms if present. The neurolysis is performed with 1 ml instilled slowly. This should be carried out again maintaining the syringe in aspiration prior to injection, to insure against vascular puncture. Halfway through the alcohol injection a control CT scan should be obtained. The pain relief is usually appreciated following the neurolysis.

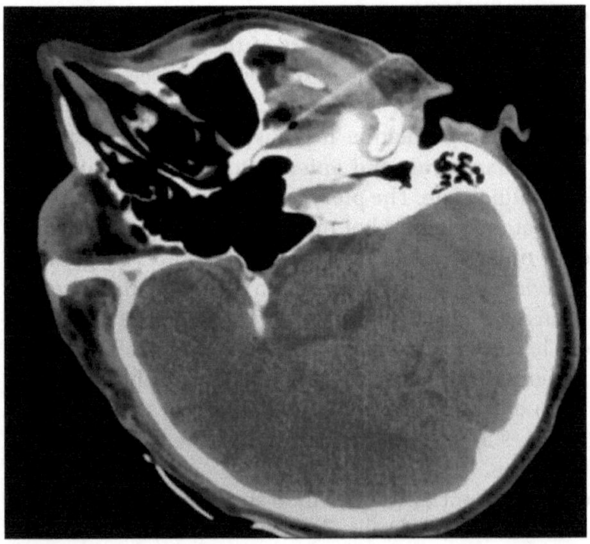

Fig. 9.7. Injection of contrast media with a local anesthetic to assure correct needle tip position on the target

RF Neurolysis

Radiofrequency is an ancient technique, whose principle has been used for many years for electric surgical knives and neurolyses when highly localized thermolysis is required without the risk of damaging any of the peripheral nerve structures. It consists in the percutaneous introduction of a needle into a lesion. By induction of an alternate RF current (400 KHz high frequency) at the conducting tip of the needle flowing into the peripheral tissues, the tissues heat up by ohmic agitation. When the tissue temperature near the needle exceeds 50–60°, a thermal lesion, normally very limited in size (equal to 1.6 the radius of the needle's diameter) appears (dry electrode principle).

- The needle is a 22 gauge, 10.5 cm RF disposable cannula for RF probes (Radionics, Burlington, MA, USA).
- The electrode is placed in the cannula and connected to the generator.
- The correct position of the needle tip at the target is determined by electrostimulation (sensory mode, 50 Hz). If the needle is in the right position, a tingling sensation in the nose will be felt at approx. 1 volt.
- A thermal lesion is created by applying heat for 60 s at a temperature 60 to of 80 °C (depending on patients' tolerance). This procedure is repeated three times, moving the cannula backwards and forwards by 1 mm each time.

Advantages and Disadvantages of the Two Approaches

- Both techniques are quite easy to perform under CT guidance on an outpatient basis under local anesthetic. Unlike fluoroscopy, CT guidance allows safe step-by-step pathway progression of the needle and precise positioning at target, reducing complications and optimizing immediate results.
- Some patients may experience epistaxis following either procedure. They should not be discharged until the bleeding has stopped completely. We however have not encountered this complication in our experience.
- A small percentage of patients will experience transient hypesthesia (lasting up to a few weeks) in the region of the soft palate.

Ethanol Neurolysis

- It is lower in cost and some authors report longer lasting effects.
- Excessive alcohol diffusion is the main drawback and cannot be fully controlled. The principal such risks are diffusion of the neurolytic agent through the inferior orbital fissure into the orbit, through the sphenopalatine foramen into the nose, and/or through the pterygomaxillary fissure into the infratemporal fossa.
- Complications can be minimized by keeping the volume of injected alcohol within 1 ml and by correctly positioning the needle tip.

RF Neurolysis

- The lesion size is adequately controlled.
- It requires an initial investment (RF generator and electrodes) and is all-in-all more costly than the ethanol method.
- It is more time consuming;
- it requires precise positioning of the needle, as facilitated by electrical stimulation and impedance control.

In our series of 38 pterygopatine neurolysis (34 alcoholizations, 4 RF) in 26 patients with unilateral facial pain [7], the global efficiency was 65.7% (25/38) with total pain relief in 60% (15/25). However pain recurred in 76% of the cases (with a 3 months mean delay). Non typical facial pains, cluster headaches and local tumoral compression appear to be the most suitable indications. Post herpetic neuralgia and atypical dental pain did not respond properly to this therapy.

References

1. Buckley FP, Moricca G, Murphy TM (1990) Neurolytic blockade and hypophysectomy. In: Bonica JJ (ed) The management of pain, 2nd edn. Lea and Febiger, Philadelphia
2. Clair C, Kastler B, Aubry R et al (1998) Neurolyse du ganglion sphénopalatin sous contrôle TDM. Radiol J CEPUR 18:405–411
3. Clair C, Kastler B, Aubry R et al (1997) Pterygopalatine ganglion neurolysis under CT guidance, scientific exhibit, Radiological Society of North America, 83th scientific assembly and annual meeting. Chicago, Dec 1997
4. Devoghel JC (1981) Cluster headache and sphenopalatine block. Acta Anaesth Belg 32:101–107
5. Hardebo JE, Elner A (1987) Nerves and vessels in the pterygopalatine fossa and symptoms of cluster headache. Headache 27:528–532
6. Hofmann E, Wimmer B (1989) Die anatomie der flugelgaumengrube im CT. Rofo 15:27–31
7. Kastler B, Cadel Gilles (2006) Pterygopalatine ganglion neurolysis under CT guidance: Results of 38 procedures in 26 patients. Scientific poster. Radiological Society of North America, 92th Scientific Assembly and Annual Meeting. Chicago November 29 – December 3. Radiology [Suppl]
8. De KersainT-Gilly A, Sonnier CD, Legend F et al (1991) Radioanatomie de la fosse infratemporale. Région ptérygomaxillaire. Ann Oto Laryng (Paris) 108:77–81

9. Kitrelle JP, Grouse DS, Seybold ME (1985) Cluster headache. Local anesthetic abortive agents. Arch Neurol 42:496–498
10. Legent F, Beauvillain C, de KersainT-Gilly A (1981) Fosse ptérygomaxillaire. Division topographique. Moyens d'exploration. Abord transmandibulaire de la région des ptérygoidiens. Ann Oto Laryng (Paris) 98:435–442
11. Lewis J (1990) The radiographic demonstration of the pterygopalatine fossa and canal. Radiogr Today 56:21–22
12. Meyer JJ, Binns PM, Ericsson AD, Vulpe M (1970) Sphenopalatine ganglionectomy for cluster headache. Arch Otol 90:475–484
13. Morton AL, Khan A (1991) Internal maxillary artery variability in the pterygopalatine fossa. Oto Laryngol Head Neck Surg 104:205–209
14. Prasanna A, Murthy PSN (1993) Combined stellate ganglion and sphenopalatine ganglion. Block in acute herpes infection. Clin J Pain 9:135–137
15. Rabischong P, Guerrier Y, Vignaud J et al (1980) Bases anatomiques de l'abord de la fosse ptérygopalatine. Anat Clin 2:209–222
16. Robert R, Legent F, Rogez JM et al The infratemporal fossa: a trial classification
17. Robert R, Lehur PA, Bordure T et al (1991) Étude anatomique de la fosse infra-temporale. Ann Oto Laryng (Paris) 108:69–76
18. Wentges RT (1975) Surgical anatomy of the pterygopalatine fossa. J Laryngol Otol 89:35–45

Stellate Ganglion Neurolysis Under CT-Guidance

10

Bruno Kastler, Démonsthène Michalakis,
Nicolas Sailley, Philippe Pereira, Bernard Fergane

Introduction

Algodystrophy or reflex sympathetic dystrophy syndrome, currently referred to as type I complex regional pain syndrome (CRPS), is a combination of a non-systematic pain syndrome, tenderness and swelling, changes in cutaneous blood flow, abnormal sweating, and stiff joints [18]. CRPS, although benign, is highly invalidating because it resists specific medication. Treatment is founded on blockades of sympathetic activity (temporary or more lasting) and physical therapy. Infiltration of the stellate ganglion is a technique whose efficacy has been known for many years and is widely used in the treatment of CRPS [1, 2, 18]. Anesthetists, who introduced the technique, use external anatomical landmarks before administering a local anesthetic by an anteriolateral tracheal approach. Such blockades are effective, even when the target is attained imprecisely because of the large quantities injected (contralateral diffusion possible [5–9]); their effect is, however, limited in time.

It has been suggested that alcohol may bring longer lasting relief in cases of severe intractable cancer-related pain arising from regional neoplasms [1–4]. But the frequent onset of Horner's syndrome as an after-effect (sometimes already present because of cancerous invasion of the stellate ganglion) can counteract the technique's efficacy.

The RF technique by radioscopic guidance was introduced in 1999 by Sluijer [20]. A recent retrospective study confirms the positive action of this technique on cervical thoracic and upper limb pain of sympathetic origin, with pain relief in 13 out of 35 patients (37%) [3].

More precise than radioscopic guidance, CT guidance offers an excellent and safe means of leading the needle to target behind the vertebral artery, which constitutes the most reliable landmark [4, 8, 10, 12, 19]. We thus use a lateral trans-scalenic approach and not the anterior one mandatory with osseous landmarks [10–14].

We will first briefly describe the anatomy of the stellate ganglion, which must precede adequate CT-slice-level positioning and make it possible to define a safe percutaneous pathway. Secondly, we will demonstrate how CT guidance allows step-by-step control of positioning the needle tip at the target for either alcohol or RF thermal ablation. Finally, we will discuss the advantages and disadvantages of each approach.

Clinically Relevant Anatomy

The stellate ganglion (or cervical thoracic ganglion) is part of the orthosympathetic chain [7, 16, 17]. It is formed by the fusion of the inferior cervical and first thoracic sympathetic ganglia. At dissection it appears as a rather large oval-shaped structure 2 cm long, 1.5 cm wide, and 0.5 cm thick oriented in the axis of the spine. On MRI, however, [6] the stellate ganglion has been seen as a smaller structure with a maximum cephalocaudad dimension of just over 1 cm.

It is situated in a concavity that is limited (Fig. 10.1):

- Medially by the portion of the vertebral column covered by the longus colli muscle
- Posteriorly by the neck of the first rib, the transverse process of the C7 vertebra, and the interspace between them
- Anteriorly by the vertebral artery near its origination from the subclavian artery (which is well displayed after bolus contrast injection)
- Laterally by the scalene muscle mass
- Inferiorly by the posterior aspect of the pleura.

The sympathetic nerves that supply the head and neck usually pass through the stellate ganglion. The ganglion, via the gray rami communicantes, also sends branches into the C7, C8, T1, and sometimes C5 and C6 spinal nerves, constituting the major part of the sympathetic supply to the upper limb. Creating a lesion of the stellate ganglion thus induces a sympathetic denervation of this structure which can be partial (RF) or more complete (alcohol).

As mentioned the stellate ganglion is a rather diffuse structure: the first thoracic and inferior cervical components are usually partially fused [1, 7]. The cranial component lies in front of the transverse C7 vertebra and the major lower component in front of the neck of the

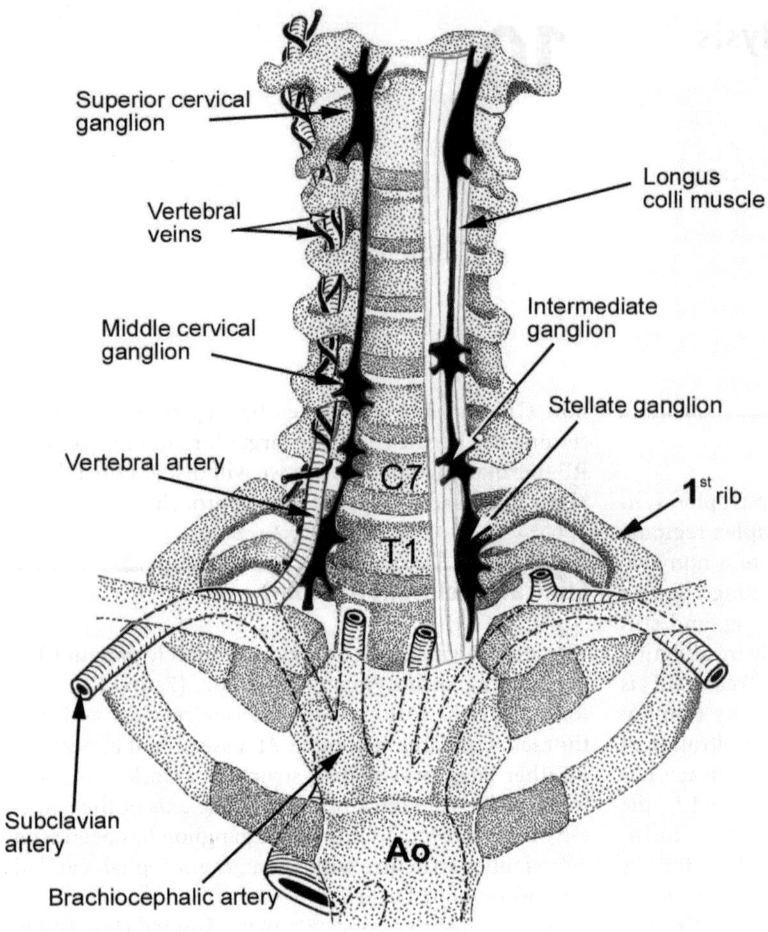

Fig. 10.1. Anatomy of the stellate ganglion and cervical sympathetic chain (see text for further explanations – drawing by Andia Hashemizadeh)

first rib (T1), (Figs. 10.1–10.4). It has been shown that a partial localized disruption (RF) of the stellate ganglion frequently produces high-quality pain relief [20, 21]. We thus aim precisely at these two targets for RF neurolysis. Moreover the stellate ganglion is close to the bony structures (0.5 cm), surrounded by adipose tissue in which the injected material diffuses particularly alcohol. For this reason an alcoholization or a simple blockade will require less precise targeting at only one C7 or T1 level.

Needle Tip Targeting at the Stellate Ganglion Under CT Guidance

Please refer to Figs. 10.2–10.4.

- The technique of stellate ganglion block under CT guidance has been previously described. For both alcohol neurolysis and RF ablation at our institution the needle tip is placed by means of a simplified approach. We will describe the technique at both C7 and T1 targets [10–12, 14].
- The patient must have normal clotting values and give informed consent for the procedure.
- The patient is placed in a supine position on the CT table with the head turned away from the side of puncture and arms at the sides.
- Axial adjoining CT slices of 5 mm in thickness are obtained from the superior aspect of the C6 vertebra through the superior level of the T2 vertebra, as determined on the scout view. A bolus injection of contrast medium is given to visualize the vertebral artery (the stellate ganglion lies immediately behind its origin) as well as to display other possible intervening vascular structures.
- As stated, the stellate ganglion lies anterior to the transverse process of the C7 vertebra and the neck of the first rib, and is targeted on these slice levels.
- A safe pathway is chosen at both C7 and T1 target levels (anterior, lateral, or preferably anterolateral) in order to avoid inadvertent puncture of the external and internal jugular veins, carotid and vertebral arteries, the pleura and branches of the brachial plexus. We thus advocate an anterolateral trans-scalenic approach, which is possible with CT guidance.

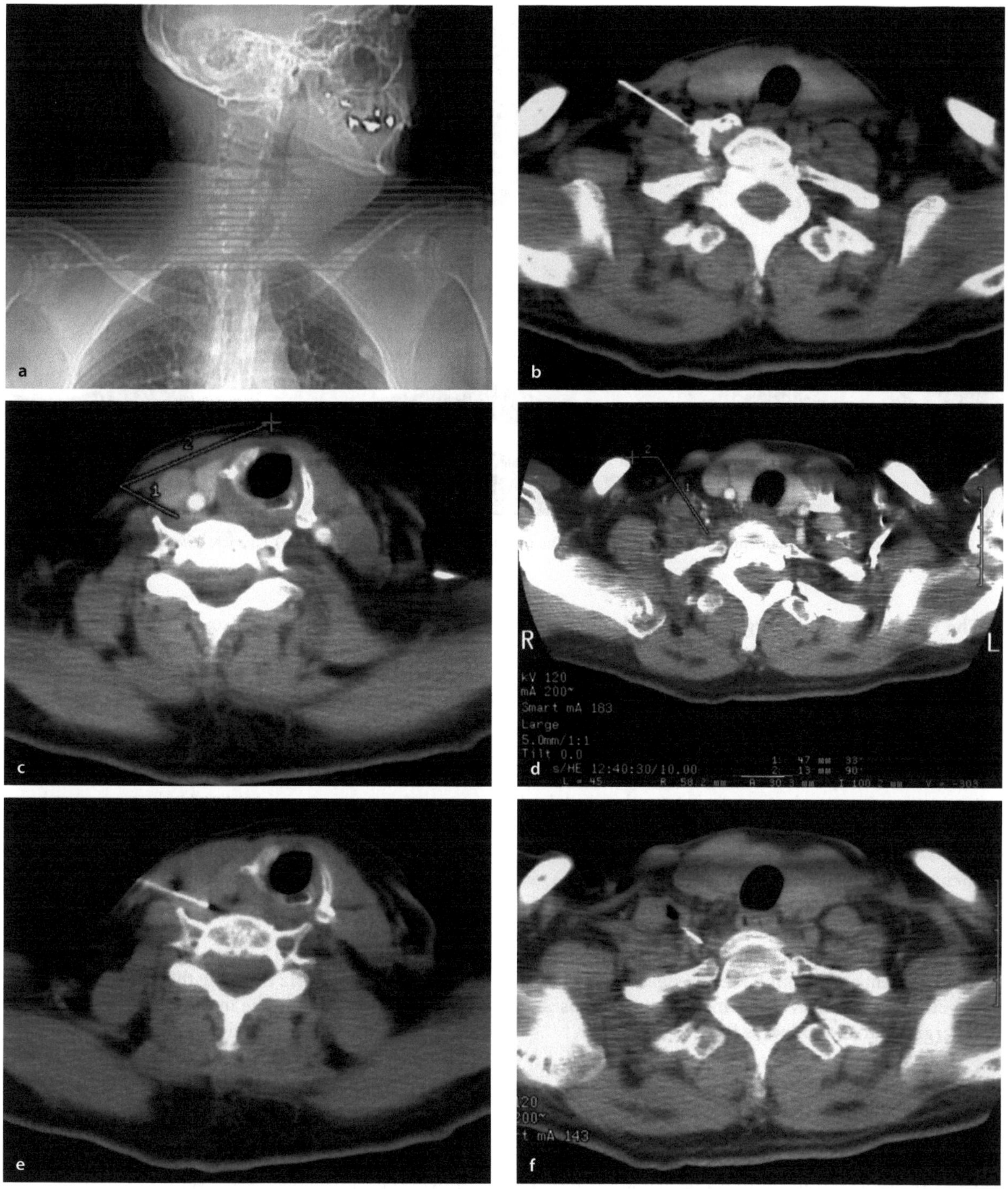

Fig. 10.2 a–f. RF neurolysis. Male patient 49 years old. RCPS type one syndrome after wrist trauma (positive scintigraphy). A good result was obtained after the procedure. **a** Slices are displayed on scout view. **b** A blockade was performed at the end of the procedure (see the contrast–anesthetic mixture diffusing around the needle tip). **c, d** Entry points and trans-scalenic pathway are displayed at C7 and T1 levels. **e, f** Needle tips on targets at C7 and T1 levels (see text for further explanations)

- Optimal entry points are determined and marked on the skin with a felt-tip pen, a long the projection of the laser light on the two reference slices (C7–T1 targets).
- The patient is draped in a sterile fashion, the skin scrubbed and sterilized, and a local anesthetic administered at the entry point and on initial presumed pathway.

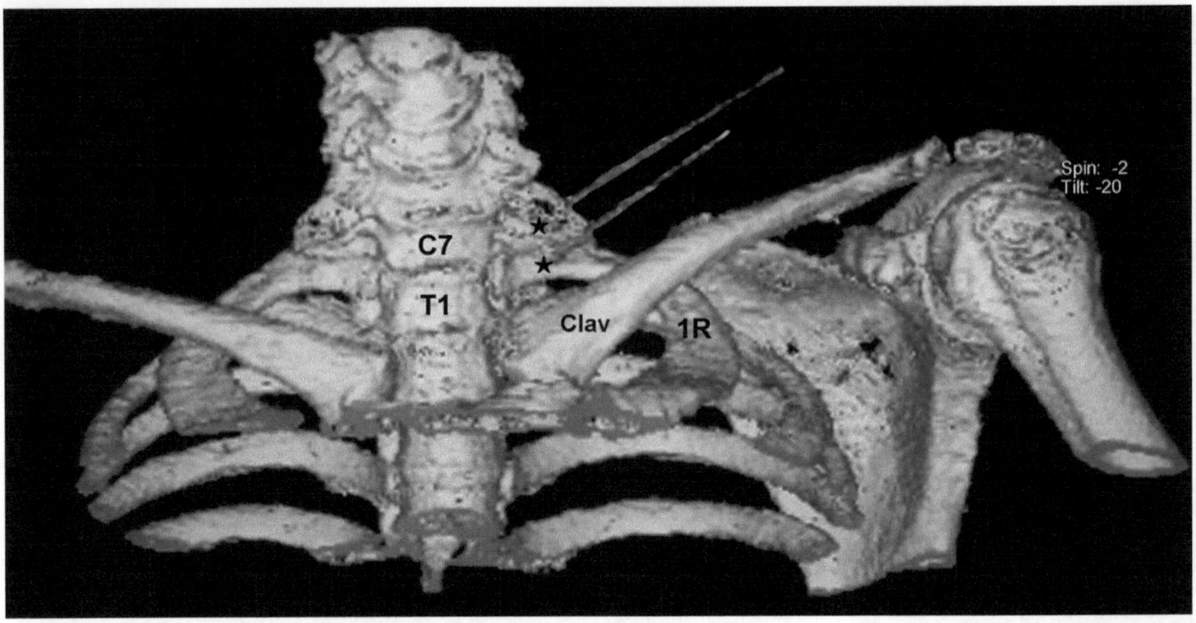

Fig. 10.3. Three-dimensional reformatted image displaying the needles at C7 and T1 targets (*stars*). Clavicle (*Clav*), 1st rib (*1R*)

- The correct needle-to-target path should be determined with respect to the skin entry point of the anesthetic needle left in place (either parallel or at a slight angle to that pathway; see Chap. 3).
- The first needle is slowly and carefully advanced step by step under CT guidance until its tip (check for the tip artifact) is positioned slightly anterior to the transverse process, just posterior to the vertebral artery, close to the junction with the vertebral body of the C7 vertebra (Fig. 10.2d). The second needle is then advanced to the second target (T1 vertebra) in front of the neck of the first rib behind the origin of the vertebral artery
- A saline injection combined with needle tip lateral displacement and rotation (bevel-edge rotation) is an effective means of averting intervening organs and enlarging narrow pathways [9] (see Chap. 3).

Stellate Ganglion Blockade

Five ml of a mixture of lidocaine 1/3 and ropivacaine 2/3 and 10% contrast medium is injected at the level of the C7 or T1 (Fig. 10.2b). Prior to injection the syringe in maintained in aspiration (under vacuum) for 5 seconds to ensure against vascular puncture This initial block may be used in the case of a doubtful diagnosis in order to ascertain that the patient's pain is indeed of sympathetic origin before later performing a more definitive blockade by RF. We also generally carry out an anesthetic block (3 to 5 ml of the same mixture at one or both levels) at the end of the RF procedure to reinforce and boost the overall effect by an immediate blockade.

RF Neurolysis

Please consult Figs. 10.2 and 10.3.

- The needles used are 20 gauge, 145 mm RF disposable cannulas for RF probe (Radionics). The electrode is introduced into the cannula and connected to the generator.
- No stimulation should be noted (as by motor fasciculations) at 2 volts 2 Hz ensuring that the cannula tip is at a safe distance from the motor nerves.
- At both levels a thermal lesion is created at a temperature of 55 to 80° C (depending on patients' tolerance) for 60 s. This procedure can be repeated up to three times, moving the cannula forward and backward by about 1 mm each time.
- At the end of the procedure a blockade (as described above) is performed at each level.
- The procedure is performed under local anesthesia and requires 45 to 60 min.
- As has been advocated [20], the C6 level can also be targeted for radio frequency ablation (if the C7 level is difficult to access safely, due to intervening vascular structures or nerves).

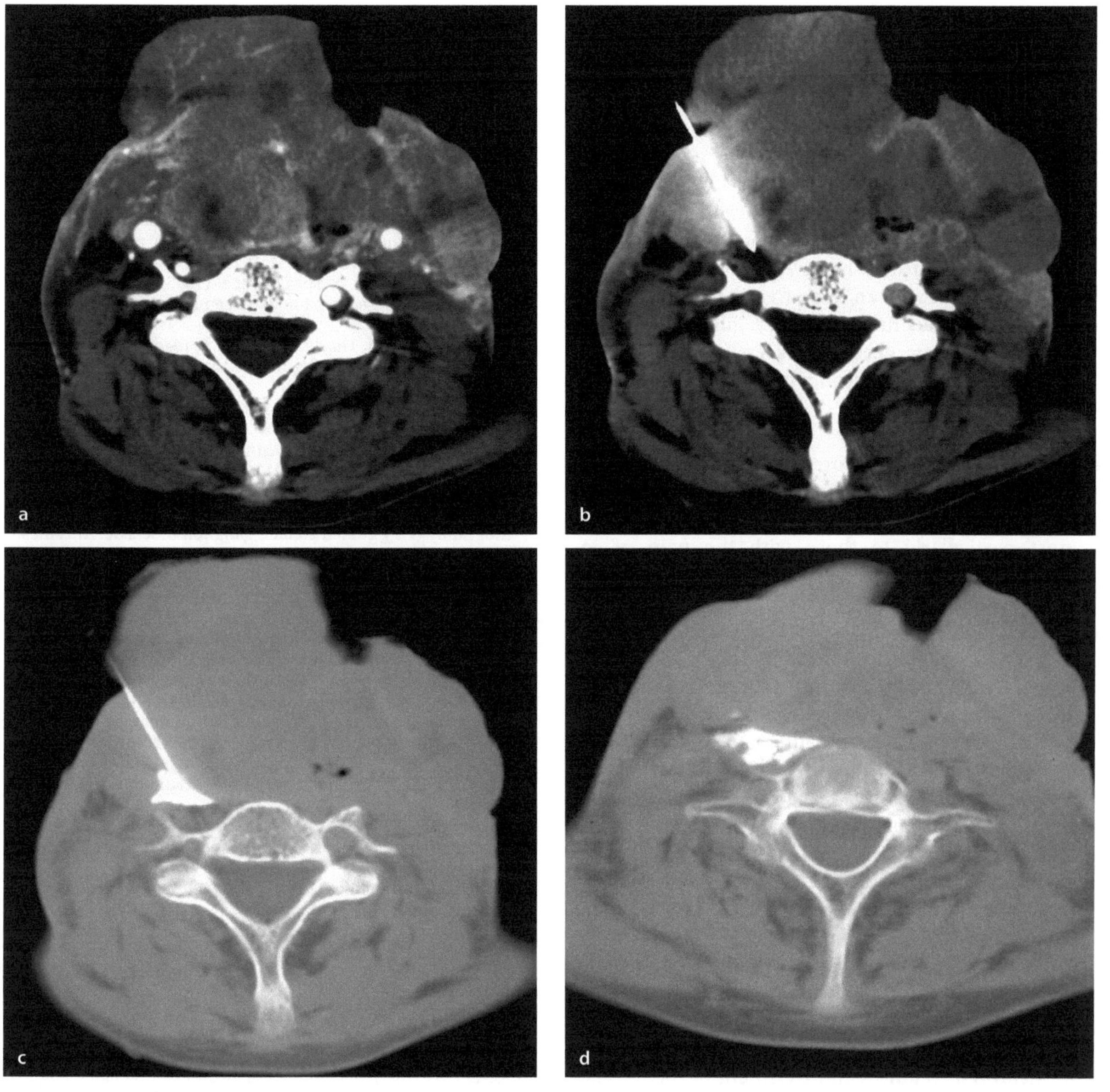

Fig. 10.4 a–d. Alcohol neurolysis. **a** Male patient 45-years-old with a vascularized mass of advanced throat cancer and suffering severe intractable cervical pain. Excellent pain relief was observed immediately following ethanol neurolysis, lasting until the patient died 5 months later. **b** An anterolateral approach at the posterolateral aspect of the mass is performed here at C7 to avoid the hypervascularized tumor. **c** Correct positioning of the needle tip at target is attested by the diffusion of a local anesthetic diluted with contrast medium showing good diffusion around and particularly behind the vertebral artery. **d** Injection of 1 ml of absolute alcohol appearing as hypodensities within the contrast medium

Ethanol Neurolysis

Please see Fig. 10.4.

- The needle used is a disposable 22 gauge, 7 cm spinal needle.
- The syringe in maintained in aspiration (under vacuum) for 5 seconds to ensure the absence of vascular puncture The correct position of the needle tip at target is determined by an injection of contrast medium diluted with local anesthetic (1:5, a total of 0.5 ml) which allows anticipation (checked by CT) of possible diffusion of the forthcoming alcohol injection, and to perform a test block.
- The patient may observes a decrease in symptoms following the anesthetic test block (not invariable). The neurolysis is performed with 1 to 1.5 ml of absolute alcohol instilled slowly. This should be carried out again maintaining prior to injection, the syringe in aspiration to insure against vascular puncture.

Pain relief is usually appreciated immediately following ethanol neurolysis.

Advantages and Disadvantages of the Two Approaches

- Needle placement on target at the level of the stellate ganglion is quite similar for RF and alcohol neurolysis. Both techniques are relatively easy to perform under CT guidance on an outpatient basis under local anesthesia. Unlike fluoroscopy, CT guidance allows a safe step-by-step needle progression and precise positioning at target, reducing complications, optimizing immediate results.

- Although it is lower in cost, ethanol neurolysis typically produces Horner's syndrome [4] and should be limited to patients with short life expectancy [1, 4], most particularly to those with the pain of intractable cancer where the benefits of pain relief outweigh the disadvantages of Horner's syndrome.
- Alcohol (both lipid and water soluble) may diffuse to surrounding motor nerves; the C8 and T1 roots of the brachial plexus are particularly exposed [13] as they are located posterior to the stellate ganglion (and the patient is supine). Possible diffusion to the epidural and subdural space is another significant drawback. These are illustrations that alcohol diffusion is not fully controllable and is not reliably predictable from that of the contrast medium because it is solely water soluble. Diffusion of the injected material to the contralateral side has been demonstrated in test blocks when large volumes are injected [9].

  These complications may be minimized by keeping the volume of injected alcohol within 1.5 ml and by precise positioning of the needle tip.

- RF neurolysis requires an investment in the RF generator and its electrodes. It is more time consuming (requiring the positioning of two needles).
- The lesion size is, however, adequately controlled. As described above, RF thermal neurolysis creates a discreet lesion that provides good pain relief and does not interrupt the entire ganglion's function. It therefore does not tend to produce Horner's syndrome [6, 20, 21]. Very precise positioning of the needle tip at the stellate ganglion is nonetheless required, but this is greatly facilitated by CT guidance in comparison with fluoroscopy.
- RF neurolysis is aimed at treating pain in benign conditions in which one must not run the risk of Horner's syndrome. We have treated 50 patients with RCPS type one with good long- lasting results on pain in 30 of them (60%), usually in one session [12, 14, 15, 16]. The procedure can, in any case, be easily repeated.

References

1. Bonica JJ, Buckley FP (1990) Regional analgesia with local anesthetics, in Bonica JJ, The management of pain. Philadelphia: Lea & Febiger, p 1941–1944
2. Brasseur L, Chauvin M, Guilbaud G (1997) Douleurs, bases fondamentales, pharmacologie, douleurs aiguës, douleurs chroniques, thérapeutiques. Paris: Maloine, p 517–527
3. Forouzanfar T, Van Kleef M, Weber WEJ (2000) Radiofrequency lesions of the stellate ganglion in chronic pain syndromes. The clinical journal of pain 16:164–168
4. Gangi A, Dietmann JL, Jeung M et al (1995) Interventional CT procedures in cancer pain management. Radiology [Suppl] 197:519
5. Guntamukkala M, Hardy PA (1991) Spread of injectate after stellate ganglion block in man: an anatomical study. Br J Anesth 66:643–644.
6. Haynsworth RF Jr, Noe CE (1991) Percutaneous lumbar sympathectomy: A comparison of radiofrequency denervation versus phenol neurolysis. Anesthesiology 74:459–463
7. Hogan QH, Erickson SJ (1992) MR imaging of the stellate ganglion: normal appearance. AJR 158: 655–659
8. Hogan QH, Erickson SJ, Abram SE (1992) Computerized tomography (CT) guided stellate ganglion blockade. Anesthesiology 77:596–599
9. Hogan QH, Erickson SJ, Haddox JD, Abram SE (1992) The spread of solutions during stellate ganglion block. Reg anesth 17:78–83
10. Kastler B, Clair C, Fergane B et al (1997) Stellate ganglion neurolysis under CT guidance. Radiological Society of North America, 84th Scientific Assembly and Annual Meeting. Chicago November 29 – December 3, 1997. Radiology [Suppl] 205:563
11. Kastler B, Clair C, Delabrousse E et al (2001) RF neurolysis of stellate ganglion in sympathetically-maintained pain syndrome of the upper limb. Scientific paper. Radiological Society of North America, 87th Scientific Assembly and Annual Meeting. Chicago, November 25–30, 2001. Radiology [Suppl] Vol. 221:616
12. Kastler B, Michalakis D, Clair C et al (2001) Neurolyse du ganglion stellaire par radiofréquence sous guidage scanographique. Étude préliminaire. JBR-BTR 84:191–194
13. Kastler B, Clair C, Michalakis D et al (2002) Interventional procedures under CT guidance in 756 patients, incidents, side effects and how to reduce their incidence. Scientific Exhibit. Radiological Society of North America, 88th Scientific Assembly and Annual Meeting. Chicago, November, 2002. Radiology [Suppl] vol. 225:724
14. Kastler B, Narboux Y, Clair C et al (2001) Neurolyse par Radiofréquence du ganglion stellaire. À propos d'un cas traité et suivi sur trois ans. J Radiol 82:76–78
15. Kastler B, Sailley N (2006) RF neurolysis of Stellate ganglion aiming at two sites C7 and T1 under CT guidance: Results in 28 patients with Complexe regional pain syndrome one of the upper limb. Scientific paper. Radiological Society of North America, 92th Scientific Assembly and Annual Meeting. Chicago November 29 – December 3, 2006. Radiology [Suppl]
16. Michalakis D (1999) Neurolyse du ganglion stellaire par radiofréquence ou alcoolisation sous guidage scanographique dans les douleurs d'origine sympathique: étude préliminaire à propos de 7 cas. Thèse de médecineBesançon, 8 décembre
17. Monnier F (1999) Neurolyses percutanées du ganglion cervicothoracique par radiofréquence sous contrôle tomdensitométrique: bases atomiques. Besançon, 15 December
18. Roberts WJA (1986) Hypothesis on the physiological basis for causalgia and related pains. Pain 24:279–311
19. Scott J, Erickson SJ, Quinn H, Hogan QH (1993) CT guided injection of the stellate ganglion: description of technique and efficacy of sympathetic blockade. Radiology 188:707–709
20. Sluijter ME, Koestveld-Baart (1980) Interruption of pain pathway in the treatment of cervical pain syndromes. Anaesthesia 35:302–307
21. Smith HP, Mc Worther JM, Challa VR (1981) Radiofrequency neurolysis in a clinical model. Neuropathological correlation. J Neurosurg 55:246–253

Percutaneous Neurolysis of the Celiac Plexus and Splanchnic Nerves

Under CT and color Doppler US Guidance

Bruno Kastler, Jean-François Litzler,
Pierre-Yves Marcy, Gérard Schmutz

11

The first description of blockades of the splanchnic nerves in the management of abdominal pain was by Kappis in 1919 [24, 25]; he relied on palpable bony landmarks. Scopic guidance was introduced in the 1950s [1, 25], followed by echographic guidance in the 1970s [21, 22].

Introduced in the early 1980s [3, 15, 35], computed tomographic (CT) guidance is currently almost exclusively used to accurately and reliably position the needle tip, thereby reducing the risk of complications and controlling the diffusion of lytic agent. Echographic guidance is less in use, but the advent of echo-endoscopy [13] and color and contrast products explain its recent return to favor in the hands of experienced echographers [32].

Clinically Relevant Anatomy

The celiac plexus, crossroads of the visceral vegetative nervous system, is made up of ganglia linked to each other on either side of the abdominal aorta (Fig. 11.1). It is supplied by thoracic splanchnic, right pneumogastric. and less often right phrenic afferents. Contrary to the initial descriptions of Hovelacque [17] and Ward [42], these ganglia vary in number, size, and topography depending on the individual. There may be 1 to 5 pairs, with size ranging from 0.5 to 4.5 cm and extending from T12 to the middle of L2 (less frequently L1).

The origin (ostium) of the celiac trunk remains the most reliable anatomical landmark [27, 39]: on the right, the ganglia are generally located 6 mm below the ostium, and on the left 9 mm below this landmark. However, it should be remembered that individual variations exist: on the right, the ganglia can be located between 5 mm above and 15 mm below the origin of the celiac trunk; on the left, between this landmark and 30 mm below. These variations can explain the ineffectiveness of the blocking procedure on some patients. Diffusion of lytic agent longitudinally diminishes the significance of this anatomical consideration.

It is important to know the relationship between the celiac plexus and neighboring organs potentially damaged by the needle or the diffusion of lytic agent (see Fig. 11.1):

- Immediately posterior: the ventral side of the aorta near the origin of the celiac trunk
- Posterior and lateral: the diaphragmatic pillars (between the spinal column and the pleural cul-de-sac)
- Posterior and further laterally: the kidneys
- Right posterolateral: the inferior venal cava
- Anterior: the pancreas.

The splanchnic thoracic nerves (splanchnic ganglia) are located posterior to the diaphragmatic pillars, and in anteroposterior orientation are at the junction of the anterior third and middle third of the vertebral bodies T11 and T12.

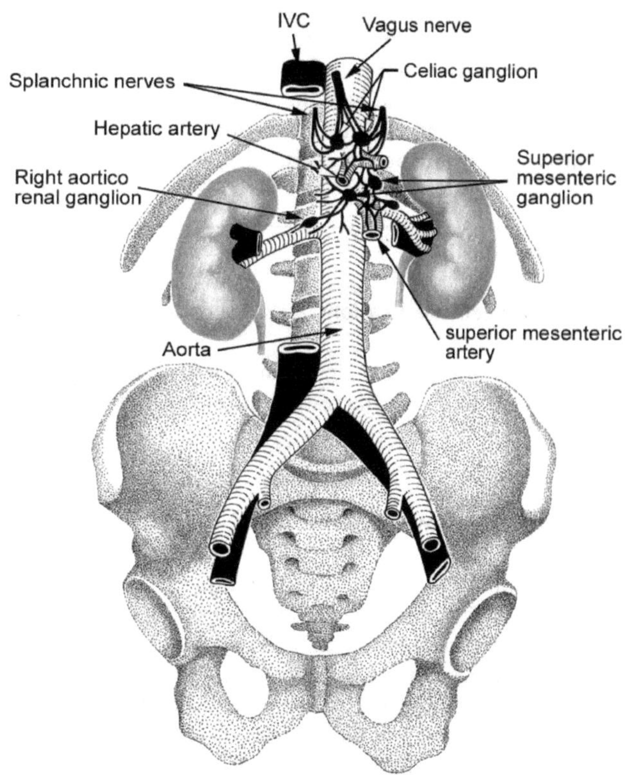

Fig. 11.1. Diagram of the celiac plexus and its relationship with the abdominal aorta, celiac trunk, and upper mesenteric artery

Indications

The indications for celiac neurolysis are varied: from neurospasms to peptic ulcer [12]. The main indications currently accepted are intolerable abdominal pain caused by visceral sub-mesocolic pathology affecting the retroperitoneum and compressing, invading or irritating on contact the celiac plexus.

Gastric and pancreatic tumors [2, 43] are the main indications. Chronic pancreatitis is another, although for undetermined reasons the efficacy of neurolysis is reduced in this condition [29, 38].

In conjunction with such pain centers or palliative treatment units as may exist, neurolysis is performed in cases of severe algic phenomena which do not respond to major analgesics, or when these are poorly tolerated or contraindicated. If applied at an early, sometimes anticipative, stage prior to massive tumoral infiltration of the retroperitoneal space, its efficacy is improved because of better diffusion at that time of the neurolytic agent. By delaying the administration of analgesic treatments (namely opiods) and making it possible to reduce the amounts administered (and their side effects), neurolysis improves the quality of the patient's terminal life.

Other indications can be visceral neuropathy of patients suffering from diabetes or Crohn's disease, and more recently, from sclerosing cholangitis of AIDS [5]. Anesthesia of the solar plexus (via 1% lidocaine) is responsible for temporarily interrupting the adrenosolar nervous axis; it inhibits the secretion of vasoactive adrenal substances and relieves the arterial spasm in the case of severe pancreatitis.

Contraindications

Absolute Contraindications

They are exceptional and transitory, including only irregular blood clotting results and severe hypovolemia (see Chap. 3).

Relative Contraindications

These influence the choice of technique:

- A posterior approach with the patient in a prone position should be avoided with patients suffering from chronic respiratory insufficiency.
- An anterior approach should be avoided when there is significant gastric stasis with distension.
- A transaortic path is excluded in aortic aneurysm, voluminous calcified parietal plaque, or mural thrombus [20, 31].

Obstructive stenosis of the esophagus or at the pylorus can be a source of potential failure of the echo-endoscopic technique which others advocate.

Technique and Material

Refer to Chapter 3 for guiding techniques.

A rapid acquisition on a multi-slice scanner reduces the duration of the initial morphological assessment carried out with an IV injection of contrast medium. The procedure is ideally carried out under cardiac and respiratory monitoring, and with appropriate anesthetic and resuscitation equipment present. Usual consumables are employed: IV contrast medium (tri-iodide or non ionic), 1% lidocaine, physiological saline.

On an ultrasound machine with color and power Doppler, the procedure is carried out under breath hold, in real time, and under permanent visual control with the help of a sterile probe.

To standard interventional radiology material is added single-use sterile material comprising several well-identified syringes (shape, size, material) and cupules and a variety of different needles (local anesthetic, neurolysis, 22 gauge spinal needle). Strict asepsis requires the use of sterile sheets, surgical garments, and gloves.

Patient Care and Preparation

The patient is informed (if possible during a preliminary consultation) about the procedure to be carried out, its expected benefits and risks, and written consent is obtained as required by regulations. After obtaining a blood-clotting analysis and information on allergy (antiallergic premedication administered as necessary), the patient is prepared.

Schematically, there are two ways to approach the celiac plexus, either anteriorly or posteriorly. After setting up a peripheral intravenous line, the patient is placed for optimal comfort in either a prone or supine position, depending on the choice of pathway.

In prone position, a pillow is placed under the patient's stomach. The head, turned to the side, is laid on the forearm or another small pillow. In supine position a pillow is placed under the knees to relax the abdomen.

Locating the Level of Slice, Trajectory, and Point of Cutaneous Entrance

After a topographic helical acquisition (5 mm/5 mm or 7/7), adjacent slices from T11 to L2 (Fig. 11.2) are obtained during the injection of contrast medium (with free breathing). At a rate of 1.5 to 2 ml per second over

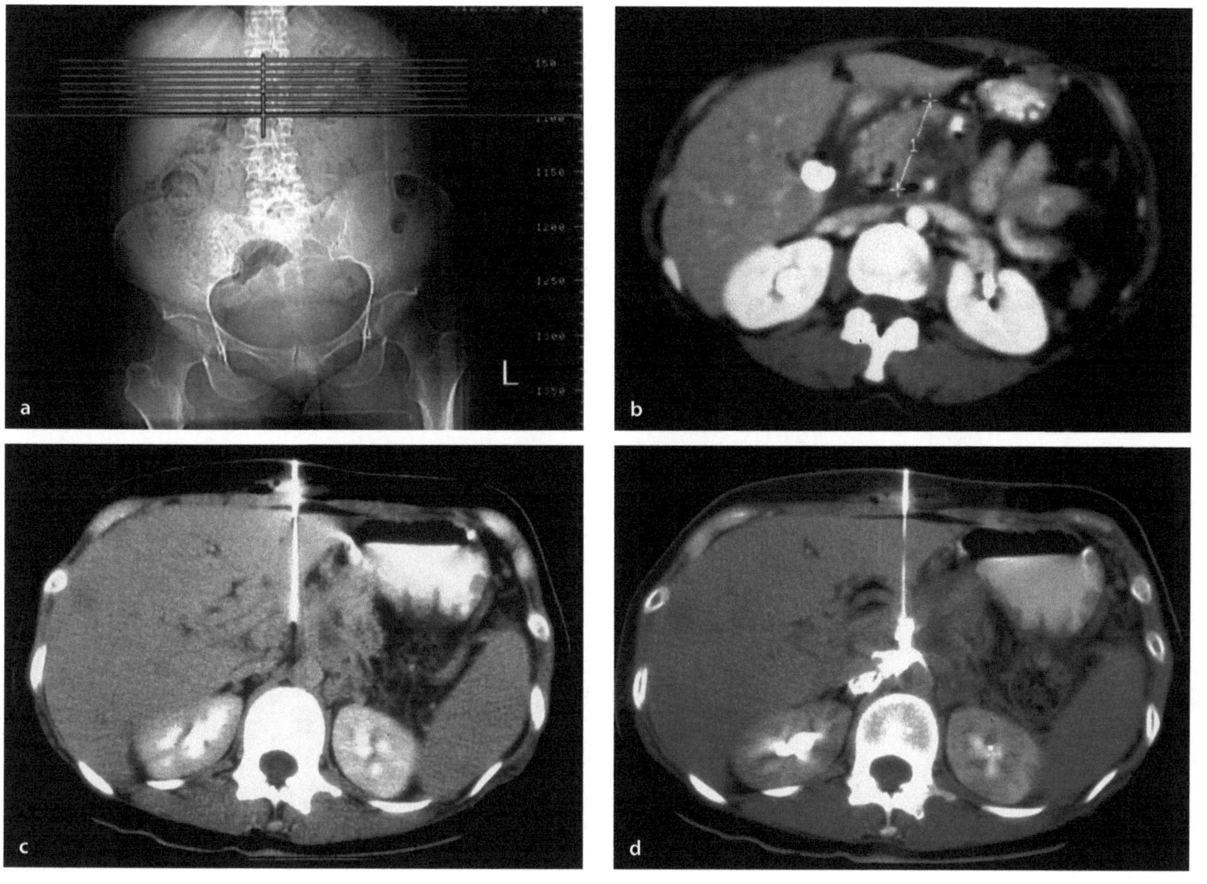

Fig. 11.2 a–d. Cancer of the pancreas, celiac neurolysis, . **a** Frontal topogram showing the adjacent slices from T11 to L2 **b** Celiac neurolysis by anterior approach. **c** The needle is positioned and oriented towards the target transhepatically (tip shown by the tip artifact). **d** Good bilateral diffusion in the celiac region (in front of the aorta)

50 seconds, 100 to 120 ml of contrast medium are introduced.

The ostium of the celiac trunk is the most reliable anatomical landmark and the ideal slice is level with this landmark or immediately below. The skin entry point must enable the needle to follow the most direct trajectory, while avoiding various organs and obstacles: colon in the case of an anterior approach; and pleural cul-de-sac, inferior vena cava, and possible bony vertebral obstacles in the case of a posterior approach.

The puncture trajectory is determined on the control panel by drawing a virtual line between a cursor positioned at the target and an appropriate entry point. The entry point(s) thus determined is/are marked by drawing a line on the patient's skin with a felt pen along the projection of the laser beam of the CT-scanner on the section initially chosen. on the section initially chosen. The distance is measured on the console in relation to a line connecting the spinous processes.

Positioning the Needle

Carried out in normal aseptic conditions (after preparation and thorough cutaneous disinfection), a local anesthetic is administered along the predetermined cutaneous and subcutaneous trajectory (See Figs. 11.2–11.4). The local anesthetic needles are left in position as a marker for control slices (see Chap. 3). The trajectory and progression of the definitive needles (22 gauge spinal) are carried out under CT guidance in biopsy mode for 3 adjoining slices from 5 to 7 mm, centered at the tip of the needle (check for the tip artifact in the middle slice), in spiral acquisition and free breathing. The frequency of control (i. e., of obtaining CT slices) is the decision of the operator and dictated besides his experience and dexterity by foreseeable anatomical difficulties or incidents (pain, obstacle).

The correct needle tip position is controlled by injecting contrast medium 10% diluted in a mixture of lidocaine 1/3 and ropivacaine 2/3 (3 ml celiac, 1 ml splanchnic). Prior to injection the syringe in main-

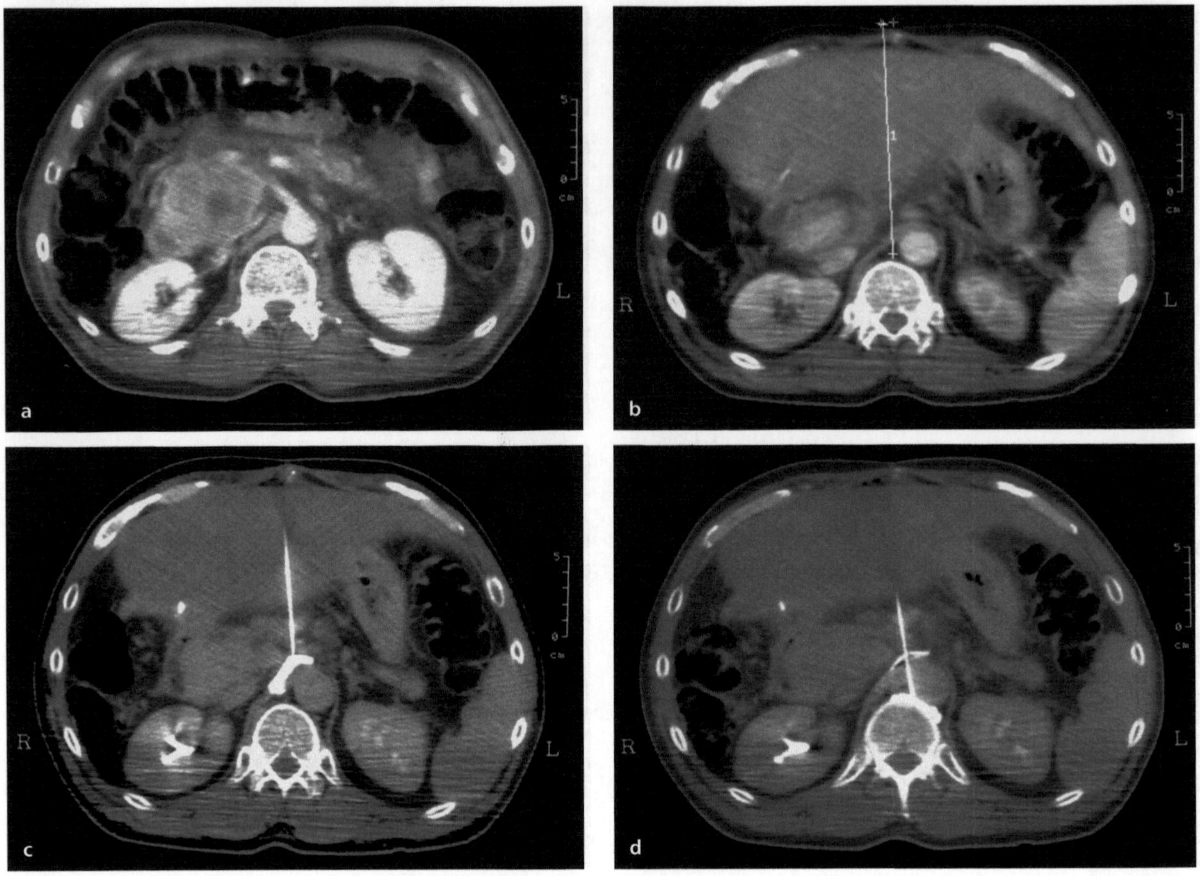

Fig. 11.3 a–d. Cancer of the pancreas. **a, b** Splanchnic and celiac neurolysis by anterior approach. Trajectory indicated (*line* **b**) for celiac and splanchnic neurolysis. **c** Celiac neurolysis. **d** Splanchnic neurolysis by approach lateral to the aorta; transaortic approach also possible (see Fig. 11.4)

tained in aspiration (under vacuum) for 5 seconds to ensure against vascular puncture . Its spread reflects the extent to which the neurolytic will be active[1]. This also enables a test block to be carried out which, by providing pain relief, bears witness to the needle's correct position as well as to the origin of the pain. This infiltration will also reduce pain accompanying the neurolysis (alcohol injection) and dilute the lytic agent (but which must remain over 66% alcohol; see Chap. 3 and 4).

During chemical neurolysis (carried out after again maintaining a pull on the syringe 5 to 10 seconds in order to insure against blood reflux and thus avoid an intravascular injection), the needle is held in place by the operator or taped at the skin entry point to avoid inadvertent progression. A syringe containing lidocaine must be ready and on hand in case of unbearable pain during the injection. Most often it is sufficient to distract the patient by asking him/her to breathe in and out deeply; the pain recedes in less than a minute, the time it takes for the nerve fibers to be destroyed.

The spread of the product injected, as well as its effect (temporary reproduction of the usual algic syndrome), are verified on each successive control slice, carried out during the injection after every 1 to 2 ml injected for the splanchnic and after every 3 to 5 ml for the celiac procedure.

At the end of the procedure, the injection of one fourth of milliliter of physiologic saline or lidocaine, just off the main site, provides relief from pain as the needle is removed. See Chap. 3 and 4 for more information.

1) It is to be remembered however that the alcohol is both hydrosoluble and liposoluble, which therefore is strictly consistent with that of the anesthetic-contraste mixture being solely hydrosoluble. Please refer to chapter 3.

Site of Injection

- For celiac preaortic infiltration, the tip of the needle is advanced to a position near the origin of the celiac trunk. When using a posterior and lateral approach

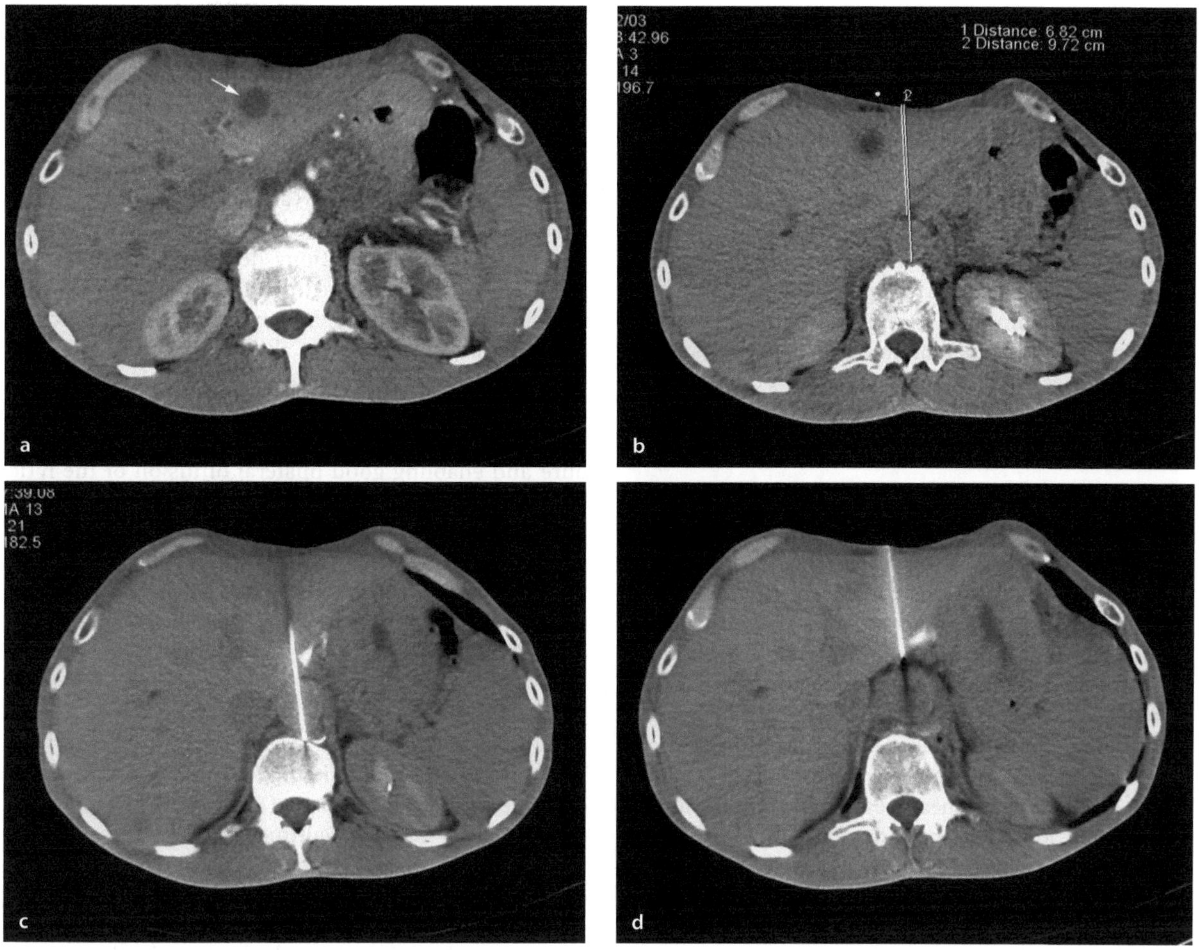

Fig. 11.4 a–d. Cancer of the tail of the pancreas with hepatic metastases, splanchnic and celiac neurolysis by transaortic anterior approach. **a** A splanchnic neurolysis lateral to the aorta is not recommended (*lines*) due to the presence of hepatic metastasis on pathway (*arrow*). **b** Trajectory indicated (*line*) for celiac and splanchnic neurolysis. **c** Transaortic passage to reach splanchnic nerves. **d** Celiac neurolysis at removal of needle

with the first needle (usually the left one), the material rarely spreads as it should bilaterally (molding the anterior aspect of the aorta, see Fig. 11.5 d and e), making a contralateral injection with a second needle necessary. Regarding this preaortic infiltration via a posterior approach, a second problem often occurs: on the right (for the contralateral injection) the inferior vena cava or another obstacle (bones, kidney) often hinders the needle's trajectory. A transaortic left approach solves these problems, enabling satisfactory preaortic diffusion bilaterally.

- As before, the splanchnic ganglia sites are retrocrural and, in anterior/posterior orientation, at the junction of the middle third and anterior third of the bodies of vertebrae T11 and T12.
- Two approaches are possible, anterior and posterior (actually posterolateral). They require CT guidance as only the anterior approach is possible with echography.

Anterior Approach

Anterior Celiac Neurolysis

This approach, made in a supine position (see Figs. 11.2–11.4), is the most comfortable for and usually the best tolerated by the patient. It requires a single puncture at the celiac level, and the infiltrate spreads to both sides, making it possible to choose the side depending on each patient's anatomy. If possible, the injection should reach a total amount of 15 to 20 ml of absolute alcohol (see Fig. 11.2). Because of its sensitivity to respiration, the transperitoneal approach is more difficult and requires multiple control slices. The transhepatic passage is ideal; and the tiny caliber (22 gauge) of the needle makes the transgastric passage possible.

Anterior Splanchnic Neurolysis

Splanchnic ganglion neurolysis can be carried out at the same time (with the same trajectory and same needle), if the patient's anatomy so allows and if planned at the outset, by a passage lateral to the aorta. Thus in general the injected material (1 ml contrast medium diluted with local anesthetics followed by 4 to 6 ml of absolute alcohol) diffuse to mainly one splanchnic site (left or right) (see Fig. 11.3). A transaortic trajectory (see Fig. 11.4), sometimes a transpancreatic, may then be necessary to allow bilateral spread.

Bilateral destruction by alcohol of only the splanchnic ganglia, using an anterior approach, is recommended by some. We, however, strongly advocate when possible carrying out concomitant celiac and splanchnic neurolysis (see Fig. 11.3 and 11.4) [39]. Splanchnic neurolysis is particularly indicated in tumors involving the lower third of the mediastinum.

Posterior Approach

Please refer to Figs. 11.5, and 11.6.

The patient is positioned in the most comfortable prone position. Slightly turned to one side if necessary. The transpleural trajectory is avoided by a not-too-lateral paramedian cutaneous access, with care taken to reduce physiological lumbar lordosis (pillow beneath the abdomen) or by first tilting the gantry to allow for a more caudocranial needle trajectory (see Chap. 3, Figs. 3.3). Contrary to measures taken using the anterior approach, for experienced operators the injection of contrast medium is not always essential because the aorta and celiac trunk are often visible without contrast, and no other vascular structures are encountered along the posterior route.

Posterior bilateral two-needle technique

A classic posterior bilateral approach with two needles includes first a splanchnic neurolysis (injection of an equivalent of 4 to 5 ml of absolute alcohol on either side). And then by directing the same needles through the diaphragm and lateral to the aorta, neurolysis can be carried out at the celiac site (with injection of the equivalent of 15 to 20 ml of absolute alcohol) (see Fig. 11.5a–c). Also refer to Chapter 3 (Fig. 3.19). As mentioned before the material rarely spreads bilaterally in front of the aorta, and/or on the right for the contralateral injection, the inferior vena cava or an other obstacle (vertebral body, kidney) often hinders the needle's trajectory (see Fig. 11.5d). A transaortic left approach solves these problems (see Fig. 11.5e).

Posterior one-needle transaortic technique

A modified posterior approach with a programmed direct transaortic passage (the route we advocate) makes it possible with the left needle to first reach the left splanchnic site enabling left splanchnic neurolysis (injection of an equivalent of 4 to 5 ml of absolute alcohol), and with the same needle pass through the aorta reach the celiac site where the celiac neurolysis can be carried (with injection of the equivalent of 15 to 20 ml of absolute alcohol) The second needle on the right is aimed at the right contralateral splanchnic ganglion for neurolysis (see Figs. 11.5d, e and Fig. 11.6). Also refer to Chapter 3 (Fig. 3.7 and 3.19). As before, an equivalent of 4 to 5 ml of absolute alcohol is used.

The transaortic passage (as well as that through the liver, stomach, or pancreas, as mentioned earlier) is subject to the contraindications described above, but is feasible because use of the tiny caliber (22 gauge) needle is not accompanied by hemorrhagic, thrombotic, or other local complications, always providing that the operator strictly avoids the aortic collaterals, in particular the visceral branches. Though perhaps bizarre, this trajectory offers the advantage of shortening the procedure and enabling good bilateral diffusion of the lytic agent in the celiac region (avoiding the need to position a second needle to the right side of the aorta). It provides a good alternative to the bilateral two-needle technique, in particular when it is difficult to position the needle to the right of the aorta (i.e., in the space bordered by the spine, kidney, and inferior vena cava).

Echography

When this method of guidance is employed, the anterior procedure is slightly faster (Fig. 11.7). The cutaneous point of entry is a few centimeters below the xyphoid, the target lying between the celiac trunk and the superior mesenteric artery. These landmarks, identical to those of the CT technique, are better visualized with an echographic view through the liver in the case of left hepatomegaly, in color mode, and possibly after IV injection of echographic contrast to underline the arterial signal of the celiac ostium. The puncture needle is visualized in real time (advantage over CT guidance), but is less clearly visible, requiring to-and-fro movements of the needle shaft, sometimes injection of in situ contrast medium when no clear echographic view through the liver is available. Clinical observation of aortic systolic pulses combined with 2D visualization of the needle tip provide correct positioning. Echogenic images generally appear, revealing the spread of alcohol bubbles in the celiac region, the diffusion volume of the neurolytic agent mirroring roughly that visualized under CT guidance (after accounting for the contrast medium).

Results

The results are identical and the risk of complications low, whatever the technique. The technique selected will depend on the patient's preference and the anatomy. The experience and dexterity of the operator should also be considered, especially in relation to the duration of the procedure.

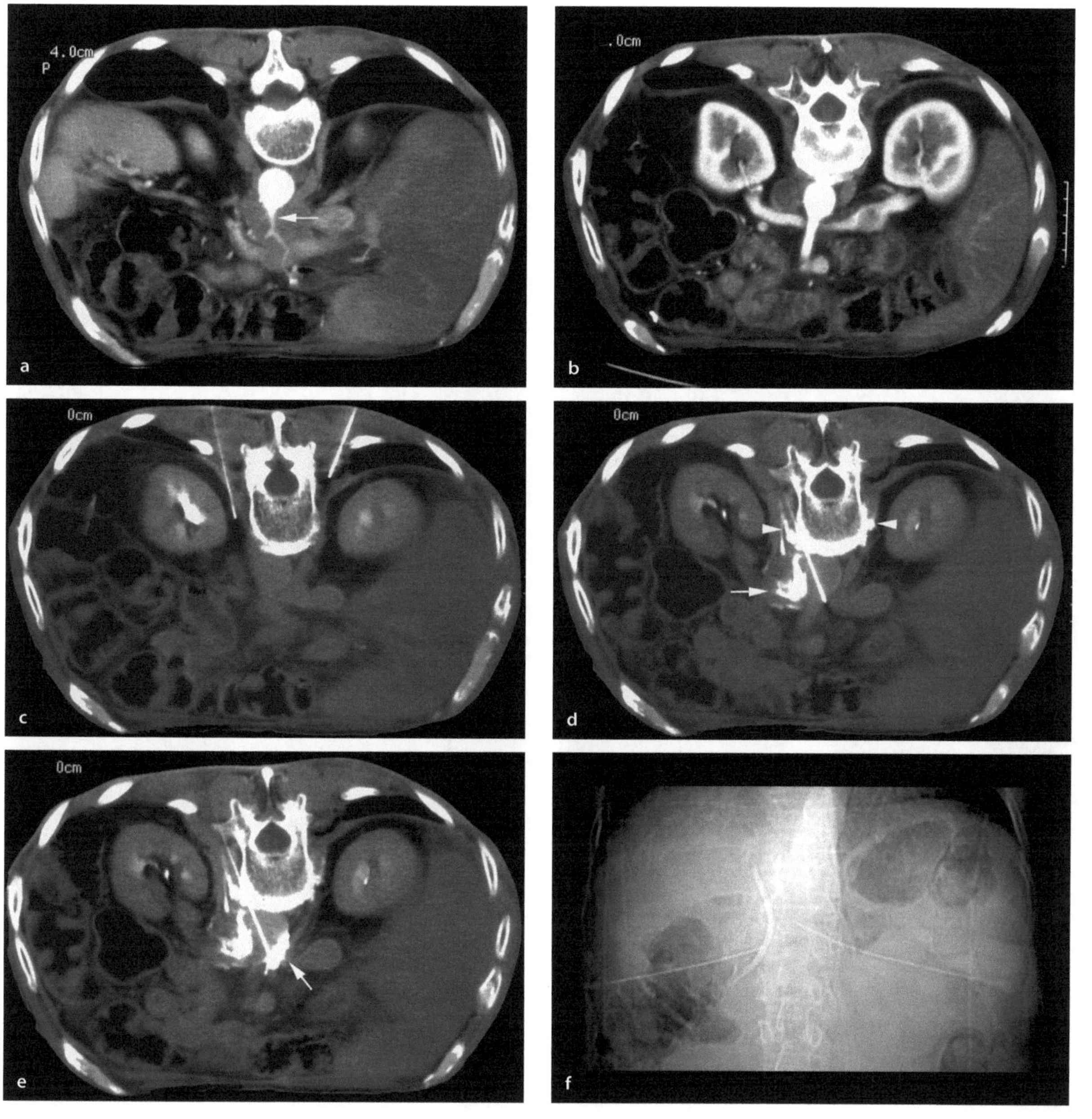

Fig. 11.5 a–f. Posterior celiac neurolysis. **a** Injection of contrast medium shows the ganglia compressing the celiac trunk (*arrow*), and thus also the celiac explaining compression of the celiac plexus. **b** Slice carried out below a showing the lower mesenteric artery (*arrow*); left renal vein passes in the aorticomesenteric angle. **c** The left and right needles advance towards the lateral vertebral splanchnic sites avoiding the pleural cul-de-sacs; note that the pathway has been enlarged on the right to allow safe needle progression. **d** Splanchnic neurolysis (*arrowhead*). Celiac neurolysis (*arrow*) carried out at to the left of the aorta does not spread at all to the right. A celiac aim to the left of the aorta is impossible because of interposition of the rib, kidney and/or spine on the trajectory. **e** A transaortic passage is selected in order to obtain good diffusion to the right and in front of the aorta (*arrow*). **f** Needles in position on the topogram

Controlling Diffusion and Injection

Tip Artifact

This must always be searched for. Ideally, by keeping the needle tip in the middle slice of the three CT control slices, the artifact enables the operator to control the needle's progression along the trajectory. It is the best indicator of the correct positioning of the needle for injection at the target.

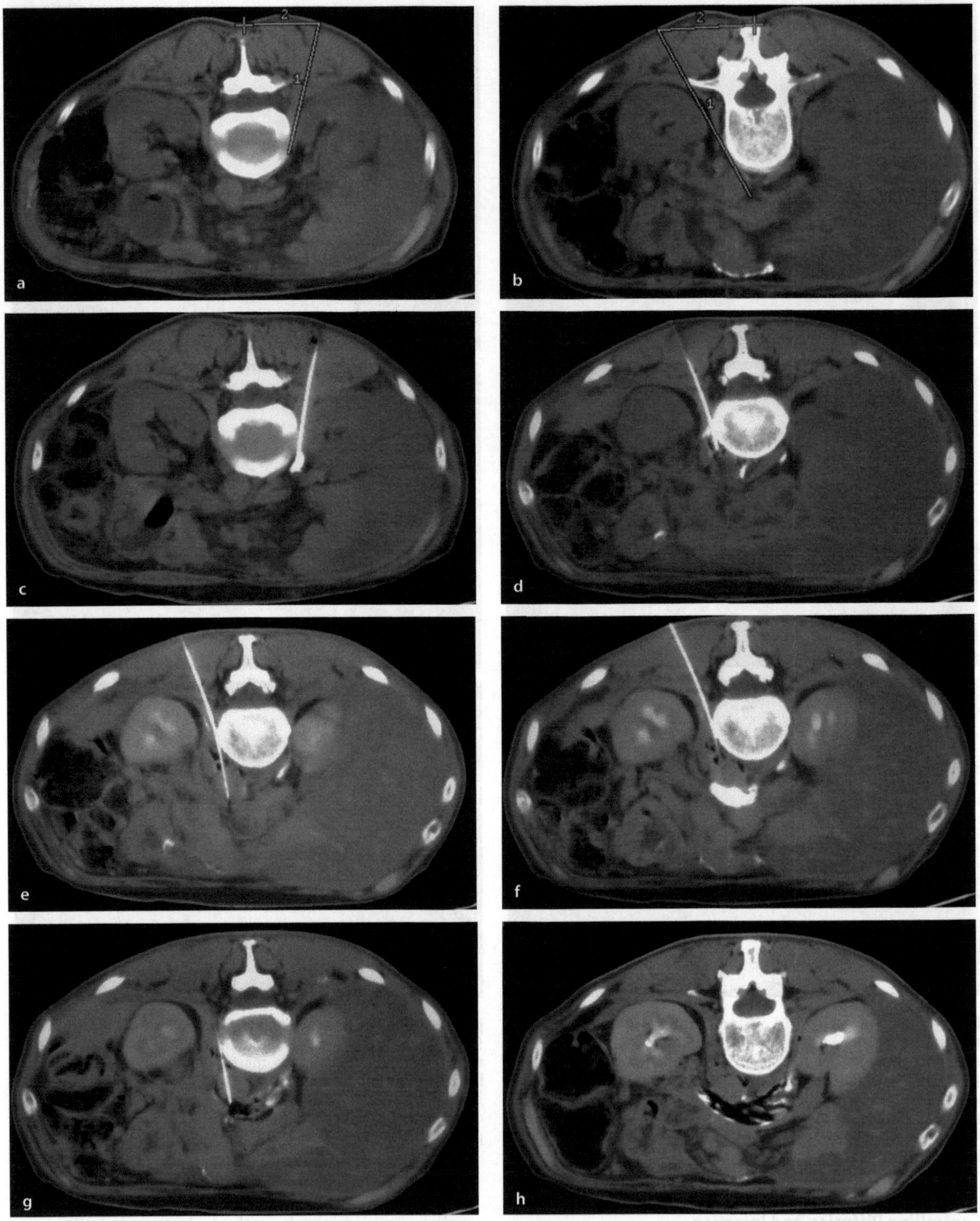

Fig. 11.6 a–h. Celiac neurolysis directly using transaortic passage. **a** Trajectory shown (*line*) for right splanchnic neurolysis. **b** Trajectory (*line*) makes it possible to carry out left splanchnic neurolysis and transaortic celiac neurolysis with the same needle. **c** Right and **d** left splanchnic neurolyses. **e** Transaortic passage of the needle to the celiac site; note that the needle tip artifact is located in front of the anterior aortic wall; injection of the anesthetic-contrast mixture (**f** good symmetrical diffusion, hyperdensity). **g** Control after injection of 5 ml absolute alcohol (hypodensity). **h** Control after end of injection of absolute alcohol (15 cc): excellent alcohol diffusion (also see Chap. 3, Fig. 3.7 and 3.19)

Lidocaine Test Block

We recommend a test block prior to the neurolysis, as do others [14, 16, 30], combining the anesthetic with contrast medium (a mixture of lidocaine 1/3 and ropivacaine 2/3 and 10% contrast medium)
in order to keep the procedure's duration as short as possible.

The contrast medium/lidocaine medium-anesthetic mixture, monitored by CT, delineates the boundaries of the injection and subsequent diffusion at the retroperitoneal (paraceliac, para-aortic) or retrocural (splanchnic, lateral vertebral) site.

The appearance of dense echoes (alcohol bubbles) is the echographic equivalent (see Fig. 11.7e). If relief be achieved by this test injection, one can be confident both that the needle is in the correct position and that the definitive procedure will succeed.

Administering the Neurolytic Agent

As the neurolytic is administered, ideally the patient's symptoms are at first reproduced, providing additional evidence that the site of injection is correct and that the procedure will be effective. The onset of unusual pain or that of normal sensory nerve distribution should prompt the operator to obtain CT control slices in order to adjust position and (hopefully) control diffusion.

Type and Dosage of Chemical Lytic Agent

Phenol glycerine (7%) and pure or 90% (180 proof) ethanol are available, packaged in 10 ml ampules. (Phenol must be stored in the dark and requires the use of a glass syringe.) We prefer to use alcohol, which is easier to inject and less toxic. It causes immediate cellular destruction by local dehydration and coagulation of intracellular proteins at any concentration over 66%. Its final concentration must be correctly calculated taking into consideration the total quantity of liquid injected, including local anesthetics and contrast medium mixture. To simplify the calculation, we inject 3 to 5 volumes of absolute alcohol after an injection of 1 volume of contrast medium-anesthetic diluted with lidocaine (see Chapter 3). As an example, the average quantities injected in the splanchnic region are 1 ml contrast/anesthetics, followed by 4–5 ml of absolute alcohol, and in the celiac region 3 ml contrast/anesthetics and 15 to 20 ml of absolute alcohol.

It should, however, be remembered that the quantities must be adapted to each patient depending on the available prevascular retroperitoneal space available for diffusion of the lytic agent. It is important not to forcibly inject the alcohol because it might then spread outside the intended space, possibly causing unwanted damage. The quantity injected must be adapted to the projected diffusion of the material, which can be controlled to some extent by obtaining a hypodense scan image after the administration of every 1 to 2 ml portion of the agent during splanchnic neurolysis, and every 3 to 5 ml for the celiac region, in the absence of any unusual symptomatology.

A like control plan can be conducted in real time when using ultrasound (see Fig. 11.7b–d).

"The more the better" is not synonymous with efficacy: on the contrary, introduction of overabundant lytic agent carries the risk of useless diffusion of the product outside the optimal site, at the very least. Careful, modest, and controlled injection prevents such mishaps. If there is massive tumoral invasion of the celiac region the quantity injected must be reduced – or even dispensed with altogether.

Complications, Side Effects

Complications

Complications are exceptional providing the procedure is carried under CT guidance and all contraindications are respected: those relative to all interventions that employ contrast media, and those relative to celiac and splanchnic neurolysis. CT guidance during the needle's progression by posterior passage should prevent renal puncture (detectable by hematuria, or subcapsular or perirenal hematoma), transpleural passage (detectable by pneumothorax or pneumohemothorax).

Serious neurological complications (paraplegia, lasting sphincter disorders) are practically inexistent under CT guidance. Epidural or subdural injections aside, such disorders can, however, arise despite the best possible control (quantity and spread of injectant both carefully attended to) if diffusion comes in contact with the dural sheath, causing a spasm of or even thrombosis of a spinal branch of the vertebral artery (most likely arising from the L1 or L2 region), or perhaps of another vessel, to cause ischemia of a portion of the spinal cord [23].

During posterior diffusion of alcohol (splanchnolysis), we have encountered two cases of transitory inguinofemoral neuropathy [26], the origin of the nerves involved being the roots of L1/L2 (see Chapter 14, Fig. 14.1). The transdigestive transperitoneal, passage has not been found to be responsible for peritonitis so long as the colon is avoided. Chemical peritonitis by alcohol diffusion along the needle's trajectory remains exceptional. If any doubt about a possible peritoneal diffusion the needle should in any case not be retrieved and one must attempt to dilute the alcohol by a subsequent

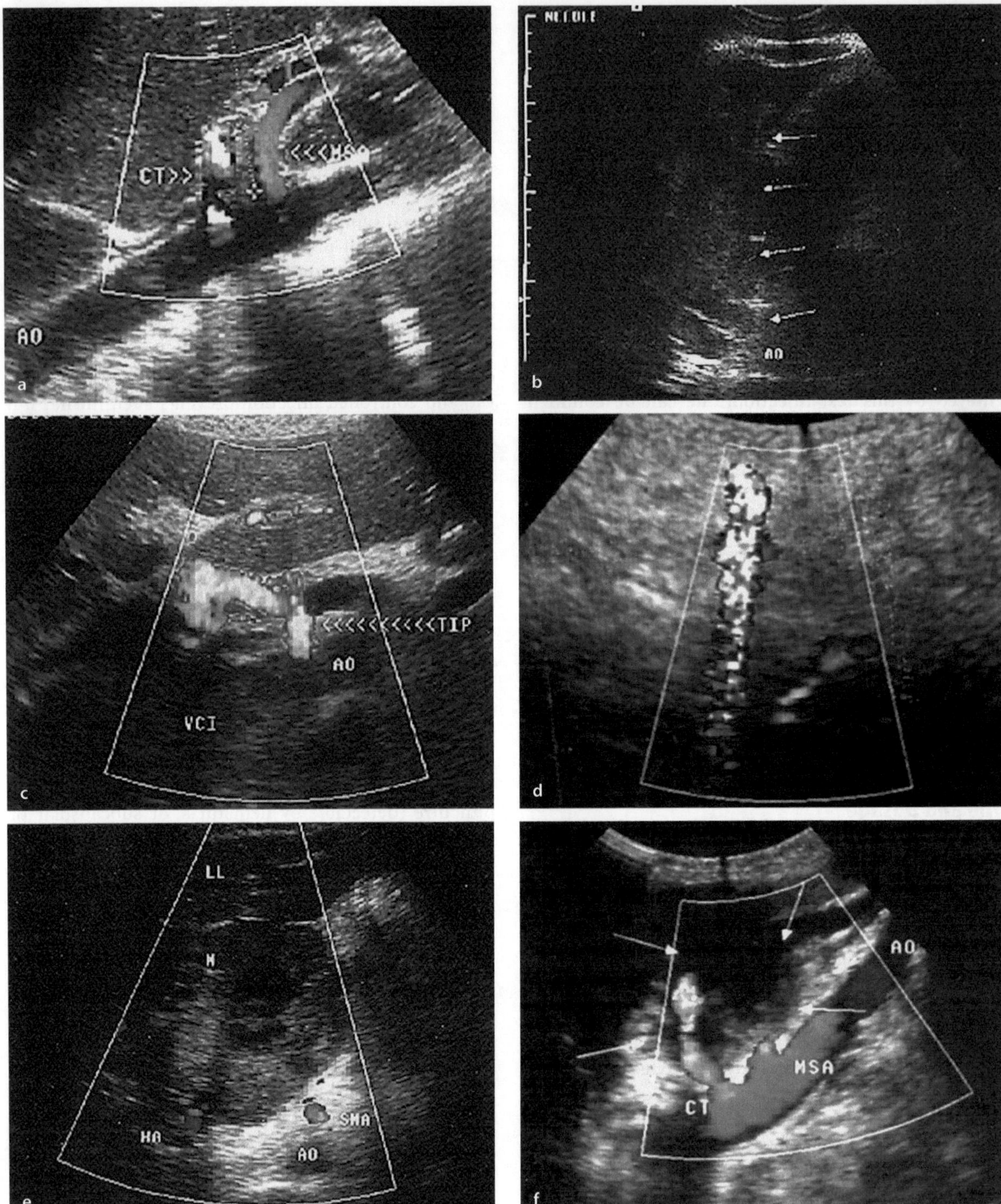

Fig. 11.7 a–f. Celiac neurolysis using echography. **a** Color sagittal slice of the abdominal aorta (*AO*) clearly showing the vascular celiac arterial and upper mesenteric landmarks. For the trajectory of the left transhepatic puncture, the tip of the needle must be between the origin of the celiac trunk (*CT*) and the upper mesenteric artery (*MSA*). **b** Transhepatic sagittal slice in gray scale, showing the trajectory of the needle (uncolored; *arrows*). **c** Axial transverse slice via the distal tip of the needle (*TIP*), between the origin of the celiac trunk and the upper mesenteric artery. The echo tip, in contact with the anterior Hepatic artery (*AH*) is colored by the to-and-fro movement of the needle in the color mode. **d** An injection into the needle's shaft makes it possible to color the needle, thereby allowing visualization of the trajectory in real time (also of the mesenteric ostium). **e** Transverse axial slice after alcoholization, in color mode. The appearance of dense echoes in front of the aorta (*AO*), behind the voluminous metastasis of the (*M*), indicates diffusion of the neurolytic agent around the superior mesenteric ostium (*SMA*). Hepatic anterior wall of aorta (*AO*), left liver (*LL*). **f** Color sagittal slice of the abdominal aorta (*AO*). Tumoral invasion (*arrows*) sheathing the ostium and the initial portion of the celiac trunk (*CT*), moving back down to the superior mesenteric ostium (*MSA*)

injection of a large volume of lidocaine. The bolus injection of contrast medium makes it possible to locate the larger vessels and thereby avoid them.

The anterior passage presents a rare risk of iatrogenic pancreatitis but one which should be considered. A transpancreatic passage should be carried out only in case of necessity (almost always for a pancreatic tumor). The transhepatic trajectory and its risks are the same as those for other liver punctures (e.g., biopsy). The transaortic passage and the occurrence of retroperitoneal hematoma, well known at the time of translumbar aortographies using 14 to 18 gauge needles (risk estimated at 0.1 to 0.5%), is exceptional when the caliber is not larger than 20 gauge.

Side Effects

The side effects encountered are local pain (particularly in the case of transdiaphragmatic passage), diarrhea (which in fact often alleviates the frequent cases of chronic constipation in these patients often under large do), and orthostatic hypotension. The respective frequency has been found to be about 96%, 44%, and 38% of cases [30].

Vasodilatation and an increase in blood flow in the mesenteric region by rapid raising of the sympathetic tonus constitute a blood bypass, which justifies surveillance of the blood pressure pre- and post-procedure and strict bed rest for 8 hours. A saline drip or administration of a vasoconstrictor (e.g., 15 to 25 mg of ephedrine) are rarely necessary. An increased transit rate (diarrhea) for 48 hours also is a regular result of the autonomic effect and is also a sign of the procedure's efficacy.

Intense stomach pains due to peritoneal or phrenic chemical irritation only last several hours but can justify the prescription of an analgesic. The rapid resorption of ethanol can lead to a rise in blood alcohol content and transitory inebriation. Side effects more rarely encountered and reported are chronic diarrhea [4, 10] (often as mentioned correcting stubborn constipation), post-neurolysis celiac gastroparesis [18], reactive pleural effusion [9], and retroperitoneal fibrosis after iterative neurolysis for chronic pancreatitis [36].

Results and Efficacy

The efficacy and success of the procedures described in this Chapter are shown by a decline in pain (visual analogical scale) and reduction in dosage or cessation of analgesics. Collation of the results remains difficult due to the plurality of techniques employed, the pain threshold of each patient, and the quantification differences among teams. Under CT guidance, positive results are reported in 75 to 95% of patients, all techniques considered. Celiac neurolysis is described as effective in over 85% of pancreatic neoplasms and in 75% for other submesocolic malignancies [33, 34, 39].

The half-life of the analgesic effect is over 4 weeks. Data including over one thousand patients suffering from malignant abdominal illnesses shows an efficacy of 89% over the first 15 days [7]. Partial or total alleviation from pain was reported for between 70 to 90% of patients after the first quarter [7]. Long-term efficacy can be less well defined due to the lack a reliable average life expectancy. Less spectacular is the case of chronic pancreatitis: 66% of good results are obtained in the short term and only 30% in the long term. The reason remains unclear, but nociceptive passages other than celiac and splanchnic may explain.

Under ultrasound guidance the results are slightly less favorable (60 to 69% good results for the most recent oncological series [32, 33]). probably due to the advanced stage of the illness (frequently infiltrated celiac region) and above all the failure to address the splanchnic ganglia as well (see Fig. 11.7f).

The failures encountered (irrespective of the chosen technique), all have in common a technical failure (poorly positioned needle tip), anatomical variations (predominant unilateral celiac ganglion), too little product injected (or finally too diluted). Above all massive tumoral infiltration (see Fig. 11.7f), which constitutes an obstacle to site accessibility, to the diffusion of the alcohol, and which affects the other nervous plexi, and thus which lastly is the main etiology for short-term recurrence. If this is the case special care should be taken to perform the best possible concomitant splanchnic neurolysis.

The two main difficulties with ultrasound are gas in the digestive tract and obesity both rare in neoplastic pathology, particularly pancreatic. These limiting factors are found in less than 10% of cases [32, 33].

The regeneration of incompletely destroyed nervous filaments is a cause of more long-term recurrence, in which case the procedure can however be repeated.

Conclusion

With results at least equal to surgical methods and a low rate of major complications, percutaneous neurolysis under CT or ultrasound guidance be largely available. It has the potential of significantly improving the quality of the terminal life of patients suffering from incurable neoplastic abdominal pathology.

Carried out almost on an outpatient basis (24 hours), this treatment reduces the length of hospital stays, and preserves the patient's quality of life and autonomy. The indication remain within a multidisciplinary context, particularly within that of pain and care center.

Although easy to carry out, the procedure is rarely renewed on patients with a rather short expectancy.

In the case of pain secondary to an inflammatory pathology, in particular chronic pancreatitis, upon which the efficacy of celiac neurolysis is reduced, the situation seems totally different. The procedure must be regularly repeated to obtain a lasting analgesic effect, thereby increasing the risks of complications. In such cases, it would seem reasonable to insist on other analgesic therapies before attempting celiac neurolysis.

References

1. Bonica JJ (1954) The management of pain. Lea and Febiger, Philadelphia, pp 229–230
2. Bonica JJ (1990) Neurolytic blockade. In: Bonica JJ (ed) The management of pain, 2nd edn. Lea and Febiger, Philadelphia, pp 2015–2020
3. Buy JN, Moss AA, Singler RC (1982) CT guided celiac plexus and splanchnic nerve neurolysis. J Comput Assist Tomogr 6:315–319
4. Chan VWS (1996) Chronic diarrhoea: an uncommon side effect of celiac plexus block. Anesth Analg 82:205–207
5. Collazos J, Mayo J, Martinez E, Callejo A (1996) Celiac plexus block as treatment for refractory pain related to sclerosing cholangitis in AIDS patients. J Clin Gastroenterol 23:47–49
6. Derhy S, Couderc J, Begon C, Roche A (1989) Neurolyse coeliaque. Abord antérieur et guidage tomodensitométrique: une technique simple et logique. Ann Radiol 32:230–233
7. Eisenberg E, Carr DB, Chalmers TC (1995) Neurolytic celiac plexus block for treatment of cancer pain: a meta-analysis. Anesth Analg 80:290–295
8. Fiore D, Ravasini R, Macchi C et al (1985) Upper abdominal pain therapy by CT guided alcohol block of the coeliac splanchnic region. Rays 10:43–48
9. Fujita Y, Takaori M (1987) Pleural effusion after CT guided alcohol celiac plexus block. Anesth Analg 66:911–912
10. Gafanovich I, Shir Y, Tsvang E, Ben-Chetrit E (1988) Chronic diarrhoea induced by celiac plexus block. J Clin Gastroenterol 26:300–302
11. Gangi A, Kastler B, Gasser B et al (1992) Tomodensitométrie interventionnelle. Imagerie nouvelle, août 1992
12. Golding S, Husband JE (1990) CT-guided celiac interventional techniques: Guided neurolysis and complications of CT guided procedures. J Intervent Radiol 5:119–123
13. Gress F, Schmitt C, Sherman S et al (1999) A prospective randomized comparison of endoscopic ultrasound- and computed tomography-guided celiac plexus block for managing chronic pancreatitis pain. Am J Gastroenterol 94:900–905
14. Haaga JR, Kori SH, Eastwood DW, Borowski GP (1984) Improved technique for CT-guided celiac plexus block. Am J Roentgenol 142:1201–1204
15. Haaga JR, Reich NE, Havrilla TR, Alfidi RJ (1977) Interventional CT scanning. Radiol Clin North Am 15:456–469
16. Herpels V, Kurdziel JC, Dondelinger RF (1988) Percutaneous CT-guided nerves block of celiac plexus and splanchnic nerves. Ann Radiol 31:291–296
17. Hovelacque A (1927) Anatomie des nerfs crâniens et rachidiens et du système sympatique chez l'homme. Doin, Paris, pp 375–397
18. Iftikhar S, Loftus EV (1998) Gastroparesis after celiac plexus block. Am J Gastroenterol 93:2223–2225
19. Ischia S, Ischia A, Polati E, Finco G (1992) Three posterior percutaneous celiac plexus block techniques. A prospective, randomized study in 61 patients with pancreatic cancer pain. Anesthesiology 76:534–540
20. Ischia S, Luzzani A, Ischia A, Faggion S (1983) A new approach to neurolytic block of the celiac plexus: the transaortic technique. Pain 16:333–341
21. Jackson SH, Jacobs JB, Epstein RA (1969) A radiographic approach to celiac plexus block. Anesthesiology 31:373–375
22. Jacobs J, Jackson S, Doppman J (1969) A radiographic approach to celiac plexus block. Radiology 92:1372–1376
23. Kaplan R (1996) Neurolytic celiac plexus block: can paraplegia and death after neurolytic celiac plexus block be eliminated? Anesthesiology 84:1523
24. Kappis M (1919) Sensibilität und lokale Anasthesie im chirurgischen Gebiet der Bauchhohle mit besonderer Berücksichtigung der Splanchnicus Anathesis. Beitr Klin Chir 115:161–175
25. Kappis M (1920) Zur Technik der Splanchnicus Anasthesie. Zentralbl Chir 47:98
26. Kastler B, Clair C, Michalakis D et al (2002) Interventional procedures under CT guidance in 756 patients, incidents, side effects and how to reduce their incidence. Scientific exhibit, Radiological Society of North America, 88th scientific assembly and annual meeting, Chicago, Nov 2002. Radiology [Suppl] 225:724
27. Kurdziel JC, Dondelinger RF (1990) Percutaneous lysis of neural structures. In: Dondelinger RF, Rossi P, Kurdziel JC, Wallace S (eds) Interventional radiology. Thieme, New York, pp 768–780
28. Lee MJ, Mueller PR, van Sonnenberg E (1993) CT-guided celiac ganglion block with alcohol. Am J Roentgenol 161:633–636
29. Lieberman RP, Cuka DJ (1991) Percutaneous celiac plexus blockade. In: Kadir S (ed) Current practice of interventional radiology. Mosby-Year Book, St Louis, pp 742–745
30. Lieberman RP, Lieberman SL, Cuka DJ, Lund GB (1988) Celiac plexus and splanchnic nerve block: a review. Semin Intervent Radiol 5:213–222
31. Lieberman RP, Waldman SD (1990) Celiac plexus neurolysis with the modified transaortic approach. Radiology 175:274–276
32. Marcy PY, Magné N (2000) Technique échoguidée du bloc cœliaque. J Radiol 81:1727–1730
33. Mathon G, d'Alincourt A, Lerat F (2001) Alcoolisation cœliaque échoguidée dans les douleurs solaires néoplasiques. J Radiol 82:41–44
34. Mercadante S, Nicosia F (1998) Celiac plexus block: a reappraisal. Reg Anesth Pain Med 23:37–48
35. Moore DC, Bush W, Burnett L (1980) Computed axial tomography: the most accurate method of performing alcohol celiac plexus block. Proceeding of the 5th annual meeting: regional anesthesia and pain. University of San Francisco, San Francisco, p 33
36. Pateman J, Williams P, Filshie J (1990) Retroperitoneal fibrosis after multiple coeliac plexus blocks. Anesthesia 45:309–310
37. Polati E, Finco G, Gottin L et al (1998) Prospective randomized double blind trial of neurolytic coeliac plexus block in patients with pancreatic cancer. Br J Surg 85:199–201
38. Romanelli DF, Beckmann CF, Heiss FW (1993) Celiac plexus block: efficacy and safety of the anterior approach. Am J Roentgenol 160:497–500
39. Sarlieve P, Clair C, Saguet O et al (2002) Alcoolisation coeliaque et splanchnique par voies postérieure et antérieure. Intérêt de la voie transaortique. Journées Françaises de Radiologie, Paris, 19–23 oct 2002. J Radiol Tome 83:1542
40. Schild H (1988) Perkutane neurolyse des plexus coeliacus. In: Günther RW, Thelen M (eds) Interventionelle radiologe. Thieme, Stuttgart, pp 405–409
41. Schild H, Gunther R, Hoffman J, Goedecker R (1983) CT gesteuerte Blockade des Plexus Coeliacus mit ventralen Zugang. Rofo 139:202–205
42. Ward EM, Rorle DK, Nauss LA, Bahn RC (1979) The celiac ganglia in man: normal anatomic variations. Anesth Analg 68:461–465
43. Whiteman MS, Rosenberg H, Haskin PH, Teplick SK (1986) Celiac plexus block for interventional radiology. Radiology 161:836–838

Other Sympatholysis

12

Bruno Kastler, Philippe Manzoni, Laurent Laborie, Hussein Haj Hussein, Jean-Yves Cornu, Florence Tiberghien-Chatelain, Bernard Fergane

Thoracic Sympatholysis

Bruno Kastler, Philippe Manzoni, Laurent Laborie, Hussein Haj Hussein

Indications

This procedure has been recommended for [27]:

- Vasomotor disorders of the upper limb, occlusive arterial disease, distal arteritis, distal arterial embolism, illness or syndrome of Raynaud
- Type 1 and 2 chronic regional pain syndromes (post-traumatic dystrophy and causalgia), frostbite, pain of sympathetic origin of the upper limb and thoracic region (neoplasm of paravertebral gutters with vertebral invasion), phantom limb
- Axillary or palmar hyperhidrosis (but see below under Alcoholization)

Clinically Relevant Anatomy

The thoracic (dorsal) sympathetic chain is an extension of the cervical sympathetic chain (the stellate ganglion being the junction between the two) [4]. It is made up of nervous filaments with ganglion relays located on either side of the vertebra in front of the ribs in the costovertebral angle, and drifting more anterior in position as one moves down the spine (but remaining decidedly more posterior than the lumbar sympathetic chain, Fig. 12.1). More specifically:

- The T2 ganglion lies at the 2nd rib neck (the T1 ganglion is fused with C8 to form the stellate ganglion; see Chap. 10).
- Ganglia T3 to T6 lie at the rib heads.
- The T7 to T10 ganglia are located at the costovertebral joints (in front of the costovertebral ligaments).
- Ganglia T11 and T12 are more anterior in a lateral position in relation to the vertebra.

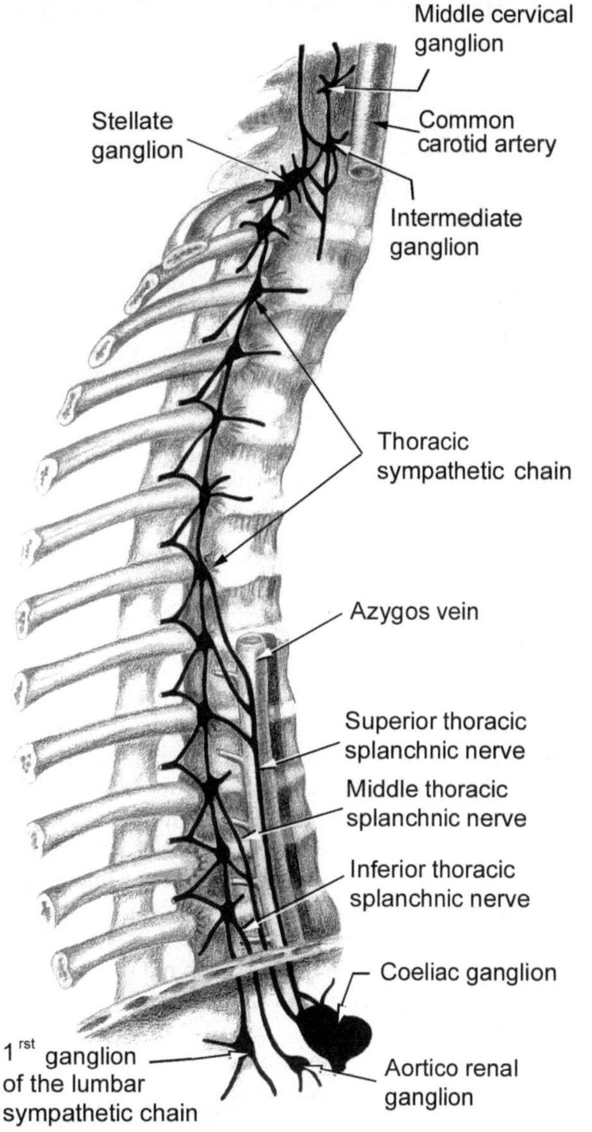

Fig. 12.1. Anatomical diagram of the thoracic sympathetic chain; the ganglion relays are located on either side of the vertebra in front of the ribs in the costovertebral angle, in a more and more anterior position as they progress further down from T1 to T12. (Drawing by Andia Hashemizadeh)

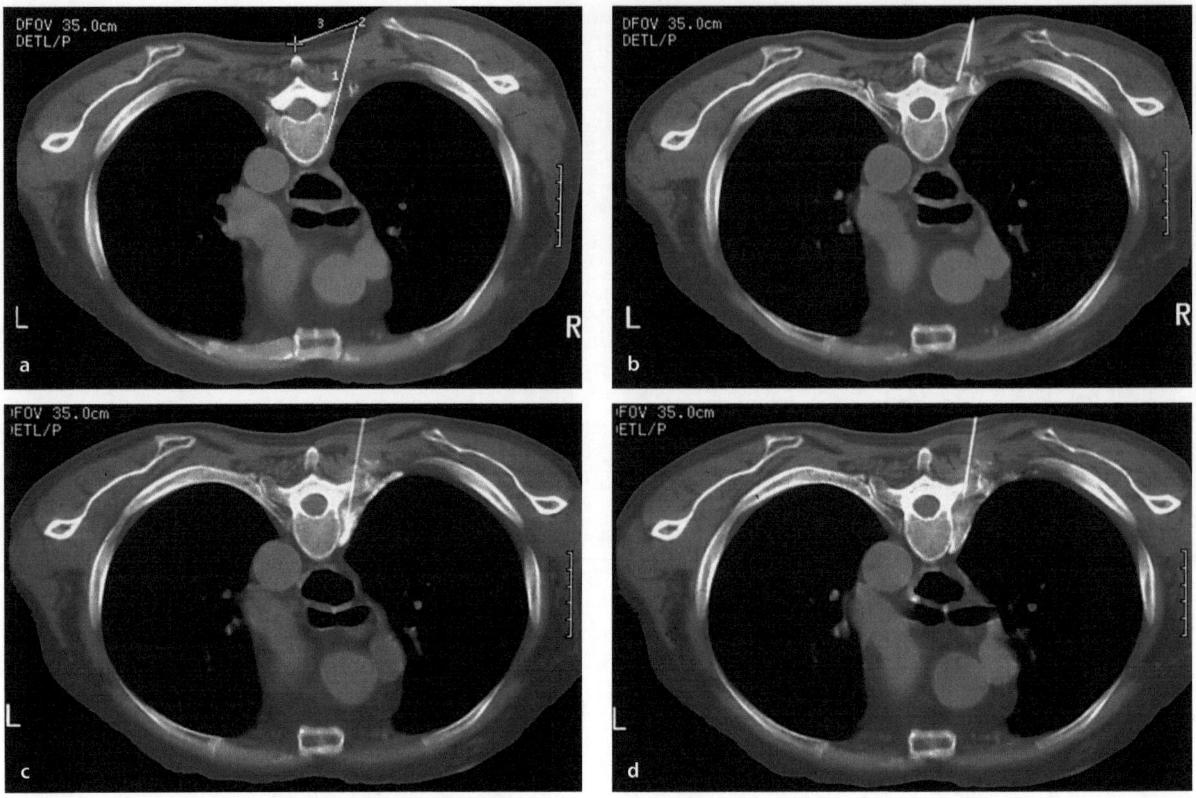

Fig. 12.2 a–d. Right thoracic sympatholysis of a patient with thrombosis of the right subclavian artery following a stent emplacement. **a** Level T3 here. The space between pleura and the lateral aspect of the vertebral body is rther narrow. **b** Guidance by the anesthesia needle left in position (see Chap. 3). **c** Widening of the channel by injection of physiological saline and contrast, thus pushing away the pleuropulmonary parenchyma (again refer to Chap. 3). **d** Injection of absolute alcohol (dilution of the contrast medium by the hypodense alcohol. Also see Fig. 3.17, Chap. 3

Technique

Please see Fig. 12.2 and Fig. 3.17, Chap. 3.

After verifying that the patient's coagulation rates are normal (see Chap. 3), the patient is informed, preferably during a previous visit, about the procedure and the potential risks, and gives consent as required by law. The patient is placed in a prone position, head turned away from the puncture side. Axial joint slices of 5 mm thickness are carried out from T1 to T3; generally two targets in T2 and T3 are selected [1, 2, 7]. The skin entry point and trajectory are determined in such manner that the pleura, vertebral body, and intervertebral disk are avoided.

The needles are progressively inserted under CT guidance until their tips are located at the costovertebral angle at the rib heads at T2 and T3 respectively. As the space between the ribs and the pleura is sometimes minute, it can sometimes be useful to enlarge it by injecting physiological saline as the needle progresses toward this point [15, 16].

Alcoholization

A 22 gauge (spinal) needle 5 to 7 cm long is used. Half a milliliter of analgesic (1% lidocaine) mixed with contrast medium is injected into each target point. A series of control slices monitor the diffusion of this mixture, making sure that it does not spread too far upward toward the stellate ganglion (remains below T1) or backward toward the intercostal nerve. The syringe is maintained in aspiration (under vacuum) for 5 seconds to ensure the absence of vascular puncture. At T2, 1 to 2 ml of absolute alcohol (2 to 3 ml for T3) are then slowly instilled, and a control CT scan is performed half way through the injection to verify the alcohol spread. (The hypodense alcohol that mixes with the contrast medium must, again, remain at a distance from the stellate ganglion). After each 0.5 ml of material is injected, the patient's homolateral pupil reflex must be checked with a torch (flashlight). In case of any weakness of the pupil reflex or of the diffusion approaching T1, the alcohol injection must be stopped.

Diffusion of alcohol to the cervicothoracic (stellate) ganglion must not occur to insure against Horner's syndrome. Ten percent of patients incur a nondisabling, delayed Horner's syndrome even in the best of circumstances [2]. This is why we use very small quantities of absolute alcohol, and then only for major indications such as particularly disabling distal ischemic arterial disease, frostbite, or neoplasm. Type I painful regional syndromes are treated by RF (heat destruction) of the stellate ganglion (see Chap. 10) [13, 17, 18]; and palmar hyperhidrosis is entrusted to surgery for a sympathectomy under video guidance. with good results [19–21].

Patients unwilling to run the risk of Horner's syndrome or surgery are treated by RF [17, 22, 30]. The very localized character of thermal ablation removes the risk of the Horner's complication [17, 18].

Radiofrequency

Needles used are 20 gauge RF, 100.5 mm single-use (Radionics). The electrode (known as "dry," with a highly restricted ablation volume) is inserted into the needle and hooked up to the radiofrequency generator (RF Radionics 3FG). A stimulation mode test is carried out, during which the patient should experience a posterior thoracic pain. No intercostal fasciculations should occur. The anesthetic (1% lidocaine, 1 ml) is injected at both targets, followed by 80° thermolysis for 90 seconds. The needle is inserted 2 mm further and a second thermolysis carried out. If the procedure is effective, the patient should experience heat in the upper limb in particular of the hand (which can be objectively confirmed by comparing with the temperature of the other hand).

A CT control scan (C7–T4) at the end of the procedure ensures the absence of complications (pneumothorax). In the case of alcoholization, the diffusion must spread from T2 (again, not beyond T1) to T3–T4, without significant posterior spread toward the intervertebral foramen. Apart from Horner's syndrome [1, 14], cervicothoracic pains, neuralgias (often transitory) [2, 14], and compensatory hyperhidrosis of another region (face, neck) can be encountered.

The procedure (alcoholization or RF) is carried out on an outpatient basis and the patient is kept under observation for one hour. Contralateral treatment (if justified) can be carried out around 2 weeks later.

Lumbar Sympatholysis

Bruno Kastler, Jean-Yves Cornu, Bernard Pergane

Indications

This procedure can be offered as an alternative to surgical sympathectomy in late stages of arteritis of the lower limbs, with excellent results [9]. Pain of the lower limb of sympathetic origin can also benefit as can type 1 and 2 chronic regional pain syndromes (of diverse origins) [10, 11].

Clinically Relevant Anatomy

The sympathetic lumbar chain is an extension of the sympathetic dorsal chain (see Fig. 12.3) [4]. It is made up of nervous filaments with ganglion relays located on either side of the vertebra of the anterolateral flank,

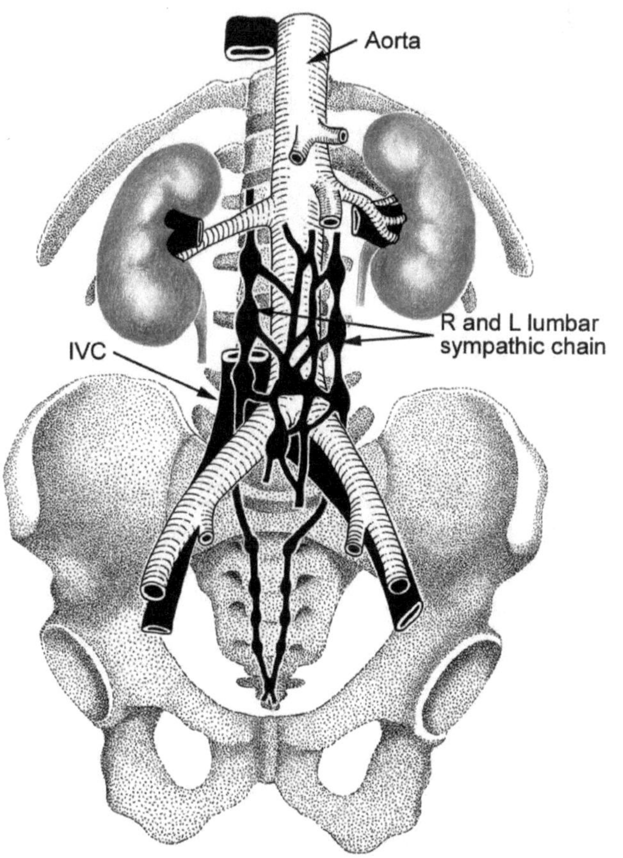

Fig. 12.3. Anatomical diagram of the lumbar sympathetic chain. The ganglion relays are located on either side of the vertebra of the anterolateral flank (much more anterior than the dorsal sympathetic chain), around the junction of the anterior and middle thirds of the vertebral body (see text for more explanations; drawing by Jean-Louis Vannson)

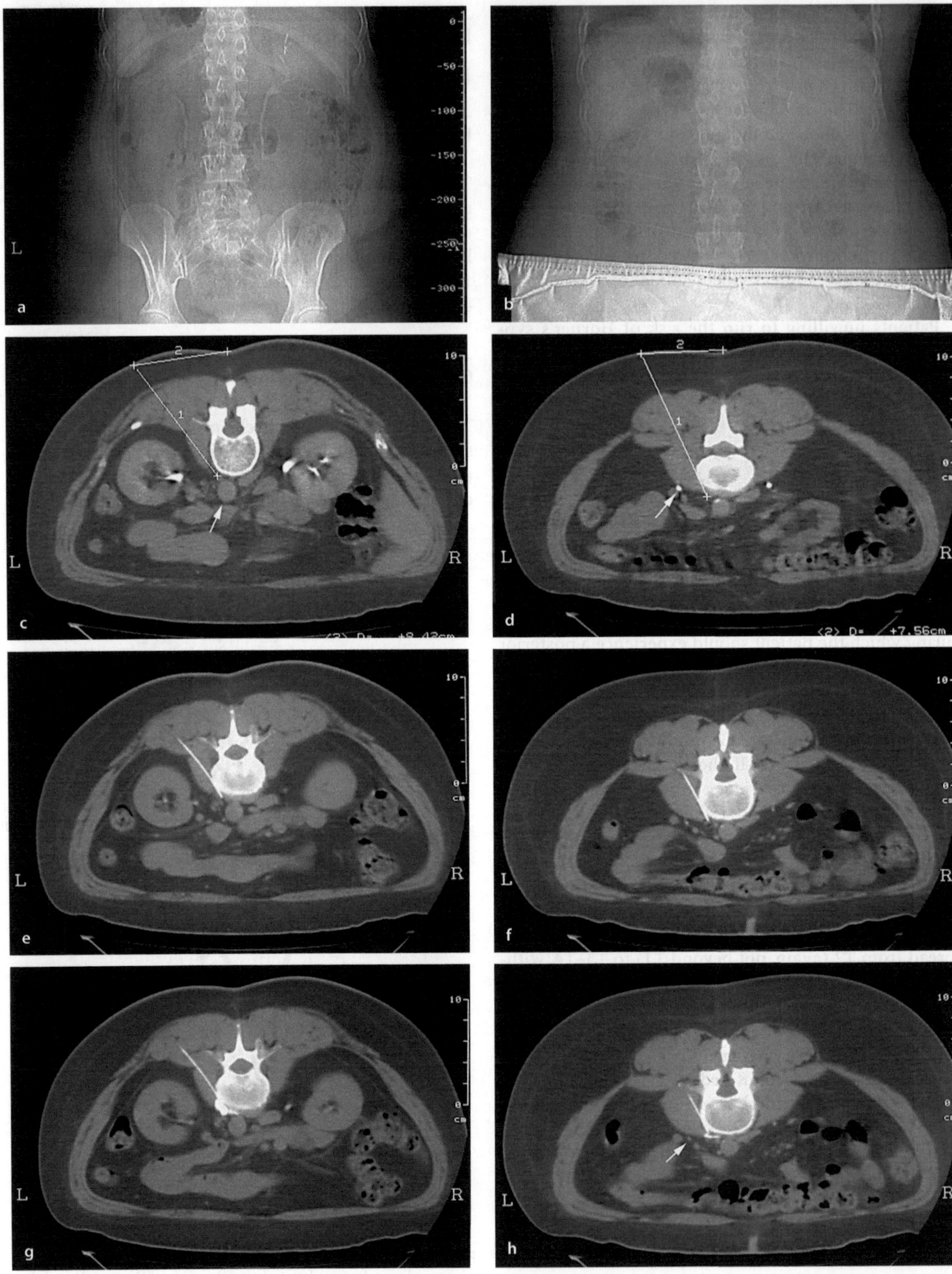

Fig. 12.4 a–h. Left lumbar sympatholysis Type 1 sympathetic reflex dystrophy following a fracture of the left ankle. **a** Scout view showing the injected ureter as it descends gradually getting closer to the spine, and thus to the targets. **b** The gonads are protected here by a lead apron. **c, d** Two targets, at L2 and L4, are selected; the lowest target must be far enough from the ureter (*arrow*) to avoid its damage. **e, f** Needles in position on both targets are in the psoas/vertebral body angle. **g, h** Diffusion of the anesthetic-contrast mixture (1 ml) which spreads locally at sufficient distance from the urethra at L4 (*arrow*); alcoholization can therefore take place (4 ml of absolute alcohol with a control scan halfway through injection). Also see Figs. 3.12, 3.14, and 3.18, Chap. 3

(much more anterior than the sympathetic dorsal chain, see above), approximately at the junction of the anterior third and the posterior two thirds of the vertebral body in the angle of the psoas muscle:

- On the right, behind the inferior vena cava
- On the left, behind and lateral to the aorta.

Technique

See (Fig. 12.4) and Figs. 3.12, 3.13, 3.18 of Chap. 3.

After verifying that the coagulation rates are normal (see Chap. 3), the patient is informed, preferably in a previous visit, about the procedure and the potential risks and is asked to give consent. An injection of 50 ml of contrast medium is intravenously administered beforehand to opacify the ureters. The patient is placed in a prone position and a lead apron applied to protect the gonads. Two axial joint slices of 7 to 10 mm thickness are carried out from L2 to L4. Two targets at L2 and L4 (or L3) are selected [8, 24–26, 31]. Two cutaneous entry points and trajectories are determined to ensure that the kidney, transverse process, vertebral body, and intervertebral disk are avoided. The two needles are inserted under CT guidance until their tips are located at the sympathetic chain.

Alcoholization

Twenty-two gauge (spinal) needles 15 to 17 cm long are used. One milliliter of analgesic mixed with contrast medium is injected into both points. A series of control slices monitor the diffusion of this mixture in order to ensure that it is not spreading toward the ureter or backward, in which case the needle is moved either backward or forward and a new diffusion control is performed after injecting a second ml of this mixture. Care must be taken as the needle is inserted to avoid the inferior vena cava to the right and the aorta to the left, and the needle should not be moved during the injection. A slight pull is maintained on the syringe for 5 seconds to ensure the against a vascular puncture (in particular of the peri-vertebral plexus; absence of contrast at the tip of the needle signifies such a puncture.) Four milliliters of absolute alcohol are then slowly instilled, and a control CT is performed at half injection at both sites to verify the alcohol spread. The hypodense alcohol mixed with the contrast medium must remain at a distance from the ureter. In the case of the slightest diffusion toward the ureter at L4, the alcohol injection must be stopped; this is also the case in the case of significant diffusion toward the rear (see chapter 14) at L1–L2 (origin of the inguinofemoral nerves), at L2–L3 (origin of the femoral and obturator nerves), or at L4-L5 (origin of the sciatic nerve). See Chap. 14, Fig. 14.1.

Radiofrequency

Twenty gauge RF, 150.5 mm single-use needles (Radionics) are used. The electrode is inserted into the needle and hooked up to the radiofrequency generator (RF Radionics 3FG). A stimulation mode test is carried out during which the patient should experience posterior lumbar pain. The anesthetic (1% lidocaine, 1 ml) is injected into both target points, followed by 80° thermolysis for 90 seconds. The needle is inserted 2 mm further and a second thermolysis carried out.

If the procedure is effective, the patient should experience heat in the lower limb, particularly in the foot (which can be made objective by comparing with the temperature of the other foot).

A CT control (around the target points) at the end of the procedure ensures the absence of complications (such as a small hematoma). In the case of alcoholization, the diffusion must spread vertically from L2 to L4. There must be no significant posterior diffusion of alcohol towards the intervertebral foramen or the ureter (for risk of ureteral necrosis see [14, 28]). Neuralgias, often transitory, of the inguinofemoral nerves, can be encountered in the case of posterior diffusion [3, 14]. Problems with erection and ejaculation appear to be more frequent when bilateral sympatholysis is carried out in a single session.

The procedure is carried out on an outpatient basis and the patient is kept under observation for one hour. Contralateral treatment (if justified) can be carried out around 2 weeks later.

Block and neurolysis of the Interiliac Sympathetic Plexus and the Ganglion Impar (Unpaired)

Bruno Kastler, Florence Tiberghien-Chatelain, Bernard Fergane

Indications

These techniques are generally recommended for pelvic pains caused by invasive of colorectal or gynecological cancer and by radiation rectitis. Chronic pain related to endometriosis can also benefit [5, 12, 29].

Coccygodynia can be treated by infiltration of anesthetics and corticoids in the pericoccygeal and completed by RF neurolysis of the unpaired ganglion (ganglion impar) [5, 12].

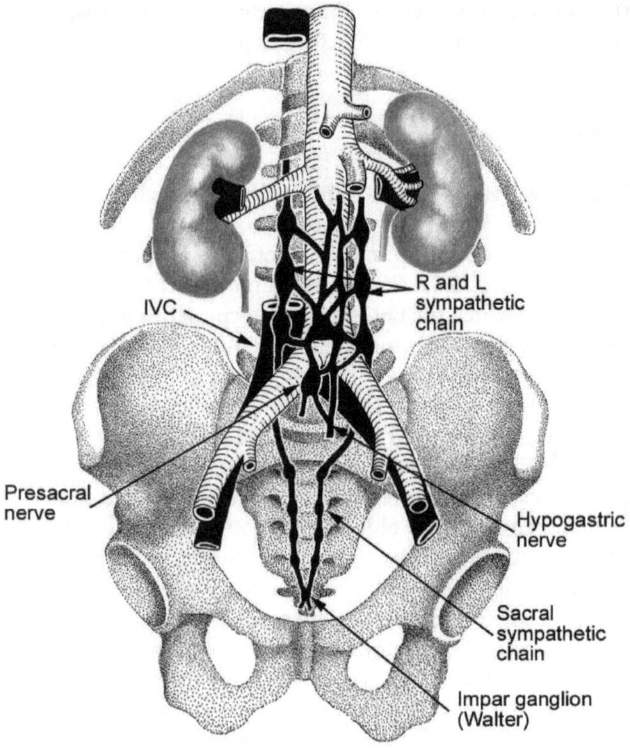

Fig. 12.5. Anatomical diagram of the interiliac plexus and ganglion impar. (Drawing by Jean-Louis Vannson)

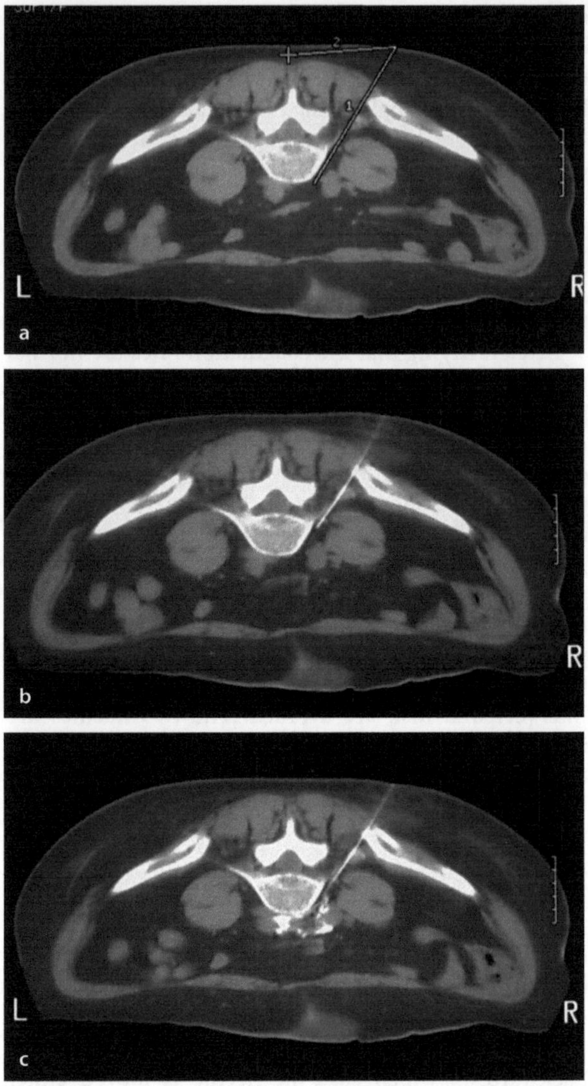

Fig. 12.6 a–c. Neurolysis of the interiliac plexus (presacral nerves). **a** Locating the trajectory, patient in prone position. **b** Progressive introduction of the needle behind the iliac vessels at the L5–S1 level. **c** Injection of hyperdense anesthetic/contrast mixture (5 ml) followed by a hypodense slow-release corticoid (ampule of cortivazol). Needle in position in frontal topogram

Clinically Relevant Anatomy

The interiliac plexus (corresponding to the presacral nerve) is located in an anterolateral position at L5–S1 below the aortic bifurcation between the common iliac arteries. It extends into the pelvis and divides into two streams that integrate with the hypogastric plexus (Fig. 12.5). Section of the presacral nerve causes hypoesthesia of the pelvic organs, vasomotor changes in women (menstrual disturbances), and ejaculatory problems in men.

The ganglion impar, also know as the Walther ganglion, amounts to an anastomosis of the caudal tip of the two laterovertebral chains. It is medially located at the anterior side of the coccyx.

Technique

After verifying that the patient's coagulation rates are normal (see Chap. 3), the patient is informed about the procedure and the potential risks and asked to give consent. In the case of the presacral nerve, a posterolateral approach is taken, the patient positioned in a prone position. The tip of a 22 gauge needle is positioned in front of L5–S1, behind the iliac vessels. An anesthetic block test (10 ml of a mixture of 1 ml contrast medium diluted with local anesthetic composed of 3 ml lidocaine and 6 ml ropivacaine) is administered, as is contrast medium to ascertain diffusion around the iliac vessels (Fig. 12.6), followed by an injection of delayed-release corticoid (cortivazol). If a more definitive neurolysis is recommended, 3 to 5 ml of absolute alcohol are injected slowly. Full neurolysis generally requires several sessions carried out at three-week intervals.

In the case of neurolysis of the ganglion impar, the approach is lateral and the tip of the needle is posi-

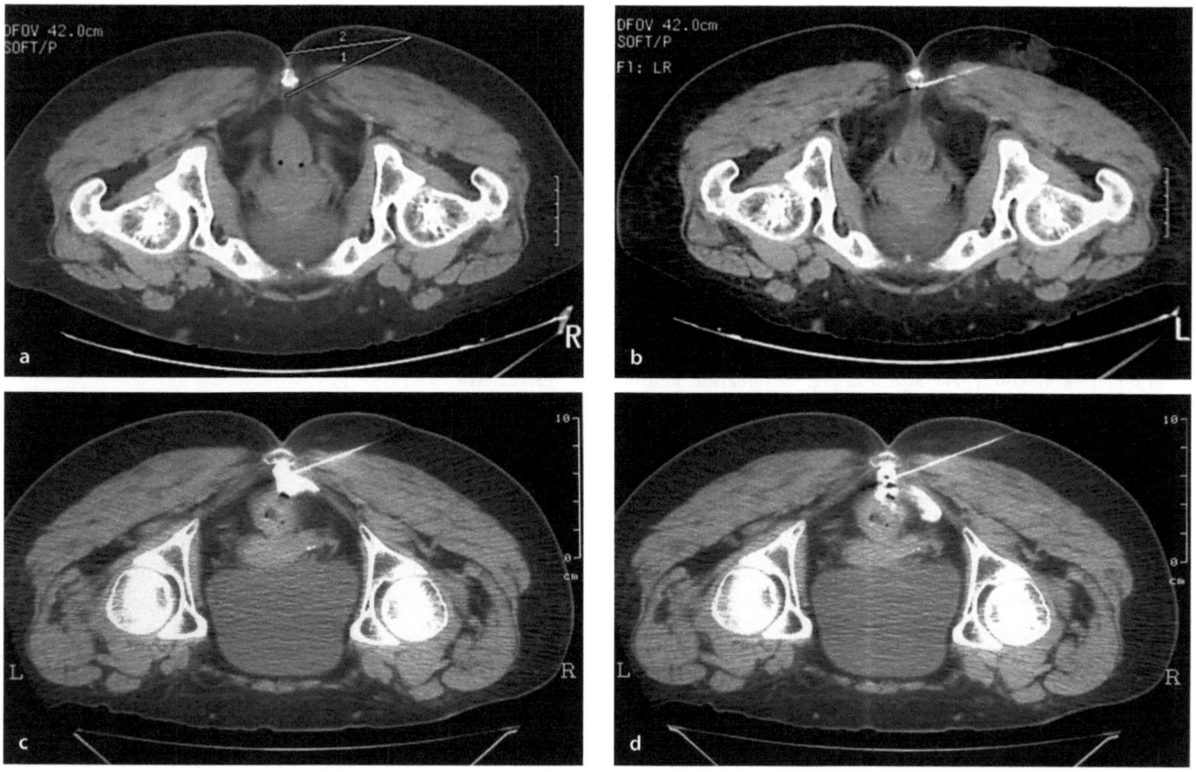

Fig. 7a–d. Neurolysis of ganglion impar (unpaired) of a patient suffering from acute coccygodynia. **a** Locating the trajectory. **b** Positioning the needle in front of the coccyx, anesthetic/contrast mixture block and slow-release corticoid injection (ampule of cortivazol). Pain relief for three weeks. **c** Second session injection of lidocaine and contrast. **d** Radiofrequency: formation of bubbles by heating; definitive pain relief

tioned in front and median to the coccyx, behind the rectum (Fig. 12.7). RF neurolysis can also be carried out at this site.

References

1. Adler OB, Engel A, Rosenbbhoer A. Dondelinger RF (1990) Palmar hyperhidrosis, CT guided chemical percutaneous thoracic sympathectomy. Rofo 153:400–403
2. Adler OB, Engel A, Sazoeno D (1994) Palmar hyperhidrosis treated by percutaneous transthoracic chemical sympathicolysis. Eur Radiol 4:57–62
3. Anand P (1986) Post-sympathectomy pain and sensory neuropeptides (letter). Lancet 1:512
4. Bonica JJ (1990) Neurolytic blockade. In: Bonica JJ (ed) The management of pain, vol 2. Lea and Febiger, Philadelphia, pp 2012–2035.
5. Clair C, Kastler B, Boulahdour Z et al (2002) Radiologie interventionnelle sous contrôle TDM dans le traitement de la douleur pelvienne. Séance thématique. Journées Françaises de Radiologie, Paris, 19–23 oct 2002
6. Dondelinger RF, Kurdziel JC (1986) Tomodensitométrie d'intervention. In: Vasile N (ed) Tomodensitométrie corps entier. Vigot, Paris, pp 603–604
7. Dondelinger RF, Kurdziel JC (1987) Percutaneous phenol block of the upper thoracic sympathetic chain with computed tomography guidance. A new technique. Acta Radiol 28:511–515
8. Dondelinger RF, Kurdziel JC (1984) Percutaneous phenol neurolysis of the lumbar sympathetic chain with computed tomography control. Ann Radiol (Paris) 27:376–379
9. Janneau D, Cormier JM (1980) La place de la sympathectomie lombaire dans le traitement des artérites diabétiques. J Mal Vascul 5:211–213
10. Janoff KA, Phinney ES, Porter JM (1985) Lumbar sympathectomy for lower extremity vasospasm. Am J Surg 150:147–152
11. Jebara VA, Saade B (1977) Causalgia: a thoracic endoscopic sympathectomy for treatment of upper limb hyperhidrosis. Lancet i:1320
12. Kastler B, Clair C, Boulahdour Z et al (2002) Traitement de la douleur pelvienne sous contrôle TDM. Séance thématique. Congrés National de la Douleur: Douleur et techniques interventionnelles. Lyon, Nov 2002
13. Kastler B, Clair C, Delabrousse E et al (2001) Neurolysis of stellate ganglion in sympathetically-maintained pain syndrome of the upper limb. Scientific paper. Radiological Society of North America, 87th scientific assembly and annual meeting, Chicago, 25–30 Nov 2001. Radiology [Suppl] 221:616
14. Kastler B, Clair C, Michalakis D et al (2002) Interventional procedures under CT guidance in 756 patients, incidents, side effects and how to reduce their incidence. Scientific Exhibit. Radiological Society of North America, 88th scientific assembly and annual meeting, Chicago, Nov 2002. Radiology [Suppl] 225:724
15. Kastler B, Couvreur M, Clair C et al (1999) Tomodensitométrie interventionnelle: suivez le guide. Feuillets Radiol 39:421–432
16. Kastler B, Gangi A, Allal R et al (1995) Optimizing interventional procedures under CT guidances: tips and hints. Scientific exhibit. Radiological Society of North America, 81st scientific assembly and annual meeting, Chicago, 26 Nov – 1 Dec 1995. Radiology [Suppl] 197:516

17. Kastler B, Michalakis D, Clair C et al (2001) Neurolyse du ganglion stellaire par radiofréquence sous guidage scanographique. Étude préliminaire. JBR-BTR 84:191–194
18. Kastler B, Narboux Y, Clair C et al (2001) Neurolyse par Radiofréquence du ganglion stellaire. À propos d'un cas traité et suivi sur trois ans. J Radiol 82:76–78
19. Kux M (1977) Thoracic endoscopic sympathectomy for treatment of upper limb hyperhidrosis. Lancet i:1320
20. Kux M (1978) Thoracic endoscopic sympathectomy for palmar and axillary hyperhidrosis. Arch Surg 113:264–266
21. Kux M, Fritsch A, Kokoschka R (1976) Endoscopic thoracic sympathectomy for the treatment of Raynaud's phenomenon and disease. Eur Surg Res 8:32–33
22. Malone PS, Duionan JP, Hederman WP (1982) Transthoracic electrocoagulation TIEC: a new and simple approach to upper limb sympathectomy. Ir Med J 75:20–21
23. Monnier G, Martin V, Parratte B (1998) L'évaluation neurophysiologique des troubles sensitifs dans le territoire des nerfs inguinofémoraux, in L'électrodiagnostic 1998: mises aux points. Conférences didactiques des 11e journées francophones d'électromyographie de Bordeaux, pp 49–53
24. Redman DR, Robinson PN, Al-Kutoubi MA (1986) Computerised tomography guided lumbar sympathectomy. Anaesthesia 41:39–41
25. Schield H, Gronniger J, Gunther R et al (1984) Transabdominelle CT-gesteurte Sympathektomie. Rofo 141:504–508
26. Schild H (1988) Percutane Neurolyse des lumbalen Sympathicus. In: Gunther RW, Thelen M (eds) Interventionelle Radiologie. Thieme, Stuttgart, pp 409–415
27. Soltesz L, Sandor GY (1957) Sympathicus-Operationsversuch zur Beeinflussung der Syringomyelic. Orv Hetil 98:740–744
28. Trigaux JP, Decoene B, van Beers B (1992) Focal necrosis of the ureter following CT-guided chemical sympathectomy. Cardiovascular Intervent Radiol 15:180–182
29. Wechsler RJ, Maurer PM, Halpern EJ, Frank ED (1996) Superior Hypogastric Plexus bloc for chronic pain in the presence of Endometriosis: CT technique and results. Radiology 105:103–105
30. Wilkinson HA (1984) Percutaneous radiofrequency upper thoracic sympathectomy: a new technique. Neurosurgery 15:811–814
31. Zagzag D, Fields S, Romanoff H et al (1986) Percutaneous chemical lumbar sympathectomy with alcohol with computed tomography control. Int Angiol 5:83–86

Pudendal Nerve Infiltration Under CT Guidance

Bruno Kastler, Christophe Clair,
Zakia Boulahdour, Julien Puget,
Marjolaine De Billy, Bernard Fergane

Introduction

Pudendal neuralgia is rare, very painful, and often disabling [2, 3, 6, 7, 9]. Infiltration has been found helpful in management, particularly during periods of acute pain. To perform the infiltration one must first have a good understanding of the anatomical relationship between the pudendal nerve and the surrounding structures to determine possible safe percutaneous pathways. We will here depict first the anatomy of the ischiorectal fossa correlated with CT on human cadavers correlated with CT cross-sectional imaging. We will then explain our technique of percutaneous infiltration of the pudendal nerve under step-by-step CT guidance at two potential sites of vulnerability on the nerve pathway.

Anatomical Background and Etiology

The pudendal nerve is formed from the fusion of the 2nd, 3rd, and 4th sacral nerves, which merge posterior to the ischial spine (Fig. 13.1). The nerve leaves the lesser pelvis over the sciatic notch, passing round the ischial spine under the sacrospinous ligament. After leaving the pelvis the nerve descends accompanied by vessels (pudendal nerve and artery) within the aponeurosis of the internal obturator muscle and the sacrotuberal ligament, forming an aponeurotic tunnel, the pudendal canal (also known as Alcock's canal) at the outer limit of the ischiorectal fossa. Branches of the perineal nerve innervate the perineum including the dorsalis nerve of the penis/clitoris, the inferior rectal nerves and the posterior scrotal/labial nerves. Anatomical studies suggest that there are two possible sites of constriction along the course of the pudendal nerve [10]. The first one is located at the ischial spine where the nerve can be entrapped between the sacrospinous and sacrotuberal ligaments (Fig. 13.2); the second is in the pudendal canal, a nonstretchable aponeurotic tunnel (Fig. 13.3). Neuralgia of the pudendal nerve usually results from its entrapment in the canal, or one of its branches near the sacrospinous ligament can become a source of pain.

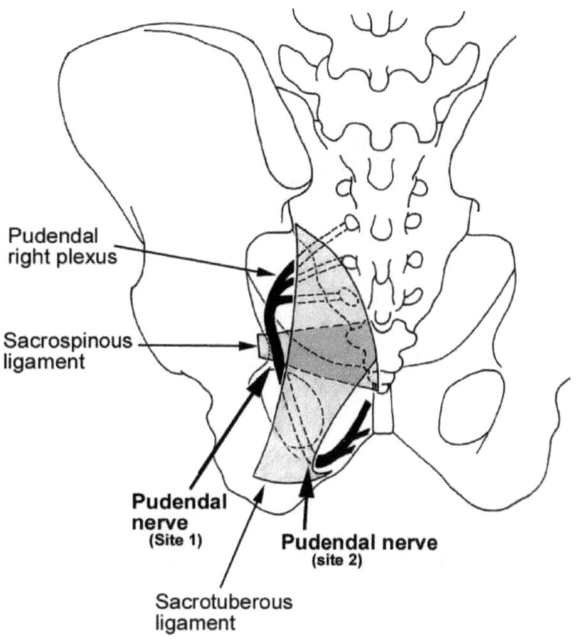

Fig. 13.1. Posterior view of pelvis .The pudendal nerve is formed from the fusion of the 2nd, 3rd, and 4th sacral nerves, which merge posterior to the ischial spine. Note the sacrospinous ligament and the sacrotuberal ligament. The two sites of possible entrapment of the nerve: (*1*) at the level of ischial spine; (*2*) at the level of pudendal canal

Bilateral pudendal neuralgia is extremely rare. It can be caused by trauma to the perineum, such as bicycling or horseback riding, or following a fall astraddle a large sharp object. Early descriptions can be found in references [2–6]. Unilateral pudendal neuralgia can have these same causes, and also can result from trauma that fractures the ischial spine (which lies just anterior to the origin of the pudendal nerve), or from perineal surgery, which can cause both direct pudendal nerve injury and traumatic scars. Additionally, a possible mechanism of entrapment of the nerve in Alcock's canal by a fibrotic process such as occurs in the carpal tunnel has been suggested.

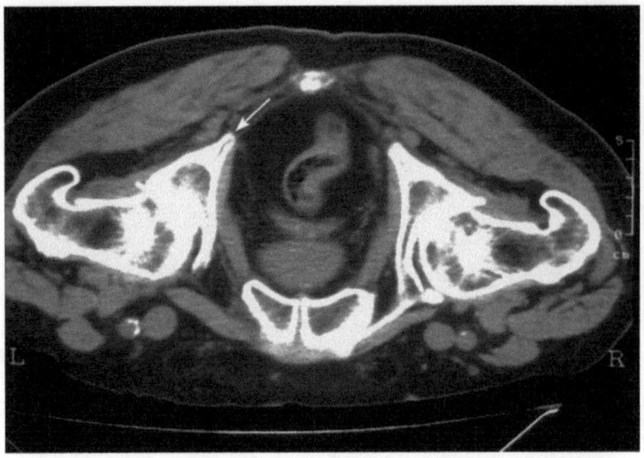

Fig. 13.2. Axial CT at the level of the ischial spines. Possible entrapment of pudendal nerve between the sacrospinous and sacrotuberal ligaments (first site; *arrow*)

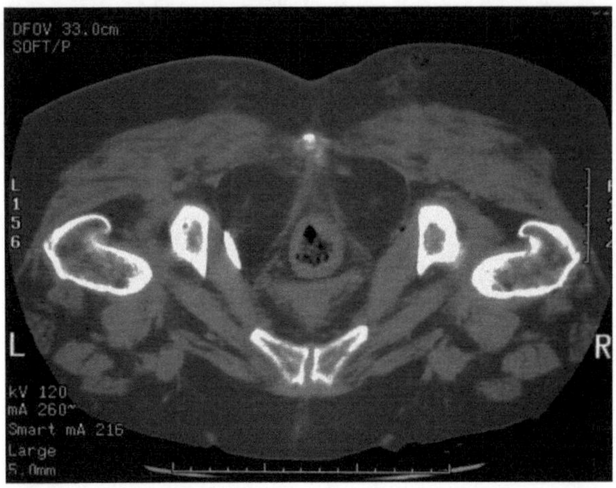

Fig. 13.3. Axial CT at the level of the ischiorectal fossa. Possible entrapment of pudendal nerve in Alcock's canal within the aponeurosis of the internal obturator muscle (second site where the hyperdense mixture diffuses)

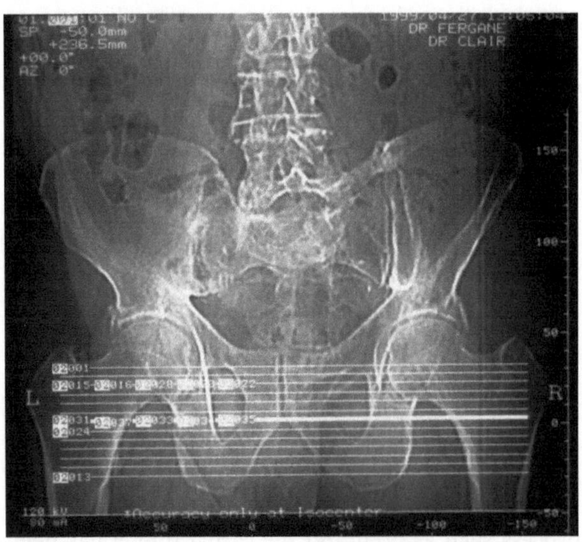

Fig. 13.4. Scout view with slices centered on the obturator foramen

Symptoms and Signs

Pudendal neuralgia, rare but sometimes disabling, is characterized [2, 3, 6, 7, 9] by chronic severe and spontaneous pain. This has been characterized as a persistent mild to severe burning pain with occasional bouts of lancinating pain; in addition, cutaneous hyperalgesia, hypalgesia, deep tenderness, paresthesia, tingling, and subjective numbness have been described. Topographically the pain may follow the course of the nerve, but it can also radiate to the entire pelvis or be circumscribed to the genitals or anus. Pain is usually exacerbated by sitting and relieved if the patient is standing or walking. It can prevent the patient from engaging in sexual intercourse.

Diagnosis

Diagnosis is made on the basis of the history and physical examination and relies on electrophysiological investigations which should demonstrate unilateral patterns and/or an increase in the distal latency of the pudendal nerve in the stimulus-detection mode [1]. Diagnosis is confirmed by a block test with injection of local anesthetic.

Infiltration Technique

References [4, 5, 8] may be consulted.

- The patient must have normal clotting values, be informed about the procedure, and give consent as required by law.
- The patient is placed in a prone position on the CT table.
- Axial adjoining CT slices of 5 mm thickness are obtained on the projection of the obturator foramen (see scout view Fig. 13.4).
- There are two targets: the first is the ischial spine, easy to visualize (Fig. 13.5); the second is in Alcock's canal (Fig. 13.6). At this second level the pudendal nerve and the accompanying vessels are seen as a small bulge or linear structure within a split in the aponeurosis of the internal obturator muscle (Alcock's canal; Fig. 13.6).
- The optimal entry points are determined and marked on the skin with a felt tip pen (vertically above the nerve) on one or both sides at the two different sites, choosing a roughly vertical course while avoiding the proximal pudendal vessels and the sciatic nerve.
- The patient is draped in a sterile fashion, the skin scrubbed, and sterilized, and local anesthesia is instilled at the entry points.

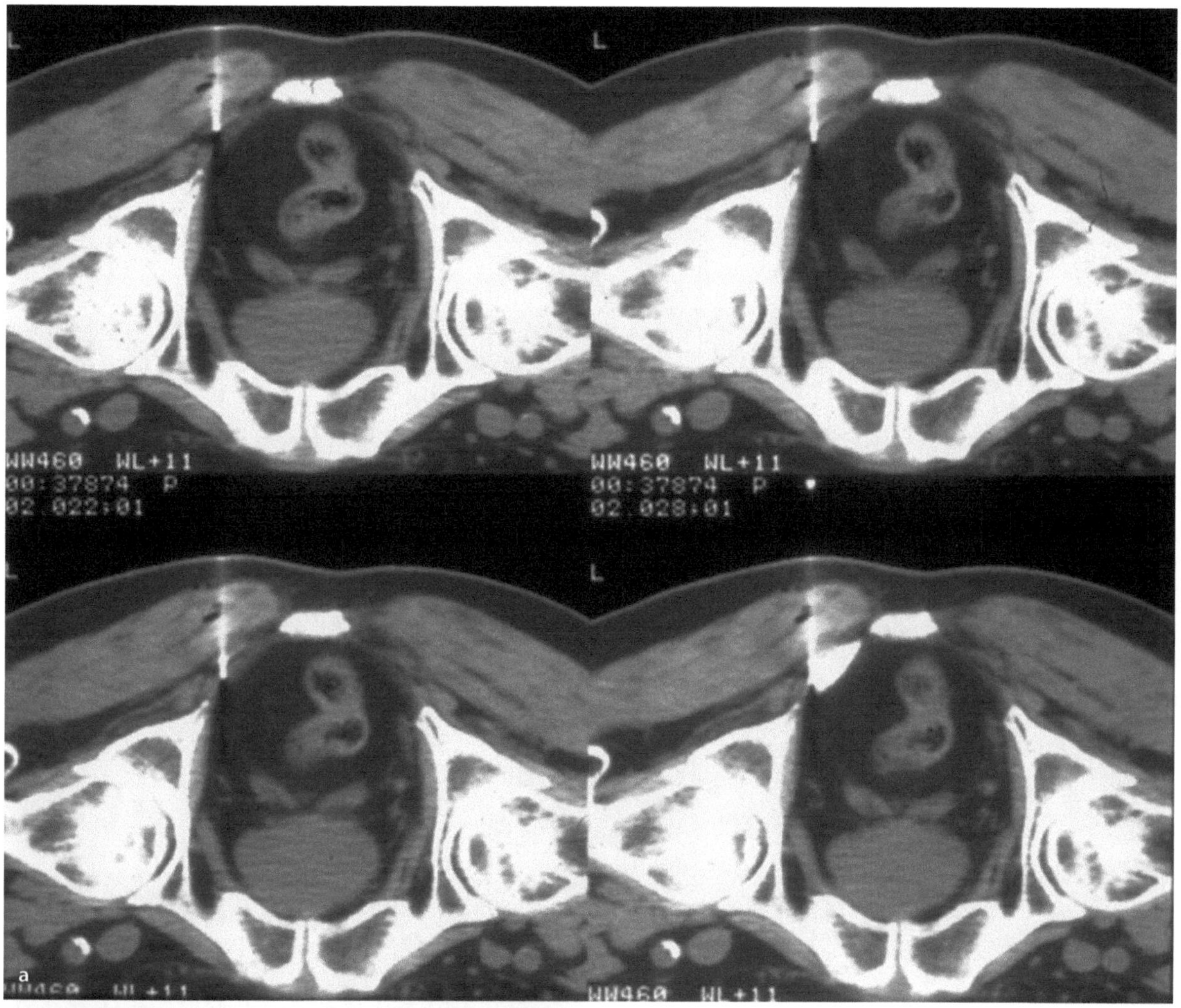

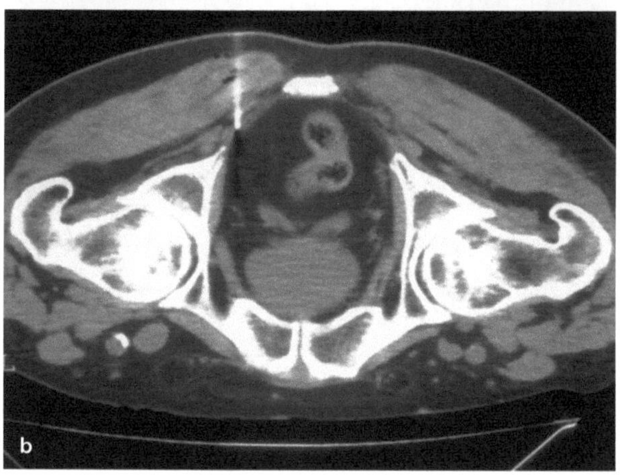

Fig. 13.5 a, b. Needle tip progressing on the right to the ischial spine between the sacrospinous and sacrotuberal ligaments (first site)

- The correct skin-to-target orientation should be determined as either parallel or at a slight angle to that of the anesthetic needle as left in place (see Chap. 3).
- Each needle is slowly and carefully advanced through the gluteal muscle under step-by-step CT guidance until the needle tip is abutting the nerve (Figs. 13.5 and 13.6). The needles used are disposable 22 gauge, 9 or 12.70 cm spin needles (BD).
- The correct position is determined by carefully moving the needle tip at the target (which may sometimes

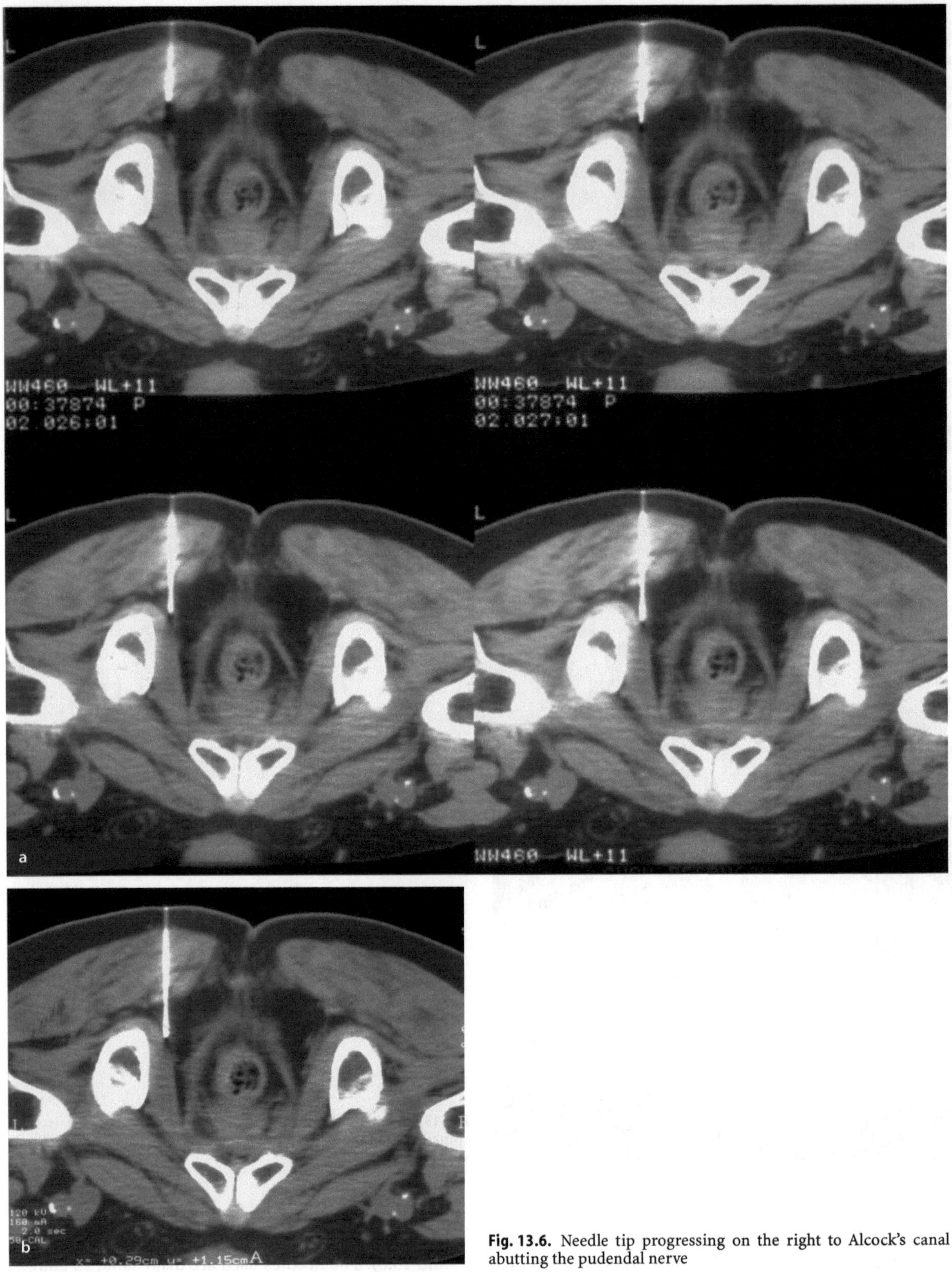

Fig. 13.6. Needle tip progressing on the right to Alcock's canal abutting the pudendal nerve

cause exacerbation of pain), followed by injection of a mixture of lidocaine 1 cc, bupivacaine 3 cc, and 10% contrast at the first site (ischial spine) and half this dose at the second site (pudendal canal). Aspiration is performed before injection to avoid accidental intravascular injection.

- Following the anesthetic block test (the patient should note a decrease in pain), the infiltration is performed with 1 ml of slow-release glucocorticoid (cortivazol 3.75 mg), which should be slowly instilled at both levels (four sites if bilateral); dose per site is 1/2 ml. After infiltration, the solution can be seen within the pudendal canal along the obturator internus muscle and within the adjacent ischiorectal fat.

Results

The patient can be discharged after one hour. He/she is seen again after a few days and if there is a pain relief the procedure can be repeated twice at 4 to 8 week intervals. Our results using one site of injection (in the pudendal canal) were 30–40% of satisfactory, comparable to others using infiltration or a surgical procedure [6]. After adding infiltration at the level of ischial spine, our good results have risen to 70 to 80% if patients present typical symptoms (with a mean sedation duration of 3 months) [8]; we thus now advocate an infiltration at both sites. Some authors have suggested that good evidence of the efficacy of surgery would be complete disappearance of pain for at least 2 weeks after the second of two infiltrations has been administered (a few weeks after the first) [11].

We believe that CT guidance allows safe needle progression and precise positioning at both targets, reducing complications and optimizing results.

References

1. Amarenco G, Ghnassia RT, Chabassol E et al (1986) Intérêt des potentiels évoqués sacrés dans l'étude des troubles vésicosphinctériens des neuropathies périphériques et des affections du système nerveux central. Étude de 110 cas. Ann Med Intern 137:331–337
2. Amarenco G, Ghnassia RT, Goudal H et al (1987) Un nouveau syndrome canalaire: la compression du nerf honteux interne dans le canal d'Alcock, ou paralysie périnéale du cycliste. Presse Med (Paris) 16:399
3. Amarenco G, Lanoe Y, Ghnassia RT et al (1988) Syndrome du canal d'Alcock et névralgies périnéales. Rev Neurol 144: 523–526
4. Clair C, Boulahdour Z, Delabrousse E et al (2001) Pudendal nerve infiltration under CT guidance: an anatomical and radiological study for aiming at two conflicting sites. Radiological Society of North America, 87th scientific assembly and annual meeting, Chicago, 25–30 Nov 2001. Radiology [Suppl] 221:692
5. Corréas JM, Belin X, Amarenco G, Budet C (1990) Infiltration scano-guidée dans le syndrome du canal d'Alcock chronique. Rev Im Med 2:547–549
6. Duhamel J, Garrigues JM, Romand-Heuyer Y et al (1982) Algies anorectales essentielles formes atypiques. Semin Hop Paris 58:392–396
7. Goodson JD (1981) Pudendal neuritis from biking (letter). N Engl J Med 304:6, 365
8. Kastler B, Clair C, de Billy M et al (1998) Pudendal nerve infiltration under CT guidance. Radiological Society of North America, 84th scientific assembly and annual meeting, Chicago, 29 Nov - 4 Dec 1998. Radiology [Suppl] 209:594
9. Robert R, Prat-Pradal D, Labat JJ et al (1998) Anatomic basis of chronic perineal pain. Role of the pudendal nerve. Surg Radiol Anat 20:93–98
10. Pradel E, Rodier B, Mot JCL (1988) Les algies anorectales chroniques. Concours Méd 111:2395–2398
11. Thoumas D, Mauillon J, Leroi AM et al Preoperative infiltration of pudendal nerve/usefulness to predict efficacy of surgical decompression. Scientific exhibit, 6th European symposium on uroradiology. Strasbourg, France, 12–16 Sept

Injection of Inguinofemoral Nerves

14

Bruno Kastler, Guy Monnier, Bernard Fergane

Introduction

Although certain inguinofemoral neuropathies are easy to identify clinically, e.g. Bernhardt and Roth's classic meralgia paresthetica involving the lateral femoral cutaneous nerve, the vast majority are difficult to diagnose, especially at the inner root of the thigh. This is due to the complexity of several nerve territories, with their possible overlapping and wide variability in anatomical distribution. In these cases, exploration by means of somesthetic evoked potentials is of some value for diagnosis [7] and the selection of an injection site, although the long-term results of infiltrative treatment remain uncertain.

We shall firstly endeavor to describe schematically the normal distribution of the nerve trunks involved, with a view to determining the territories concerned [7]. We shall consider the sensory areas from the outer to the inner aspect of the thigh. The distribution at the lateral surface of the thigh is relatively well defined, essentially deriving from the lateral femoral cutaneous nerve (3CL in Fig. 14.1 and Fig. 14.2), together with a small area in the proximal part deriving from the lateral cutaneous ramus of the iliohypogastric nerve (1CL, Fig. 14.2), which is to be considered when we study this nerve.

The distribution at the root of the thigh, at its anterior aspect and especially at its medial aspect (the inguinal region and the scrotum) is less clearly defined because of the overlapping. In terms of the genital branches, it is particularly fortunate that a neuropathic conditions associated with two or three nerves can be treated at a single injection site. The injection sites will be noted once the anatomy of the inguinofemoral nerves has been described. More information on the distribution of the sensory territories of the inguinofemoral nerves is given in reference [7].

From among the many possible iatrogenic causes of transitory inguinofemoral neuropathies, we have reported three cases, two of which were associated with celiac neurolysis and one with lumbar sympatholysis (all subsequent to excessive diffusion of alcohol; see Chapters 11 and 12) [3].

Lateral Femoral Cutaneous Nerve

Relevant Anatomy

This nerve arises mostly from the L2 root and partly from the L3 root of the lumbar spinal nerves (3CL in Fig. 14.1) [7, 8]. It emerges on the lateral margin of the psoas muscle and crosses the iliac muscle obliquely, reaching the anterosuperior iliac spine (ASIS) and passing under or through the inguinal ligament, which extends from the ASIS to the pubis (Fig. 14.1). It may produce a gluteal ramus before crossing the parietal aponeurosis of the fascia transversalis (3F, Fig. 14.2). It typically then divides in front of the sartorius muscle into an anterior branch (3A, Fig. 14.2), innervating the skin of the anterolateral region of the thigh as far as the knee, and a posterior branch (3P, Fig. 14.2), giving rise to nerve filaments in the lateral region of the major trochanter (Fig. 14.3).

Clinical Characteristics

Refer to references [1, 3]. At the inguinal ligament the lateral femoral cutaneous nerve exhibits its maximum angulation, with risk of damage. This point is approximately 1.5 cm from the ASIS on a line between it and the pubic tubercle (1.58 ± 0.87 cm) [8]. Meralgia paresthetica is idiopathic in 50% of cases. It manifests as pain (paresthesia, dysesthesia, burning sensation) in the territory of this nerve in the lateral aspect of the thigh, exacerbated by a standing position and sometimes occurring on compression of the nerve in the vicinity of the inguinal ligament. Obesity, pregnancy, chronic stretching (excessively tight belt or clothing) or iatrogenic stretching (on scar following inguinal herniorrhaphy, cholecystectomy, hysterectomy, iliac graft removal, etc.) have been reported as factors in causation.

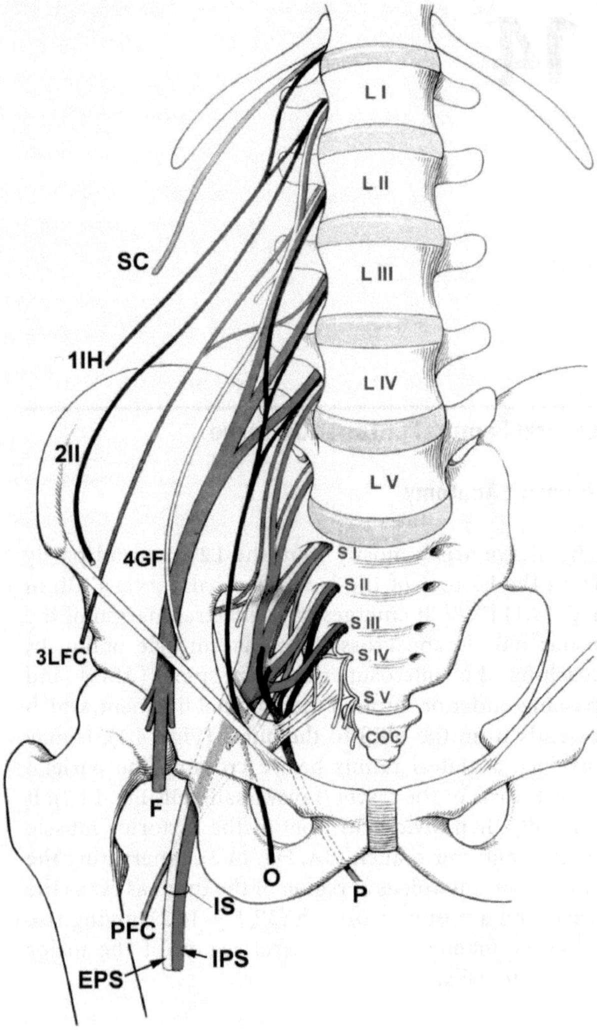

Fig. 14.1. Anatomical diagram of lumbar plexus (Jean-Louis Vannson). 12th subcostal nerve (formerly intercostal nerve; *SC*), iliohypogastric nerve (*1IH*; origin root L1), ilioinguinal nerve (*2Il*; origin root L1), genitofemoral nerve (*4GF*; origin root L2, anastomosis possible with L1), lateral femoral cutaneous nerve (*3CL*; origin roots L2 and L3), femoral nerve (*F*; origin roots L2, L3, and L4), posterior femoral cutaneous nerve (*CPC*), ischial nerve (formerly sciatic nerve; *IS*; origin roots L4, L5, S1–S3), fibular nerve (*Spe*, formerly external popliteal sciatic nerve), tibial nerve (*Spi*, formerly internal popliteal sciatic nerve), obturator nerve (*O*; origin roots L2, L3, and L4), pudendal nerve (*P*; origin roots S1–S3)

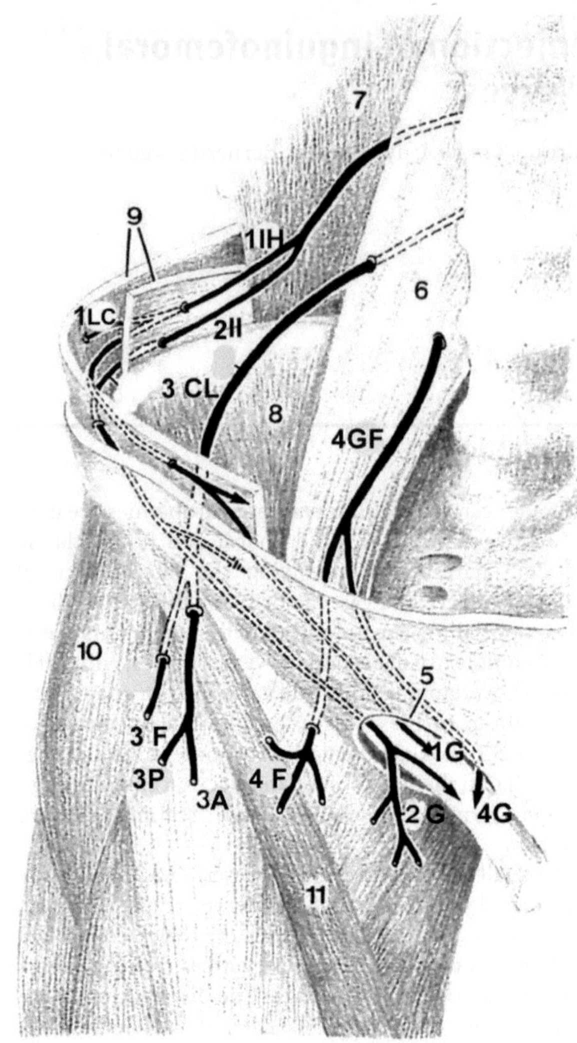

Fig. 14.2. Anatomical diagram of deep distribution of inguinofemoral nerves. Iliohypogastric nerve (*1IH*), lateral cutaneous branch (*1CL*), genital branch (*1G*); ilioinguinal nerve (*2II*), genital branch (*2G*); lateral femoral cutaneous nerve (*3CL*), gluteal branch (*3F*), anterior (*A*) and posterior (*P*) terminal branches; genitofemoral nerve (*4GF*), femoral branch (*4F*), genital branch (*4G*); superficial orifice of inguinal canal (*5*); psoas muscle (*6*); quadratus lumborum muscle (*7*); iliac muscle (*8*); external transverse (the deeper) and oblique abdominal muscles (*9*); tensor fascia lata muscle (*10*); sartorius muscle (*11*)

Technique

See references [1, 3]. Injection treatment is given in addition to specific medication. An anterior approach is used with the patient supine. Contiguous axial sections 3 to 5 mm thick are made around the ASIS; it is necessary (especially in young patients) to protect the gonads from irradiation with a lead apron. The tip of the 22 gauge needle is placed approximately 1.5 cm inside the ASIS on a line between it and the pubic tubercle. An anesthetic block test (5 ml of 1/3 lidocaine and 2/3 ropivacaine)) is conducted in conjunction with the use of a contrast medium (10%) in order to assess diffusion between the vessels (see Fig. 14.4). After aspiration is performed to avoid intravascular injection, this is followed by a delayed-release corticosteroid injection. Neurolysis by RF may also be performed at this point after ensuring that the needle is correctly positioned in the stimulation mode.

If there is radiation of pain (arising in the lumbar region, and exacerbated by an erect posture, in either

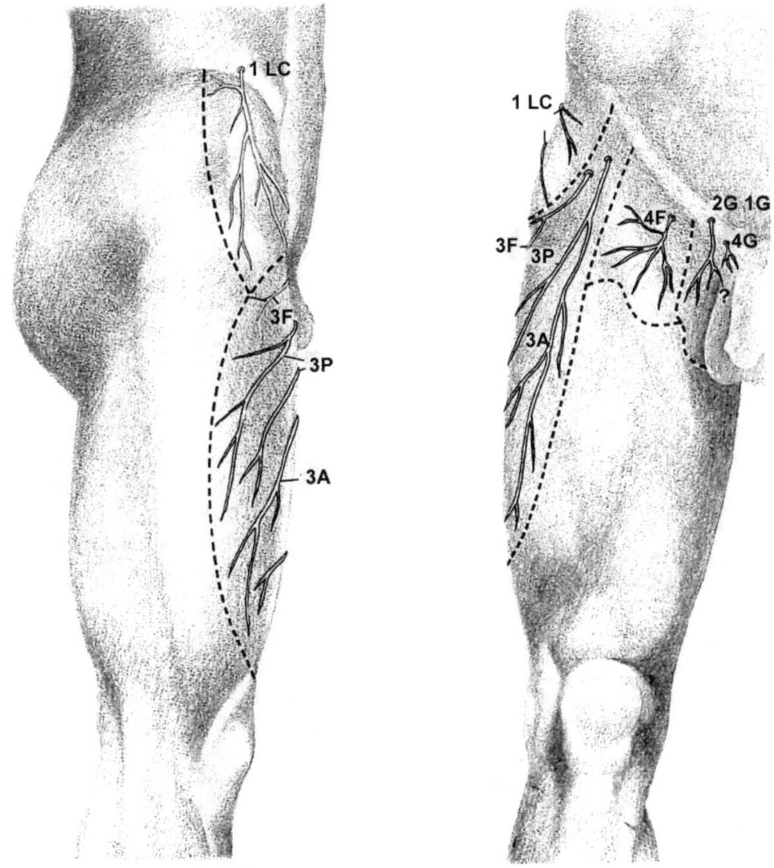

Fig. 14.3. Diagram of distribution and superficial sensory innervation territories of the inguinofemoral nerves. Iliohypogastric nerve (*1IH*, see Figs. 14.1 and 14.2); lateral cutaneous (*1CL*) and genital (*1G*) branches of the iliohypogastric nerve; genital branch (*2G*) of the ilioinguinal nerve; gluteal (*3F*), anterior (*3A*), and posterior terminal (*3P*) branches of the lateral femoral cutaneous nerve; femoral (*4F*) and genital (*4G*) branches of the genitofemoral nerve

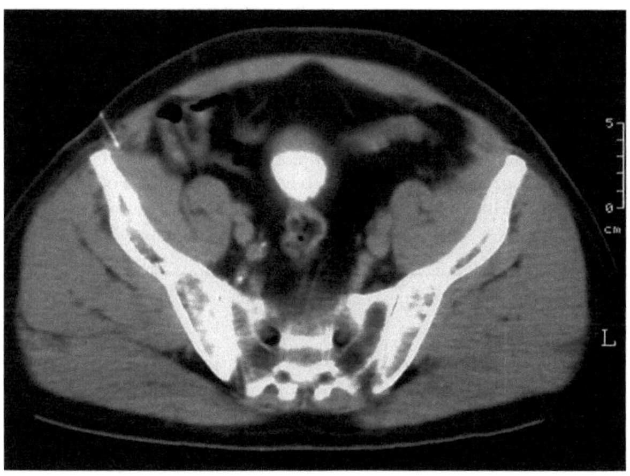

Fig. 14.4. Infiltration of lateral femoral cutaneous nerve; placement of needle where the problem originates in the inguinal ligament, inside and below the ASIS

direction along the nerve path), a supplementary injection to the near the roots of L2 (and/or L3) may be indicated. In this event the patient is placed in a lateral reclining position so that the injection can be given at both anterior and posterior sites.

Genitofemoral Nerve

Relevant Anatomy

This nerve arises from root L2, possibly anastomosing with that of L1 (see 4GF, Fig. 14.1), penetrates the psoas muscle and emerges from it at the level of disc L3–L4 (see Fig. 14.2) [7]. It passes obliquely in front of this muscle, where it is visible beneath its sheath. It then usually divides into two branches:

- A femoral branch (4F, Fig. 14.2) that follows the external iliac artery to the external part of the femoral ring and emerges in Scarpa's triangle in front of the femoral artery; after 2 to 3 cm it enters the cribriform fascia and innervates the anterior and superior region of the thigh (Fig. 14.3)
- A genital branch (4G, Fig. 14.2; external pudendal nerve) that a short way beyond its origin enters the deep inguinal ring and follows the inguinal canal on the inside of and behind the funiculus. In the inguinal canal it gives rise to a motor branch (responsible for the cremasteric reflex) and terminal fibers intended for the skin of the scrotum or labia majora.

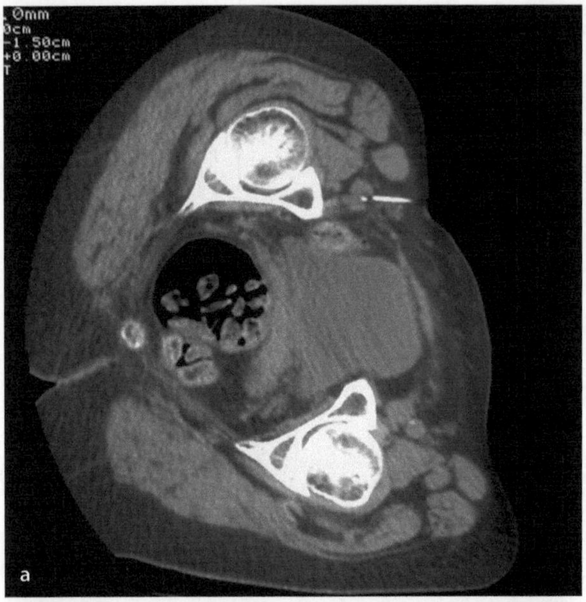

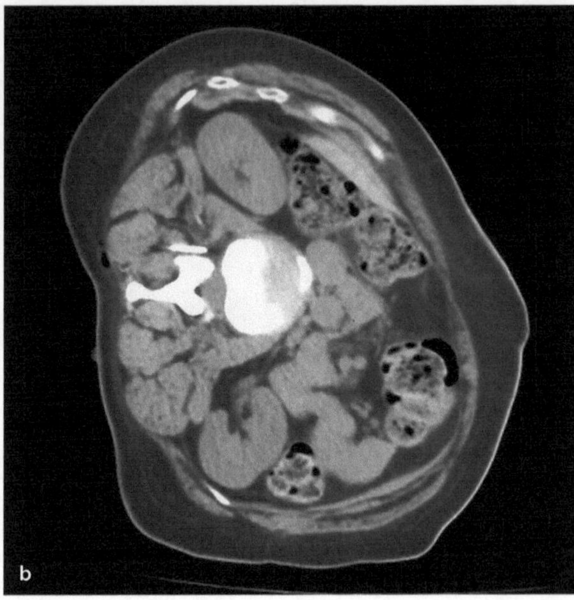

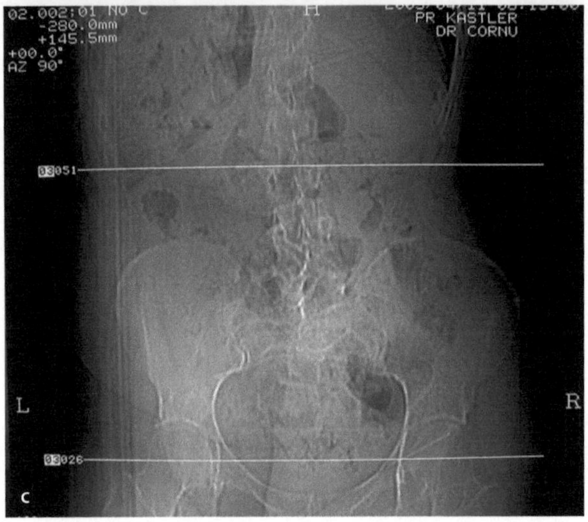

Fig. 14.5 a–c. Infiltration of genitofemoral nerve in a patient aged 53 years. **a** Placement of needle at the first site (femoral branch) in front of the femoral artery. **b** This patient had pronounced lumbar radiation and was also given an injection at the origin of the nerve at L2. **c** Topogram showing the two levels of incision. For injection of the genital branch, see technique Fig.14.6c

Clinical Characteristics

Please see references [1, 2, 7]. If the genitofemoral nerve is affected, pain occurs in nerve areas anterior and superior region of the thigh for the femoral branch, and in the inguinal region and scrotum or labia majora for the genital branch). The pain is caused by compression (e.g., clothes too tight, cycling) or may be of iatrogenic origin (e.g., appendectomy scar), and also occasionally occurs if the lumbar region of the spinal column is affected ("testicular" radiation of some lumbar radicular pains is a familiar phenomenon). In addition to pain in the specific area, examination may show loss of the cremasteric reflex. Nevertheless, it is difficult or even impossible to clearly distinguish effects involving the genitofemoral nerve from those of the ilioinguinal and iliohypogastric nerves.

Technique

Please see references [1, 2]. The injection is given in addition to specific medication. An anterior approach is used with the patient supine. Contiguous axial sections, 3 to 5 mm thick, are made at the level of the inguinal ligament; protection of the gonads from irradiation is to be afforded. For the femoral branch, the tip of the 22 gauge needle is placed in front of the femoral artery; for the genital branch it is placed in the inguinal canal. An anesthetic block test of 5 ml of 1/3 lidocaine and 2/3 ropivacaine at the femoral level and 3 ml in the inguinal canal (Fig. 14.5 c is given by slow instillation in conjunction with a contrast medium (10%) in order to assess diffusion in the funiculus (see Fig. 14.5). After aspiration to avoid introduction intravascularly, this is followed by injection of a delayed-release corticosteroid.

Neurolysis by RF may also be performed at the femoral level after ensuring that the needle is correctly positioned in the stimulation mode.

If there is radiation of pain (arising in the lumbar region, and exacerbated by an erect posture, in either direction along the nerve path), a supplementary injection may be indicated near the L2 root, the patient being placed in a lateral reclining position so that the injection can be given at both anterior and posterior sites (see Fig. 14.5a and b).

Iliohypogastric Nerve

Relevant Anatomy

This nerve, 1IH on Figs. 14.1 and 14.2, arises from the L1 root, descends behind the posterior parietal peritoneum on the quadratus lumborum muscle and, 3–4 cm from its external margin, perforates the transverse muscle of the abdomen, passes between the transverse (on the inside) and lesser oblique (on the outside) muscles and inside the ASIS (see Fig. 14.6b). At about this position it divides to produce an abdominal branch that penetrates the lesser oblique muscle and courses to the pubic insertion of the of the lower anterior abdominal wall muscles, and a genital branch (1G, Fig. 14.2) that accompanies the genital branch (2G) of the ilioinguinal nerve (2II) [7]. The two genital branches (1G and 2G) pass along the inguinal canal to become subcutaneous at the level of the superficial orifice and be distributed (see Fig. 14.4) to the inguinal region, the pubis, the anterior surface of the scrotum/labia majora, and the median part of the upper reaches of the thigh. In 18% of individuals the two latter zones arise from the genitofemoral nerve.

In the proximal lateral part of the lower limb the lateral cutaneous branch of the 1IH (1CL, Fig. 14.2) is involved. This wholly sensory branch [4, 6], arising immediately before the transverse abdominal muscle is crossed, only becomes superficial in the immediate proximity of the crest either via a purely aponeurotic orifice 5 to 10 mm above the bony edge or via a groove in the iliac crest. This ramus then ends a few centimeters below the iliac crest, innervating a variable sensory territory either close thereto, or extending as far as 10 cm beyond the major trochanter.

Clinical Characteristics

If the iliohypogastric nerve is affected, pain occurs in its territory, i.e., the anterosuperior or laterosuperior gluteal region of the thigh (lateral cutaneous branch), and pubic region, inguinal region, and labia majora/scrotum (genital branch) [1, 3]. From the etiological standpoint there may be compression phenomena (clothing too tight, especially regarding the lateral cutaneous branch), compression or invasion by iliac metastasis (see Chap. 17, Fig. 17.2), or iatrogenic factors (e.g., inguinal hernia repair) Other causes, compressive or otherwise, may be obesity, pregnancy, and injury at the lumbar level of the spinal column. The pain is often triggered by standing erect, by coughing, or by otherwise subjecting the trunk to tension. Apart from the specific painful area, examination may show that a weakness in the muscles of the abdominal wall is exacerbated in the standing position. In any event, it is difficult to clearly distinguish between an effect on the iliohypogastric nerve from one on the genitofemoral nerve or the ilioinguinal nerve (especially if the lateral cutaneous branch of the 1CL is unaffected).

Technique

Again please refer to references [1 and 2]. This technique is used in addition to specific medication. An anterior approach is used with the patient supine. Contiguous axial sections, 3 to 5 mm thick, are made at the level of the inguinal ligament. Protection for the gonads, especially for the young, is supplied. At the first site the tip of the 22 gauge needle is placed in front of and on the inside of the ASIS between the transverse muscle of the abdomen and the lesser oblique muscle; and for the genital branch it is placed in the inguinal canal (Fig. 14.6). An anesthetic block test (5 ml 1/3 lidocaine and 2/3 ropivacaine at the ASIS and 3 ml in the inguinal canal by slow instillation) is performed in association with a contrast medium (10%) in order to assess diffusion in the funiculus (see Fig. 14.6c). After aspiration to avoid intravascular injection, delayed-release corticosteroid is introduced. Neurolysis by RF may also be performed at the ASIS level after ensuring that the needle is correctly positioned in the stimulation mode.

If there is radiation of pain (arising in the lumbar region, and exacerbated by an erect posture, in either direction along the nerve path), a supplementary injection may be indicated near the L1 root. For this the patient is placed in a lateral reclining position so that he injection can be given at both anterior and posterior sites.

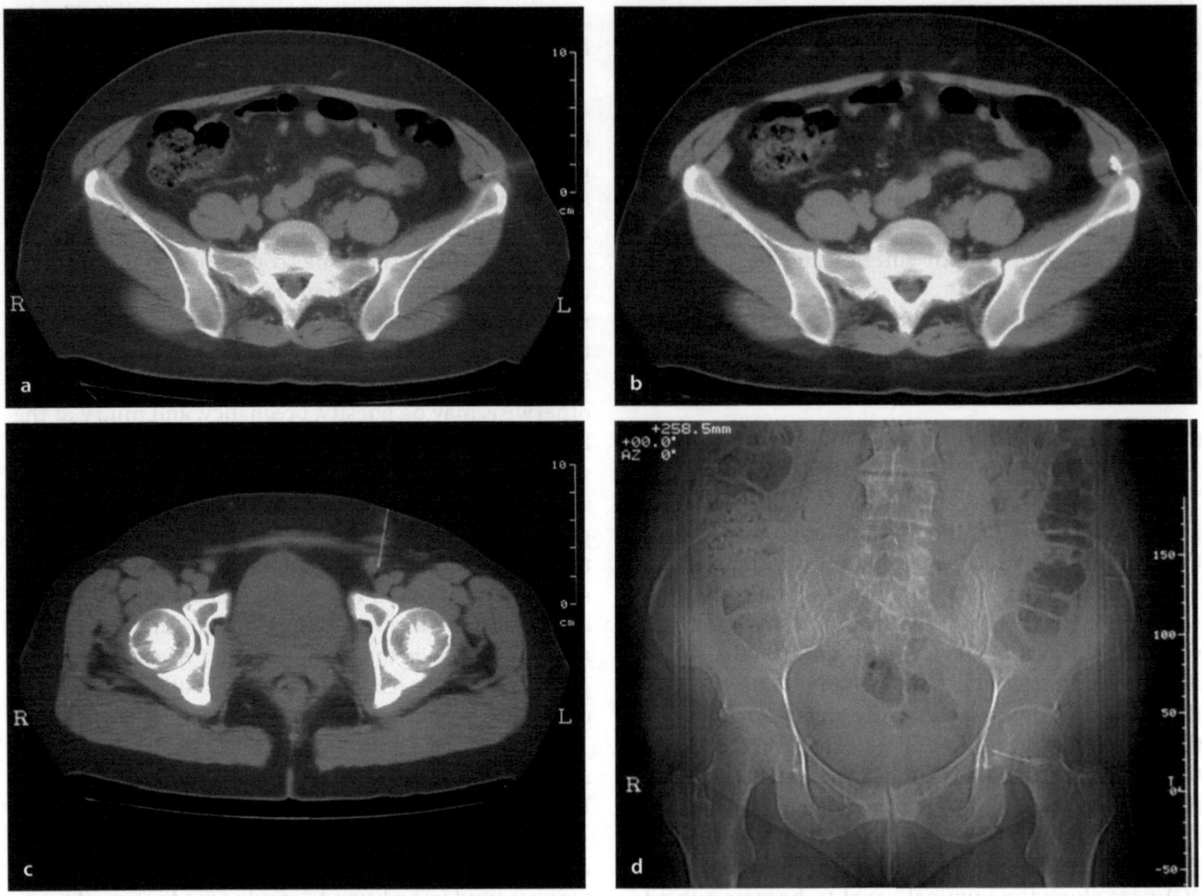

Fig. 14.6 a–d. Infiltration of iliohypogastric nerve. **a** Placement of needle at the point where the problem originates in the region of the ASIS between the transverse and internal oblique abdominal muscles. **b** Injection of hyperdense anesthetic/contrast mixture (5 ml) followed by a slow-release corticosteroid (one ampule cortivazol). **c** Injection at the second site in the inguinal canal. **d** Frontal topogram of needles in place

Ilioinguinal nerve

Relevant Anatomy

The ilioinguinal nerve (2II on Fig. 14.2) is sometimes absent. In 30% of cases it forms a common trunk with the iliohypogastric nerve [7, 8]. If they are separate, still their initial paths from their origin in L1 are identical (see Fig. 14.1). As with the iliohypogastric nerve, the ilioinguinal nerve descends behind the posterior parietal peritoneum on the quadratus lumborum muscle, perforates the transverse abdominal muscle, passes between the transverse muscle (on the inside) and the lesser oblique muscle (on the outside; see Fig. 14.2), and divides into an abdominal branch (sometimes absent) and a genital branch (2G, Fig. 14.2) that accompanies the genital branch (1G) of the iliohypogastric nerve (1IH). The two genital branches (1G and 2G) pass along the inguinal canal to become subcutaneous at the level of the superficial orifice and to be distributed (Fig. 14.4) across the inguinal region, the pubis, the anterior aspect of the scrotum/labia majora, and the median part of the upper limits of the thigh. In 18% of cases the latter two zones arise from the genitofemoral nerve.

Clinical Characteristics

If the ilioinguinal nerve is affected, pain occurs in its territory as described immediately above. Causative factors may be compression phenomena as from clothing too tight, obesity, or pregnancy, compression or invasion by iliac metastases (see Chapter 17, Fig. 17.2), iatrogenic factors (e.g., inguinal hernia surgery), and injury affecting the lumbar spinal column [1, 3]. The pain is often triggered by an erect posture, coughing, or otherwise subjecting the trunk to tension. In any case, it is difficult to clearly distinguish among effects on the ilioinguinal, genitofemoral, and iliohypogastric nerves (except in the event of a concomitant attack affecting the lateral cutaneous branch of the latter nerve).

Technique

The technique and the injection sites are the same as for the iliohypogastric nerve, as described above [1, 2].

Conclusion

The difficulty of diagnosing inguinofemoral neuropathies is linked to the wide anatomical variability of the nerves found there. Diagnosis can be improved by studying somesthetic evoked potentials [7], and can be confirmed by injection at the sites indicated in the present chapter. This should lead to improved care and treatment of inguinofemoral neuropathies, the results of which are generally viewed as disappointing, especially in the long term. In our experience, neurolysis by RF seems to give better and sometimes definitive long-term relief.

References

1. Clair C, Kastler B, Boulahdour Z et al (2002) Radiologie interventionnelle sous contrôle TDM dans le traitement de la douleur pelvienne. Séance thématique. Journées Françaises de Radiologie. Paris, 19–23 Oct 2002
2. Kastler B, Clair C, Boulahdour Z et al (2002) Traitement de la douleur pelvienne sous contrôle TDM. Séance thématique. Congrès National de la Douleur: Douleur et techniques interventionnelles. Lyon, Nov 2002
3. Kastler B, Clair C, Michalakis D et al (2002) Interventional procedures under CT guidance in 756 patients, incidents, side effects and how to reduce their incidence. Scientific Exhibit. Radiological Society of North America, 88th scientific assembly and annual meeting. Chicago, Nov 2002. Radiology [Suppl] 225:724
4. Maigne JY, Maigne R, Guerin-Surville H (1986) Anatomic study of the lateral cutaneous rami of the subcostal and iliohypogastric nerves. Surg Radiol Anat 8:251–256
5. Mandelkow H, Loeweneck H (1988) The iliohypogastric and ilioinguinal nerves. Distribution in the abdominal wall, danger areas in surgical incisions in the inguinal and pubic regions and reflected visceral pain in their dermatomes. Surg Radiol Anat 10:145–149
6. Martin V, Parratte B, Tatu L et al (1997) PES du nerf fémorocutané. Stimulations sous l'épine iliaque antérosupérieure et à la cuisse. Résultats chez 20 sujets témoins. Neurophysiol Clin 27:353–354
7. Monnier G, Martin V, Parratte B (1998) L'évaluation neurophysiologique des troubles sensitifs dans le territoire des nerfs inguinofémoraux, in L'électrodiagnostique 1998: mises au point. Conférences didactiques des 11e journées francophones d'électromyographie de Bordeaux, pp 49–53
8. Sürücü HS, Tanyeli E, Sargon MF, Karahan ST (1997) An anatomic study of the lateral femoral cutaneous nerve. Surg Radiol Anat 19:307–310

Vertebroplasty and Cementoplasty

15

Fabrice-Guy Barral, Benoît Russias, Philippe Tanji, Jean-Sébastien Billiard, Bruno Kastler

Introduction

Vertebroplasty and cementoplasty consist of injecting acrylic cement percutaneously into bone lesions, most often into osteolytic zones. The initial aim is analgesia by consolidation of bony parts that were previously fragile.

Historically, the first vertebroplasties were performed in 1987 by Galibert and Deramond on seven vertebrae with angiomatous lesions. After a while, the indications included metastases in vertebrae, myelomatous lesions, and osteoporotic spinal compression.

Later, this technique was proposed for osteolytic lesions, mainly those associated with metastases in extramedullary portions of the spine, and most of all for metastases to regions difficult to approach surgically, such as the pelvis and sacrum. The rapidity of analgesia and consolidation have conferred an important role upon cementoplasty among different anti-neoplastic treatments, such as radiotherapy and chemotherapy.

Vertebroplasty

Indications

The principal indications for vertebroplasty are osteolytic metastases in vertebrae, myelomas, vertebral angiomas, and painful osteoporotic spinal compression. The decision to perform this procedure should be made in a multidisciplinary environment to allow appropriate evaluation before undertaking surgery, radiotherapy, medical treatment, and/or other forms of therapy. These different choices should be based on many elements besides the strict medical history, current general medical status, and review of systems. These include his or her life expectations, level(s) of the spinal column affected, and the particular significance of pain for the patient.

Vertebral Angioma

Vertebral angiomas or hemangiomas [3, 5, 6, 9, 11, 12, 14, 22, 23, 27] are very frequent benign tumors of the spinal column, usually found by coincidence. When they are painful and when one can be sure the pain is caused by them, they represent a good indication for vertebroplasty. Angiomas can be responsible for medullary and/or spinal nerve root compression. They can even arise in the framework of angiomatous conditions involving a dermatome s (COBB syndrome), then being called aggressive angiomas.

The aims of cement injection in these cases are consolidation of vertebrae, pain treatment and epidural angioma reduction. Sometimes it is necessary to inject cement, by a direct approach, into elements of the posterior arch and to combine cementoplasty with purposive arterial embolization. These procedures together facilitate decompressive surgery, allowing for laminectomy instead of subtotal somatectomy.

Osteolytic Metastases and Spinal Column Myeloma

These represent the most frequent indications for vertebroplasty. The analgesic affect of cementation can not be explained only by the consolidation of a fragile, fractured or pre-fractured bone piece, because there is no correlation between the quantity of cement injected and the rapidity of pain reduction. Injected cement has a cytotoxic effect that is by nature chemical and thermal; the polymerization phase induces a significant elevation of local temperature. The analgesic effect usually occurs in the first 48 h, and permits the reduction of major analgesic agents, whereas radiotherapy for such neoplastic problems requires 1 to 2 weeks to manifest its efficacy.

The consolidation effect diminishes the risk of fracture and shortens the immobilization period significantly and rapidly, while the outcome of radiotherapy only becomes obvious much later, after 2 or 3 months.

Osteoporotic Spinal Compression

In general, osteoporotic spinal compression [2, 5, 14, 15, 18, 21–23, 25, 26, 29] reacts very well to medical treatment and rest, but in case of persistent pain, even after 6 weeks, and when there is significant risk of spinal compression, vertebroplasty has much to offer. In these cases, it is important to clarify the quality of the vertebrae above and below the actual vertebra that may eventually be cemented in order to prevent secondary compression by an imbalance of pressure forces above and below this new point of resistance. The procedure may also be considered as preoperative, before eventual surgical fixation.

Contraindications

Regarding local complications, absolute contraindications are represented by blood coagulation disorders, because the needles generally used in this procedure have a large caliber. These also represent a problem if bone infection exists, because they pose an increased risk of causing local/regional dissemination. In osteolysis with medullary or spinal nerve root compression, injection of cement is contraindicated to avoid the transformation of "soft" into "hard" compression.

Relative contraindications are rupture of the posterior wall and the risk of epidural leakage. That is why it is possible to limit this leakage by changing the viscosity of the cement injected. "Flat" spinal compression (pancake type) also presents a problem for the introduction of a large trocar.

Technique

In general, patients should be able to undergo general anesthesia with spontaneous ventilation, or a single major sedation, or analgesic sedation.

The choice of technique depends on several factors. Those related to the patient are the general health status (and more particularly that of respiration with regard to choice of anesthesia).

The region of the spine to be addressed and degree of vertebral damage determines the approach and the material to be used. Also to be chosen is the radiological monitor, i.e., CT, fluoroscopy, or a combination of the two.

Fitting the Approach to the Spinal Region

Cervical Spine

From C2 to C5

The preferred approach here is anterolateral. (It is identical to the approach we use for disc puncture inside the jugulo-carotid vascular sheath; Fig. 15.1 a.) The patient is placed in the supine position to allow a bilateral approach in case of incomplete filling of the vertebral area in question by instillation from one side. For C2 vertebra, a posterolateral approach is proposed if the vertebral body is affected (Fig. 15.2).

For C6 (and Often for C7)

An anterolateral approach is possible in slim patients with a long neck and in patients where it is possible to lower the scapular girdle. In others, it is preferable to use a trans-pedicular approach because the intercostal–transverse approach is generally extremely difficult due to the length involved and the obstructions presented by the transverse process, the posterior arch of the ribs, and scapula. For these two vertebrae patient positioning can be challenging; a supine position generally being preferable to prone or lateral.

Thoracic Spine

For the thoracic spine, all approaches are possible, the posterolateral, the intercostal–transverse, and the trans-pedicular (Fig. 15.3). The intercostal–transverse approach in our experience has several advantages (Fig. 15.4):

- It permits the use of small caliber needles (18 gauge), which is particularly helpful in major osteolysis, especially when there are pedicular lesions. It permits real-time surveillance of needle progression on fluoroscopy or scanography. (Small caliber needles are undeniably best for patients with blood coagulation disorders.)
- It permits a real-time adaptation of needle's path to patient anatomy in that needle inclination can be modulated in three dimensions: cranio-caudal, equatorial, and antero-posterior. Primarily, the needle has to follow the inclination of the intercostal space, and then has to pass between the transverse process and the costotransverse joint, now above the needle. Finally, it has to penetrate the vertebral body in an orientation from bottom to top, outside to inside, and from behind to front.
- Finally, it is particularly adapted to the laterally reclining patient position, which is very helpful for patients in whom the prone position is impossible or contraindicated. The obliquely prone position is not always easy, especially for maintain stability during the procedure. For extremely fragile patients, general anesthesia is preferable.

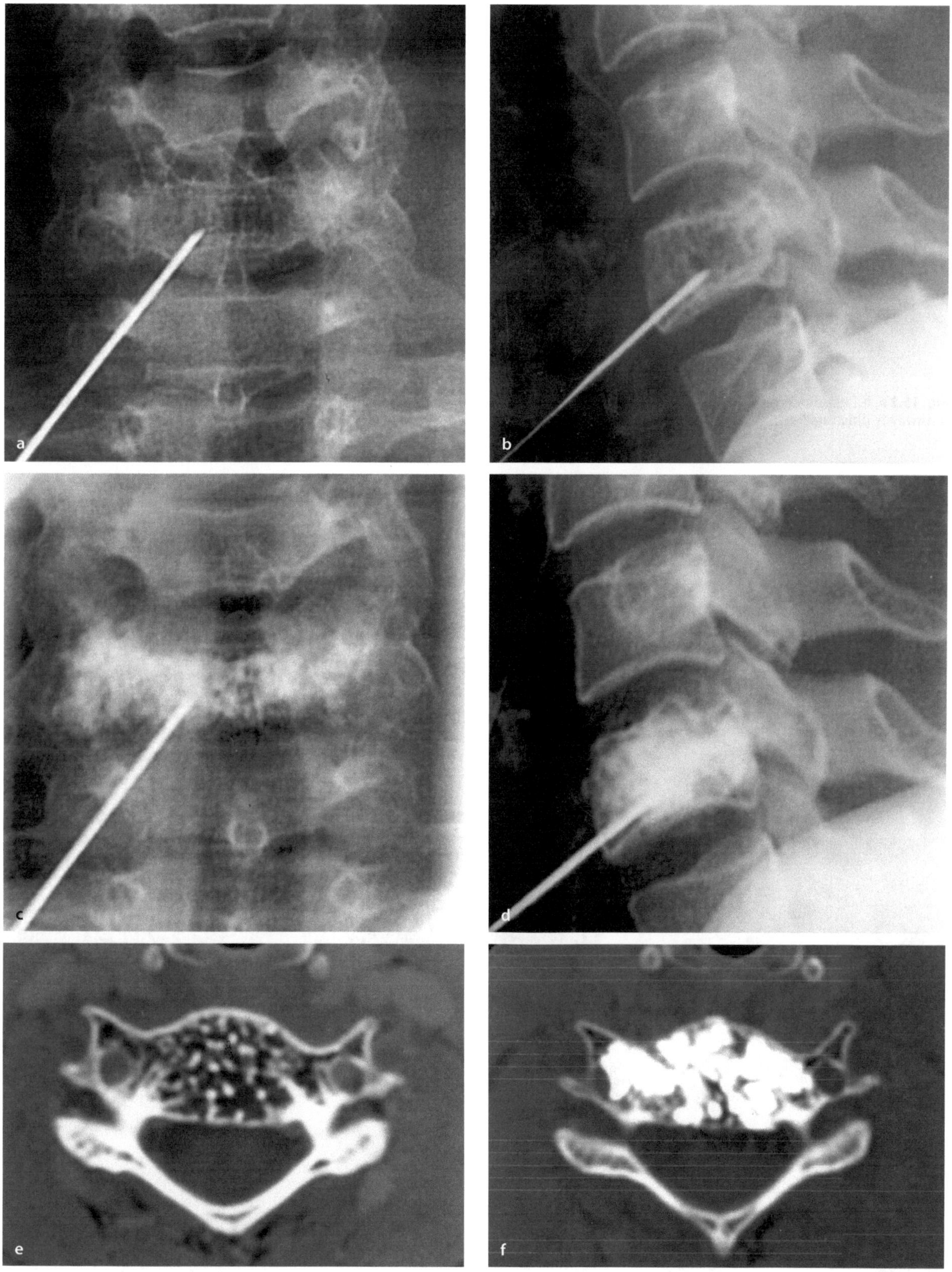

Fig. 15.1 a–f. Angioma of the vertebral body of C5. **a, b** Right anterolateral approach with 18 gauge needle, frontal and lateral views. **c, d** Injection of cement under fluoroscopic guidance, frontal and lateral views. **e, f** CT scan before and after injection confirming the filling of the angioma

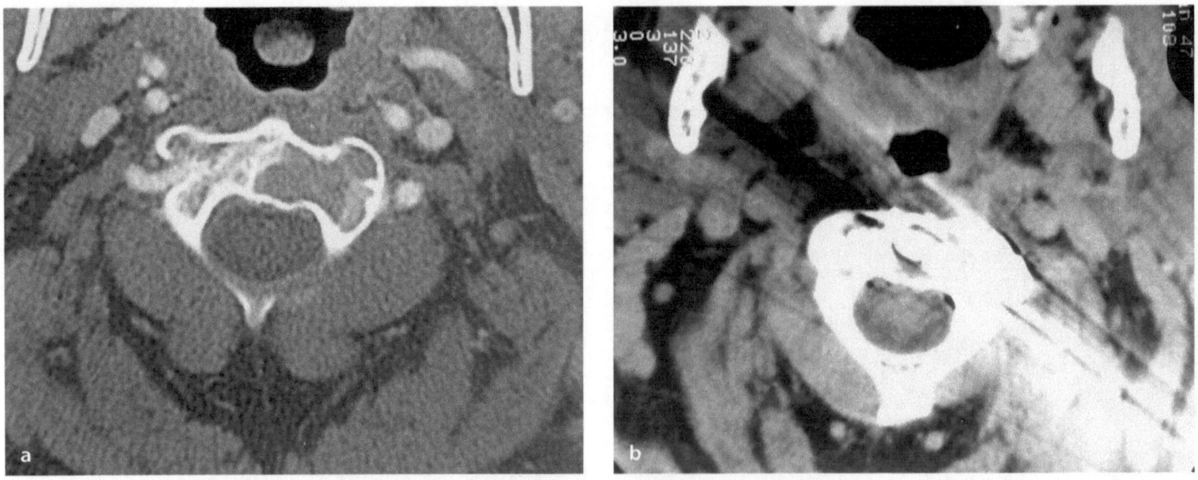

Fig. 15.2 a, b. Plasmocytoma of the C2 vertebral body. Posterolateral approach. The value of CT scan for choosing the best needle pathway is illustrated

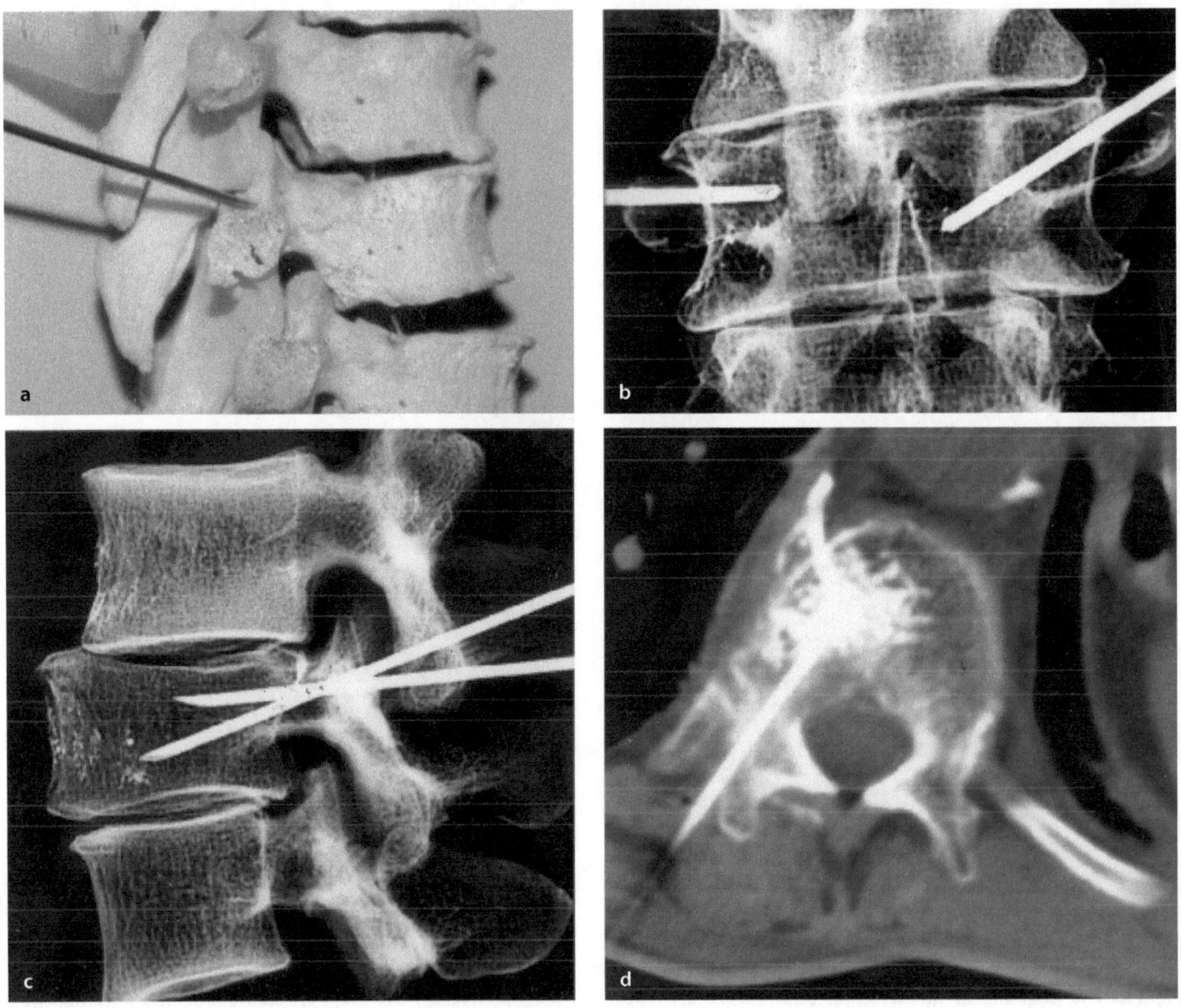

Fig. 15.3a–d. Transpedicular approach. **a** Preliminary approach, thoracic spine. **b, c** Frontal and lateral X-ray views. **d** CT scan of a thoracic vertebra cementoplasty

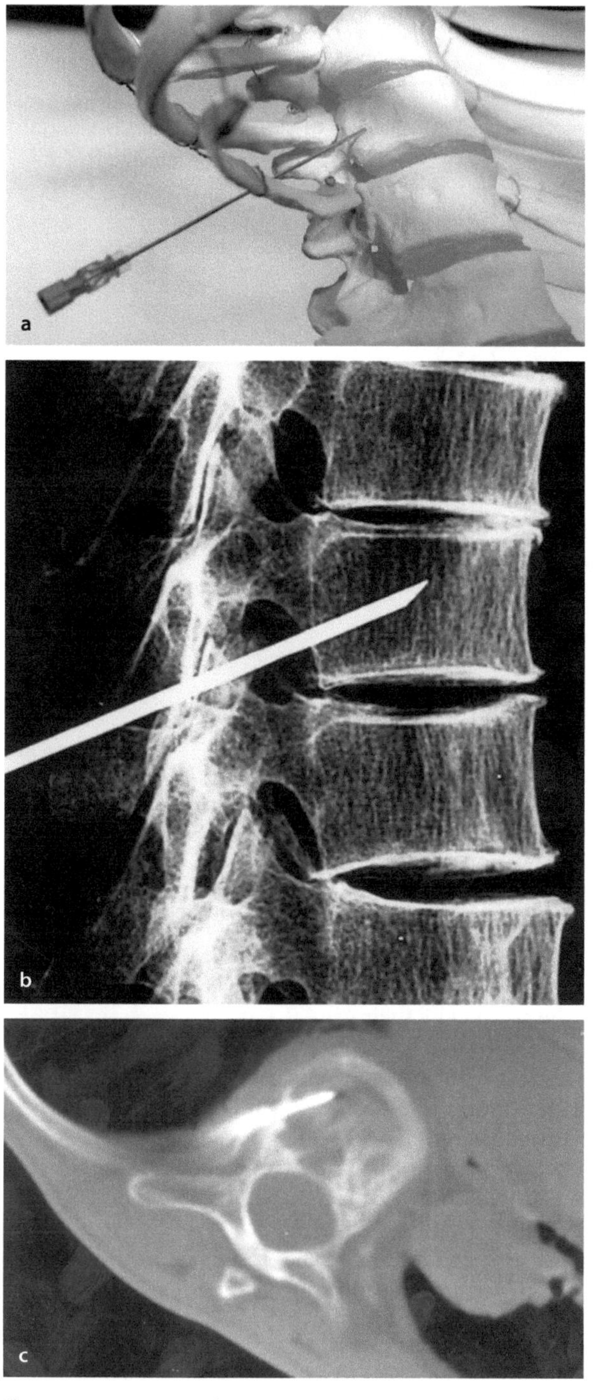

Fig. 15.4 a–c. Intercostal-transverse approach. **a** Preliminary approach with an 18 gauge needle. **b** Lateral X-Ray view of anatomical pieces. **c** CT scan checking concentric tube biopsy device

Lumbar Spine

For the lumbar spine, the trans-pedicular approach is always possible, but the posterolateral approach is not difficult either. This latter approach is usually used for all percutaneous interventions on the disks, foramina, and vertebral bodies. Needle inclination is 45° in all three dimensions, with entry point into the skin at 4 to 5 finger breadths from the medial line (Fig. 15.5).

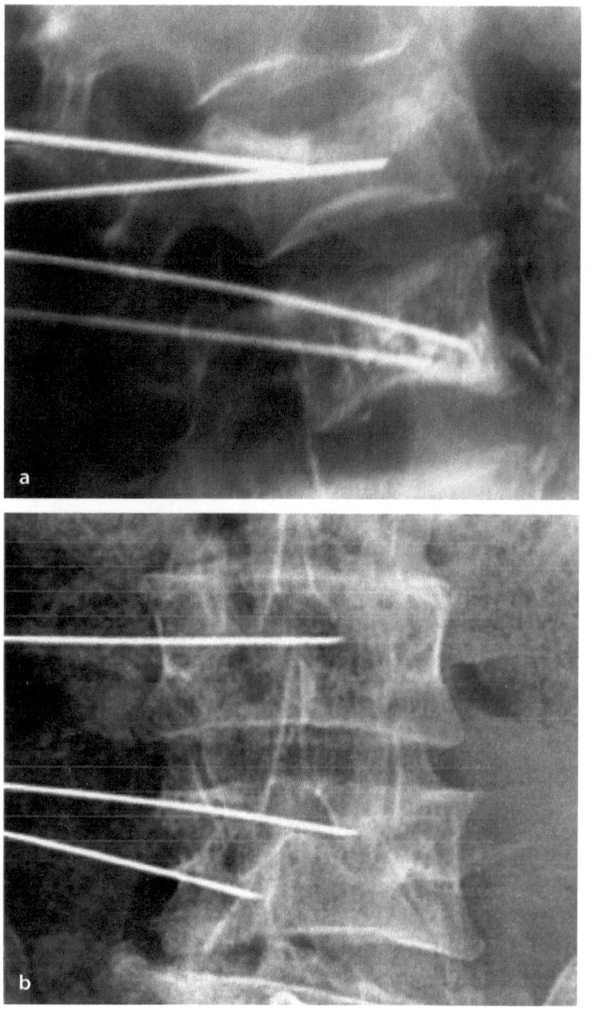

Fig. 15.5. **a** Lumbar approach, 18 gauge needles, osteoporotic vertebral crush fracture (myeloma). **b** Lateral view

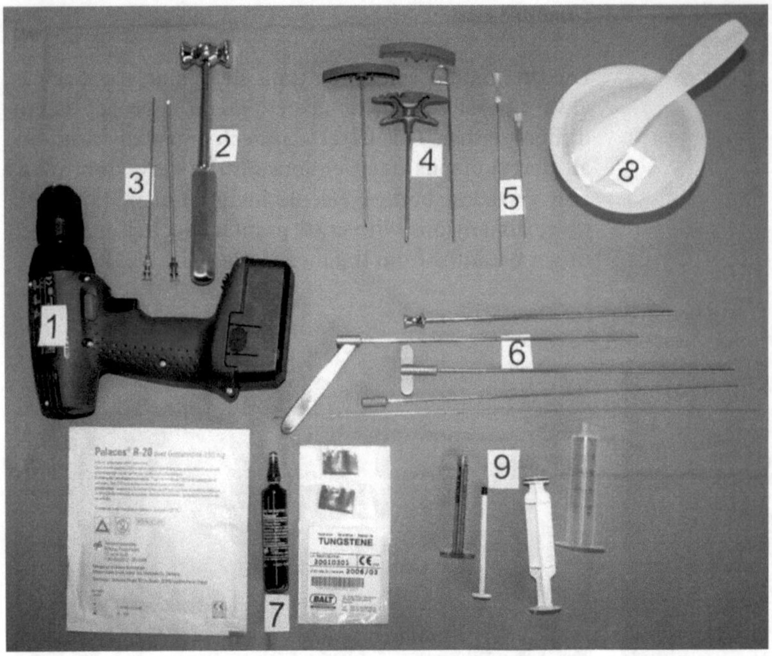

Fig. 15.6. Instruments: *1* electric drill handle. *2* surgical mallet. *3* Escoffier needles. *4* Biopsy trocars (Biomid). *5* 18 gauge spinal needles (BD). *6* Bard Trocars. *7* Palacos Gentamycine cement (Biomet) and tungsten metal powder (Balt, Montmorency, France). *8* single-use dish. *9* 20 ml and 1 ml syringes

Choice of Material

Reference here is principally to the type of trocar to be used for cementation [1, 16, 21, 23]. We employ two main types (Fig. 15.6):

- Spinal needle type of 18 gauge 3.5 inch (9 cm) and 18 gauge 6 inch (16 cm; see Fig. 15.6, no. 5)
- Cementation trocar with the adjustable Escoffier needle (10 and 14 gauge and 10–15 cm length; see Fig. 15.6, no. 3)

The choice of trocar depends on several factors:

- Status of the vertebra (degree of damage, remaining height, integrity of the pedicles, etc.)
- Location on the spine (cervical, dorsal or lumbar)
- Blood coagulation status
- Unalterably chosen approach
- Necessity of a biopsy.

The advantages of 18 gauge needles are:

- They are better for patients with coagulation abnormalities because they are less invasive.
- They are easy to manipulate manually without the need for a hammer or power pliers.
- They permit very delicate maneuvers such an intercostal-transversal approach, allowing entrance into narrow passages.
- They facilitate the filling of extensive or multifocal osteolytic zones, because they are more selective and because it is much easier to position two or three of these needles in a vertebra than to insert a single large caliber needle (see Fig. 15.5).

The advantages of Escoffier needles are:

- Their progression can be assisted; they can even be advanced by a small surgical hammer or by adapting a motorized handle (which is very beneficial for the trans-pedicular approach).
- Their caliber permits the use of higher density cement, in the final phase of polymerization, and in that way its diffusion can be limited. Most importantly, extra-corporal, venous, and/or epidural leakage can be avoided by their use.

If biopsy of a vertebra is necessary, it is logical to do so at the time of the procedure and avoid multiple invasions. Limiting cortical perforations is important.

Actually, in all of these cases cement leakage is frequent. Two solutions for reducing the likelihood of such incidents are suggested:

- After the biopsy sample has been taken, the cementation trocar can be introduced into the trocar that carries the biopsy kit and that is already placed inside the vertebra.
- Inversely, the catheter that carries the bone biopsy kit can serve as a trocar for cementation. It is slid down over the biopsy trocar that is now used as a guide for access to the osteolytic lesion, and the trocar is removed after the biopsy sample has been taken.

Two types of material are employed for biopsy:

- Sets that can be used more than once, such as the Bard type or the Masabraud trocar (see Fig. 15.6, no. 6).
- Sets for single use only, mainly Biomid (Gallini, Mantua, Italy) (see Fig. 15.6, no 4).

In some circumstances, and especially in situations where the approach can be a hazardous (with the intercostal-transverse approach, for example) it can be of value to use the (Laredo and) Bard biopsy set. It functions by first sliding coaxially along a long metallic trocar needle (at least 30 cm long) so that the tip comes to lie in the center of the target. A trocar, the carrier, is then placed over this needle, its conical distal extremity functioning as an entry point for the dilator.

Choice of the Environment

Several installation types are possible for vertebroplasty under the safest conditions, but it seems important to simultaneously monitor progression from at least two dimensions [13, 19, 23, 26].

Two-dimensional Installation

- Two-dimensional fluoroscopy helps one follow the trocar's progression in two orthogonal dimensions.
- Cementation can be stopped as soon as it as evident that the cement is being injected in the wrong direction and/or to the wrong location. In some highly osteolytic lesions (in cases of hypervascular metastasis or in hemangiomas) phlebography can be undertaken before the cementation procedure to better evaluate the lesion's extent, to predict cement distribution, and to look for dangerous drainage.

The following are fundamental for programming or technique change:

- Adaptation of trocar caliber
- Alteration of cement density
- Complementary arterial or percutaneous embolization by another approach

Scanography (CT)

The advantages of scanography in interventional radiology are already well known and used worldwide. Scans permit the visualization of spinal lesions deep in the equatorial plane. They can be analyzed in three dimensions, especially for distance from the skin surface, with visualization of both vertebrae and surrounding soft tissues. They are thus indispensable in insuring that vascular, visceral, and neurological structures are avoided. The major inconvenience has been the delay their use has imposed, and until the last couple of years, it was not possible to directly visualize trocar progression.

With the latest multislice generation of CT scanners (6 images per second) this inconvenience is largely avoided. The newer ultra-rapid scanners deliver virtually real-time image reconstruction, with a speed almost that of fluoroscopy, thus allowing trocar progression to be followed as with fluoroscopy. It is also possible thereby to follow the "real-time" diffusion of cement into bone parts. Another advantage is the significantly reduced procedure time. It is becoming no longer necessary to bring the patient from the scanner tunnel to below the scopic arch, making the procedure easier to perform and reducing the quantity of anesthetic needed.

Best Working Arrangement

The best system at present, and one that is generally very accessible, is the use of fluoroscopy and scanography at the same time, with the possibility ridding the operative room and scanner gantry of the mobile tube. After determination of pathway with scanner help, the trocar is placed under fluoroscopic control and is monitored from several equatorial projections. Finally, its target position is confirmed by the scanner. The cement is injected under fluoroscopic control, and its diffusion is monitored again by new scan slices.

Procedural Stages

References that may be consulted under this topic include: [6, 7, 8, 10, 13, 16, 19, 20, 23, 29].

Patient Preparation

All patient preparation from pre-interventional consultation, pre-anesthesia consultation, compiling a complete iconographic and medical file, to the correction of metabolic and/or blood coagulation disorders, are already well known and discussed under interventional procedures in radiology; hence, they will not be discussed here

Patient Positioning

Rigorous aseptic conditions must be respected as in all interventional procedures for osteoarticular radiology. They will not be detailed here.

Patient positioning on the examination table or on the scanner table depends on the approach chosen:

- The trans-pedicular approach is the most comfortable with the patient in the prone position.
- The intercostal-transverse approach is most comfortable when the patient is in the lateral position, but certain authors prefer the three-quarter supine position (called the "carried shadow technique").
- The posterolateral approach is most comfortable with the patient in the lateral position (when it is unilateral), but the prone position is most comfortable when the approach is bilateral.

- The antero-lateral approach for the proximal part of the cervical spine is the most comfortable when the patient is in the supine position.

These notions of comfort can be modified with regard to the performing radiologist's habits, and more importantly, the patient's condition. Actually, in certain cases the prone position is not recommended, and adapting to a "three-quarter prone" or lateral position may be necessary.

The patient's condition can also influence the choice of anesthesia, that is, general anesthesia with controlled respiration, general anesthesia with spontaneous respiration, analgesic sedation, or simple sedation.

Needle Placement

First, local anesthesia is provided with a 22 gauge needle, from skin to bone. The needle should follow the path chosen during preliminary study.

The importance of local anesthesia is threefold:

- Patient participation in analgesia during and after the procedure permits, among other things, a reduction of anesthetic drugs.
- The needle delivering local anesthesia becomes a trocar guide for either cementation or bone biopsy (for details on needle support, see Chap. 3);
- Injected lidocaine infiltrates soft tissue and separates its structures, forming a passage for the cementation trocar. Pleura can thus be displaced in a thoracic approach, or a spinal nerve root during an intercostal-transverse approach, permitting easy trocar passage (see Chap. 3).

For the anterolateral approach to cervical vertebrae, the posterolateral approach to lumbar vertebrae, and the intercostal-transverse approach to thoracic vertebrae penetration into the vertebral bodies is not difficult and can be elegantly performed manually by screwing down the needle. This technique is very important considering that metastasis or angiomas make the affected vertebrae friable. In case of resistance (partially compressed metastasis or rare compacted forms of myeloma), trocar progression can be facilitated with the help of a surgical hammer or an electric drill.

With the trans-pedicular approach, trocar progression is facilitated in the same way, with surgical hammer or by adapting a motorized handle on the proximal extremity of the trocar (see Fig. 15.6, 1 and 2).

Cement Injection

The cement injected (see Fig. 15.6) into vertebrae is an acrylic glue used in orthopedic surgery to cement prostheses.

It is a mixture of methyl-methacrylate powder (several commercial products available) and a diluting liquid monomer. The acrylic powder is mixed with tantalum or tungsten powder to accentuate its radio-opacity for visualization under fluoroscopy. We prefer Palacos Gentamicine (Biomet, Warsaw, IN, USA) cement, which combines the advantages of a low-viscosity cement with those of gentamicin for very precise properties, and for minimization of the possibility of bone infection.

The mixture polymerizes in 20 to 50 seconds. Polymerization time can be changed by increasing or reducing the liquid monomer. The mixture should be injected during the polymerization phase, while it is still in a paste (creamy) state. It is important to reintroduce the mandrin into the trocar if the trocar is to be reused, because the cement becomes a solid mass very quickly. That is why the exact quantity of cement in the trocar must be known when the mandrin is repositioned.

In vertebroplasty of myelomas, metastases, or primary tumors, analgesic effect is attained with approximately 2 to 3 ml of cement. In case of osteoporosis or hemangioma, it is necessary to inject a larger quantity (3 to 5 ml) to gain analgesic and consolidation effects.

During the solidification phase, the significant increase in local temperature (± 90 °C) is responsible for part of its anti-tumor effect. The rise in local temperature also explains the brief increase in pain and the brief hypotension that occur.

The injection phase should be monitored at all times by scan to allow its immediate interruption if epidural or paravertebral leakage occurs. It is strongly recommended that the injection be monitored by a strict profile view if a single-dimension radiographic device is used.

There are several delicate phases in cement preparation and injection. It is important to obtain a very homogeneous mix of methyl-methacrylate and tungsten powders. During mixture with the liquid monomer, rapid homogenization is imperative for injection as a creamy mass. The second delicate phase is the duration of injection, which can be minimized in several ways:

- Some authors use a syringe under pressure.
- Others adapt a force handle on their syringes.
- Finally, some employ small 1–2 ml syringes that are connected to a Luer-lock previously filled with a bigger syringe, to be able to apply stronger and more regular pressure on the piston. The latter technique is specially recommended with 18 gauge needles; already prepared kits are very practical as they contain a syringe under pressure for a single use only (recommended for 18 gauge needle).

Complications, Secondary Effects, and Surveillance

References [4, 5, 7, 10, 15, 17, 20, 22, 23, 25, 27, 29] are recommended for consultation.

Cement Leakage

The main complications is cement leakage from the vertebrae.

Posterior Leakage into the Epidural Space

This is the most dangerous complication because of the risk of spinal cord or nerve root compression (Fig. 15.7a). The compression effect may be transient if it is caused by an inflammatory reaction (increased cement temperature) that can be easily resolved with anti-inflammatory drugs. On the other hand, compression by the cement itself may be definitive and may require emergency decompressive surgery (with the usual rigorous aseptic conditions applicable). Such complications, especially those that warrant emergency surgery are rare in the literature. Epidural leakage can be due to rupture of the posterior wall, but can also occur via the foramina of basal vertebral veins. It can be avoided or limited by respecting all contraindications (that regarding epidural tumor expansion is particularly important), and if cement injection is stopped, the beginning of overflow can be seen at the posterior wall. Viscosity of the cement and its polymerization time can be modified. First, very thick cement is injected to create a protective barrier where the posterior wall is destroyed. Then, during the phase of trocar withdrawal, more liquid cement can be eventually injected for better filling of the osteolytic zone.

Vein Leakage

Leakage via the epidural and emissary veins (see Fig. 15.7b and c) can also cause spinal nerve root compression that generally stops with local therapy. Vein leakage, especially if the cement is too liquid, can elicit a pulmonary embolism (0.4% in the literature). For vertebrae with good vascularization, such as seen in renal and thyroid metastases and in vertebral hemangiomas, vertebral phlebography is recommended before cement injection. This permits choice of the best trocar position, depending on the architecture of vein drainage, and modification of cement polymerization time so that the largest drainage veins can be occluded rapidly and proximally.

Leakage into the Neural Foramina

Leakage into the foramina (see Fig. 15.7d), which can evoke irritation and spinal nerve root compression, usually stops rapidly after radiologically-guided infiltration of lidocaine plus prednisolone.

Leakage into Adjacent Disks

Leakage into adjacent disks (see Fig. 15.7e), which is generally not symptomatic, can modify the surgical strategy in osteoporotic vertebrae. It seems logical to cement the adjacent vertebra to prevent spinal compression, the cemented disc core acting as a pivot.

Leakage into Perivertebral Soft Tissues

This leakage is relatively frequent (see Fig. 15.7f), especially if a biopsy is done before cementation (but can be guarded against by using a concentric tube system when the two procedures are undertaken together.). These leakages can occur during trocar withdrawal: progressive removal is advisable after introduction of the mandrin, especially in very friable vertebrae. These perivertebral leakages are asymptomatic in the majority of cases.

The Risk of Bone Infection

Bone infections are limited with the implementation of draconian aseptic conditions. As with all procedures in osteoarticular interventional radiology, they should be implemented in a rigidly controlled environment. Some cements (Palacos Gentamicine, for example) already contain an antibiotic that acts locally.

Secondary Effects

These all appear immediately: in the form of short hypotension episodes during the procedure and as cardiac rhythm disorders during cement injection. The episodes are generally transient (and they occur most often when a large quantity of cement is used).

Immediately after the procedure, the combination of sedation and a prolonged prone position can evoke hypoventilation with the risk of pulmonary infection. Increased local temperature during the polymerization phase can induce an inflammatory reaction in the first hours after the procedure, with pain accentuation and a slight to moderate fever. These symptoms disappear within 2–3 days with the administration of anti-inflammatory drugs.

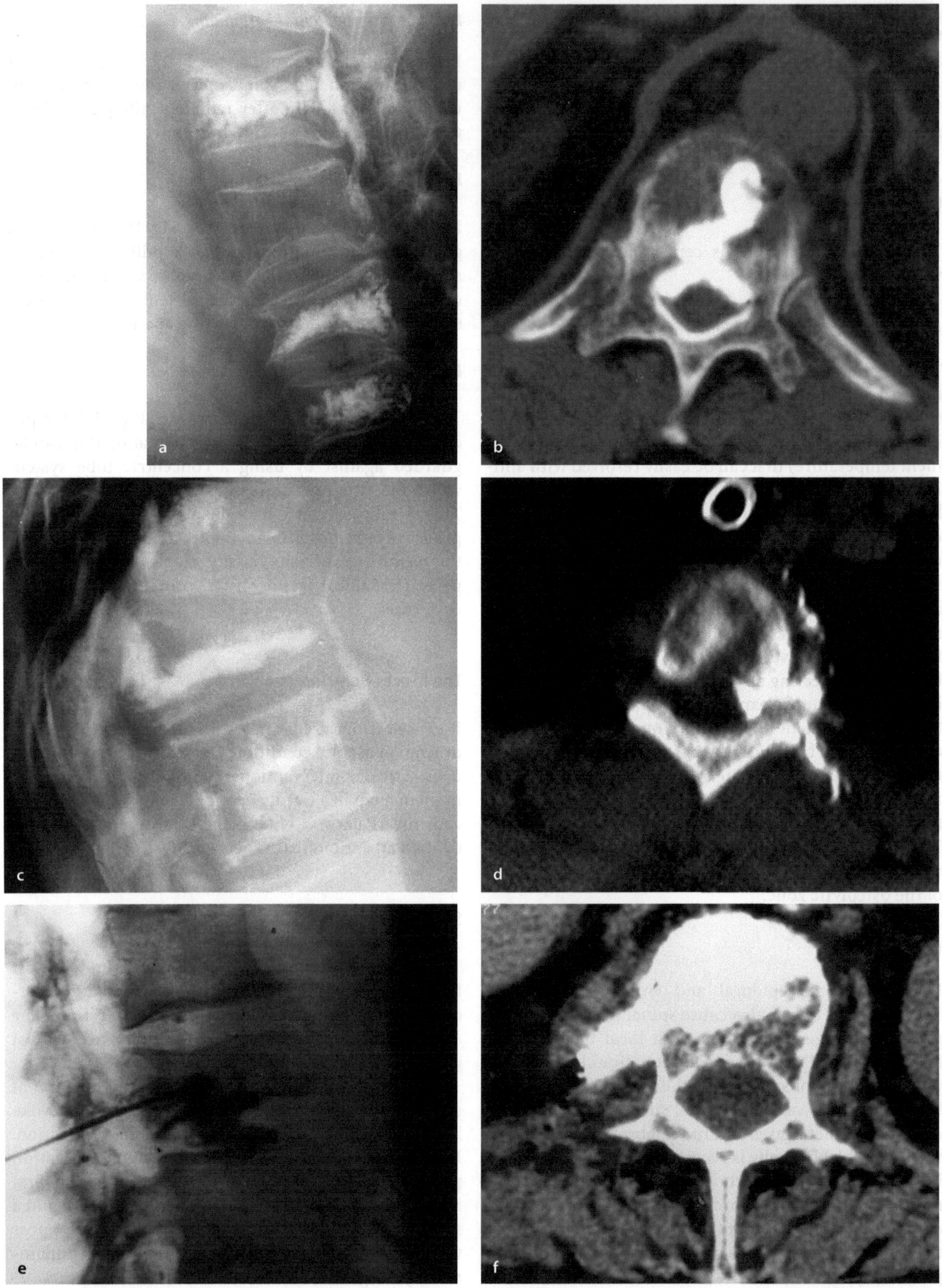

Fig. 15.7a–f. Cement leaks. **a** Posterior wall destruction. **b** Epidural vein. **c** Emissary vein. **d** Foraminal leak. **e** Intervertebral disk. **f** Paravertebral soft tissues leak

Results

The efficacy of vertebroplasty lies in its pain reduction (evaluated on a subjective scale). This analgesic effect, which appears between 16 and 72 h (average 36 h), and allows the standing position in the majority of cases, also diminishes complications when lying down. The latter point is especially noteworthy among patients in a generally bad state with poor life expectations. The analgesic effect can be quantified by a decrease in use of analgesic drugs, and often later by complete abstinence from them. Studies in the medical literature indicate that 70 % of patients with vertebral metastasis or myeloma greatly appreciate this complete disappearance of pain or very significant pain reduction. The number is even higher among cases of hemangioma or osteoporotic fracture, going up to 90 %.

The mechanism of pain reduction by cementation is not yet fully understood.

- Stabilization of vertebral fractures, usually small and multiple, partly explains the procedure's efficacy
- The procedure certainly intervenes in the destruction of sensitive fibers via mechanical, vascular, chemical and thermal factors.

For metastasis in vertebrae, there does not seem to be a correlation between the analgesic effect and the quantity of cement injected. In fractured vertebrae, the principal mechanisms are consolidation and stabilization of bony tissue by the cement. In these cases, cementation can be viewed as preventing further breakage, particularly of vertebrae surrounding the fracture zone.

Conclusion

Vertebroplasty nowadays occupies an extremely important place in vertebral pain management and permits, in a short time period, normal daily activities, with minor risks of complications, if all possible contraindications are respected.

Its indications in cancer are complementary to other antineoplastic therapies, particularly radiotherapy and chemotherapy. They can work in synergy, because the effect of radiotherapy is not obvious until after 2 to 3 weeks. The consolidation outcome is not satisfactory until at least 2 to 3 months.

Locally, vertebroplasty can be complemented by other analgesic percutaneous treatments to address situations in which metastases in vertebrae have effects outside of bone. It is quite possible to consolidate what is left of vertebral bodies and to inject ethanol into the fleshy extra-medullary part of a metastasis or combine vertebroplasty with RF ablation, see Chap. 17. Research into the material used for vertebroplasty is continuing with substances that participate in bone formation, such as coral polyphosphate cement and pearl powder.

Percutaneous Cementoplasty

Introduction

Percutaneous cementoplasty techniques derive directly from vertebroplasty. The importance of pain suppression and re-establishing functional capacity, with complications minimized, has enlarged the number of indications for percutaneous treatment of fragile bone lesions.

Indications

Please consult references [31, 32, 34, 36, 37, 39–44].

The aim of percutaneous cementoplasty, under consideration primarily in cancer patients whose precarious medical status precludes surgery, is twofold. It is first to obtain a rapid analgesic response in highly painful situations caused by bone fragments that resist medical treatment. Second, it induces a consolidation effect where osteolytic lesions have reduced functional capacity, and also in lesions where there is a risk of fracture with destruction of the carrier bone part.

Indications in Oncology

These are:

- Diffuse and deep osteolytic zones for which surgical treatment is not advisable
- Osteolytic lesions in bone pieces, especially of pelvis and sacrum, for which surgical procedures would be too destructive
- Osteolytic zones where the risk of fracture is significant and which compromise the stability of part of the skeleton or the ability to stand upright, such as the acetabular region or the femur neck
- Long bone lesions with major functional impact on the legs, compromising the standing position and walking
- Osteolytic lesions resistant to radio/chemotherapy.

These procedures are generally palliative, with an aim only to make the last days of life more comfortable. They harmonize well with chemotherapy and radiotherapy. Finally, it is possible to re-cement an already treated zone if the lesion spreads or pain reappears.

Other Indications for Percutaneous Cementoplasty

Percutaneous cementoplasty can be performed as acrylic plastic surgery for posttraumatic pseudoarthrosis. Some authors propose it as a preventive consolidation of benign tumors with large cysts, such as essential cysts and aneurysmal cysts, when injection of sclerosing agents, such as Ethibloc (Ethicon, Somerville, NJ, USA), is not possible. Finally, many practice percutaneous cementation in osteonecrosis of joints such as the knee or hip.

Contraindications

As in vertebroplasty, general contraindications depend on the anesthesia or analgesia technique. Contraindications are:

- Coagulation disorders that are difficult to correct
- Sepsis in or near the area to be cemented
- Anatomic situations in which visceral, vascular, or nerve structures cannot be avoided.

Relative contraindications are diffuse tumor lesions, as in the sacrum, in which the passage of nerve roots cannot be ruled out, and where there is a risk of definite nerve compression (these problems are also encountered in percutaneous alcoholization)

Technique

The choice of technique depends on the type of anesthesia possible and the location and size of the lesion. References [32, 35, 36, 39, 44] may be reviewed. After the best needle pathway has been determined for approaching the bone in as nearly a perpendicular manner as possible, local anesthesia should be delivered from skin to bone.

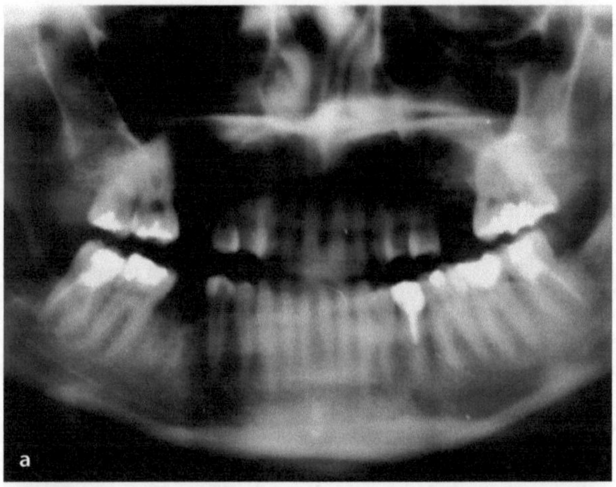

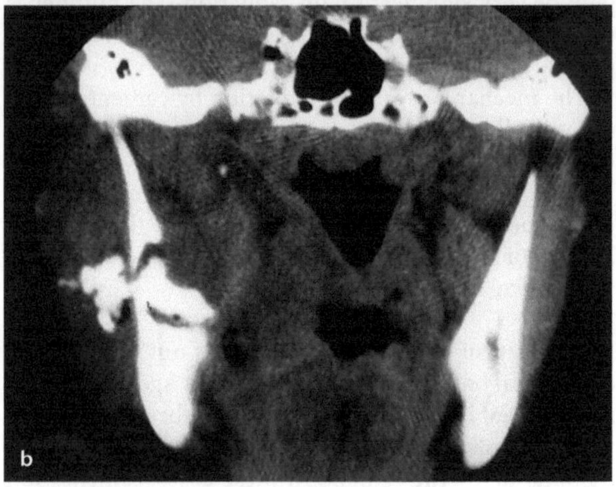

Fig. 15.8. **a** Mandible. Metastasis of a temporal hemangiopericytoma. **b** CT monitoring scan

Approach

The approach is conditioned by patient anatomy. Material, environment, and patient position differ from patient to patient as in vertebroplasty, and be reminded that aseptic conditions should be draconian and in an environment reserved for osteoarticular interventional radiology.

- When the procedure is to be performed in the face region, the preferred technique is with fine needles (18 gauge, 3.5 inch) under fluoroscopy plus scanner (see Fig. 15.8).
- For the clavicles, the procedure should be conducted with fine needles (18 gauge, 3.5 inch) in the vascular radiology room (Fig. 15.9).

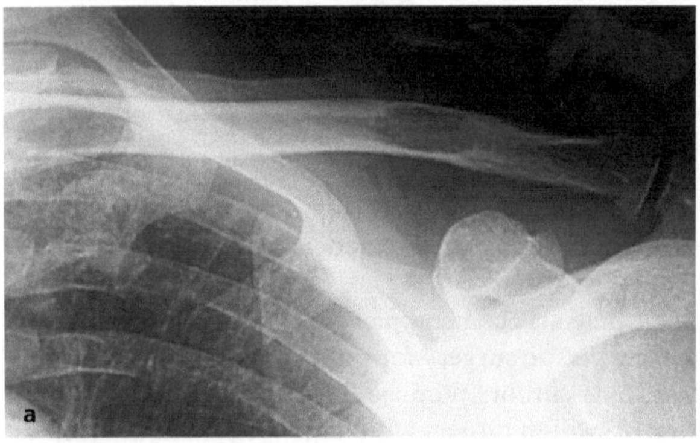

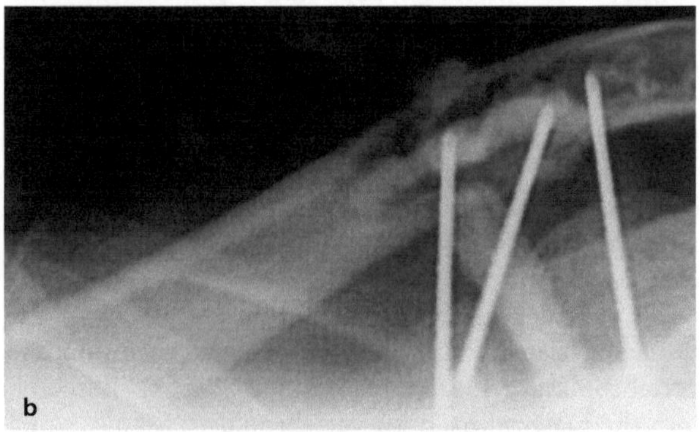

Fig. 15.9a, b. Clavicle with osteolytic metastasis from a breast neoplasm. **a** Before cementoplasty. **b** Check after insertion of three needles

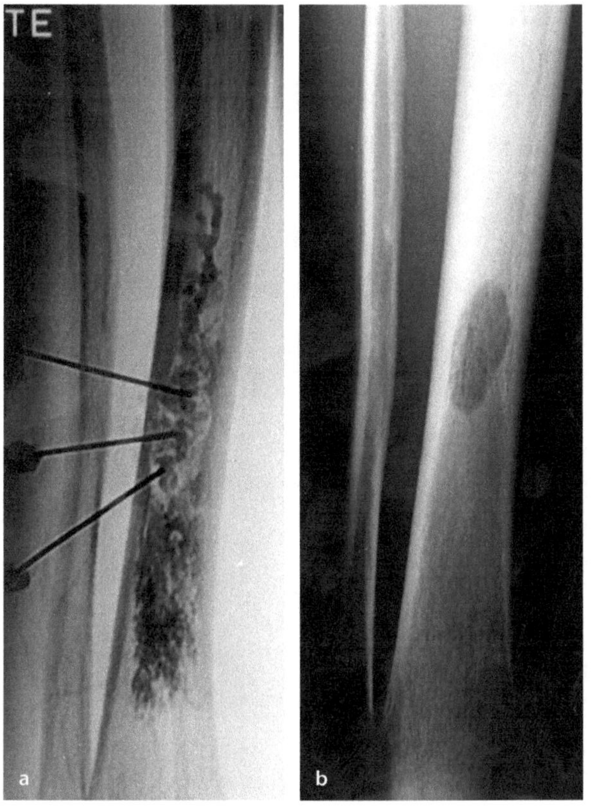

Fig. 15.10. **a** Tibia with osteolytic metastasis from a breast neoplasm. **b** Cementoplasty of the lesion with spread of the cement into the marrow

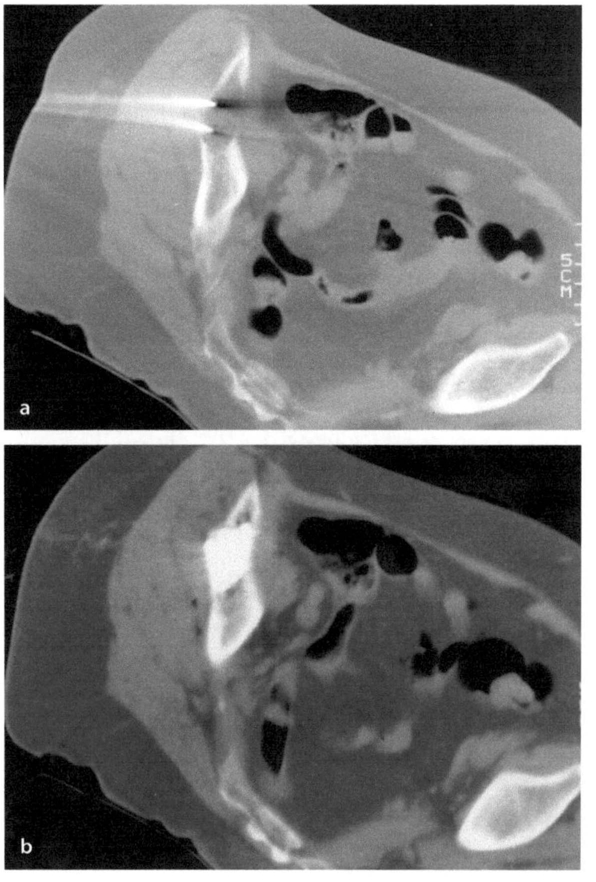

Fig. 15.11 a, b. Iliac wing with osteolytic metastasis from a renal neoplasm. Cementoplasty with two Escoffier needles

- For lytic zones in the limbs, the patient should be in the supine position and the technique undertaken with fine needles in the vascular radiology room, with the possibility of a 360° exploration field. If it becomes evident that the osteolytic zone is not well visualized by fluoroscopy, the procedure should be performed using CT scan (Fig. 15.10).
- For iliac wings, the patient is in the obliquely supine position and fine needles (18 gauge, 6 inch) are used under fluoroscopy plus scan (Fig. 15.11).
- For the acetabular region, the anterolateral approach should be taken with the patient in the supine position. If the osteolytic zone is relatively limited, an Escoffier needle of 10 or 14 gauge should be used. If the lesion is spread, 18 gauge, 6 inch needles will permit coverage of the entire osteolytic surface with minimal invasiveness (the number of needles placed can total up to 10 or 12; Fig. 15.12);
- For the pubic and obturator region, the patient is in the obliquely supine position, with an anterior approach and the use of fine needles (Fig. 15.13);
- For the ischium bone region, the patient is in the prone position, with fine needles used under fluoroscopy plus scanner.
- For the sacral wings, with bilateral and widespread lesions, the patient is in the prone position with 18 gauge, 6 inch needles used (Fig. 15.14). For extremely lateral lesions of the sacral wings, the trans-ilium homolateral approach is preferred with the patient in the supine position. It is very simple to perform and permits excellent preservation of the sacral nerves. An 18 gauge, 6 inch or 14 gauge Escoffier needle is chosen, depending on extension of the lesion.
- For the superior extremity of the femur, the vascular radiology room should be reserved if the lesion is visible, or CT scan should be used if it can not be seen on fluoroscopy. Patient position (prone or supine) and needle size should be chosen according to lesion location and size.
- For lesions of the femur head, the approach is transcervical with (a) 10 gauge Escoffier needle(s), and the patient in the obliquely supine position under fluoroscopy and scanner (Fig. 15.16).

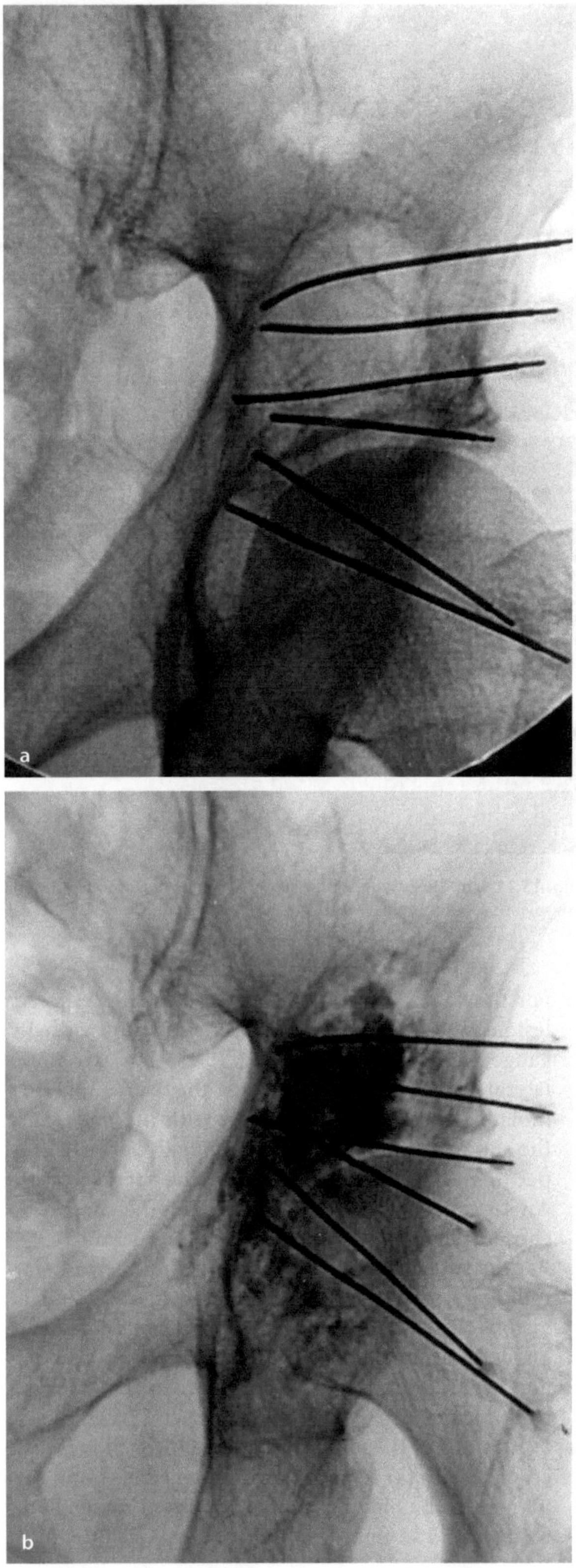

Fig. 15.12 a, b. Acetabular region metastasis of a gastric neoplasm. **a** Insertion of six 18 gauge needles and **b** nearly complete filling of the osteolytic area

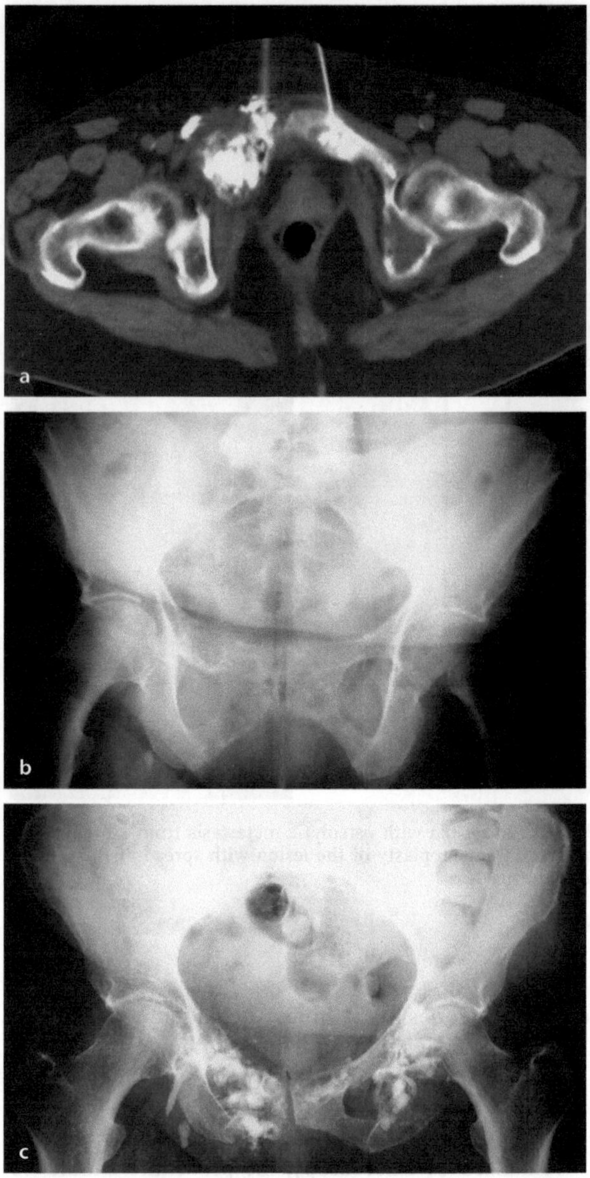

Fig. 15.13 a–c. Pubis with metastasis of a breast neoplasm. **a** CT-scan-guided cementoplasty procedure with 18 Gauge needles. **b** X-ray before and **c** after

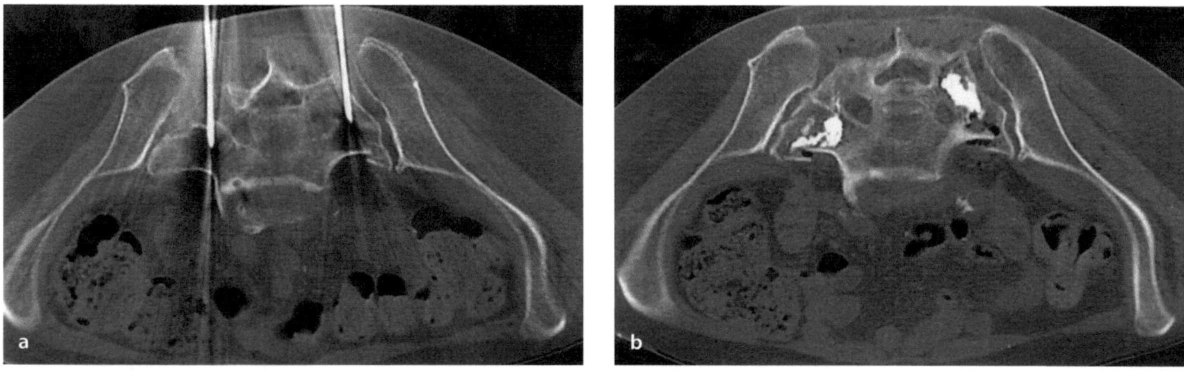

Fig. 15.14 a, b. Sacrum: cementoplasty with a double posterior approach of an osteoporotic fracture

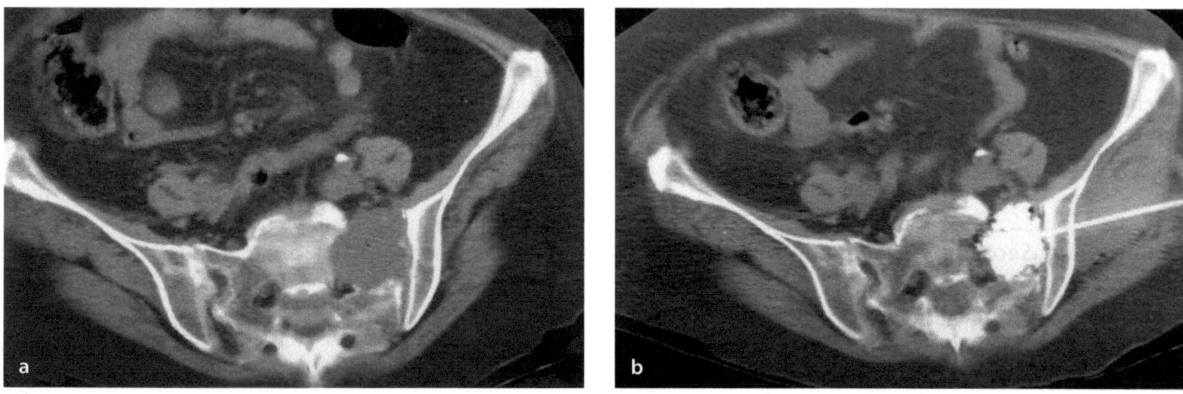

Fig. 15.15 a, b. Sacrum: transiliac approach. CT-scan-guided cementoplasty of a myeloma

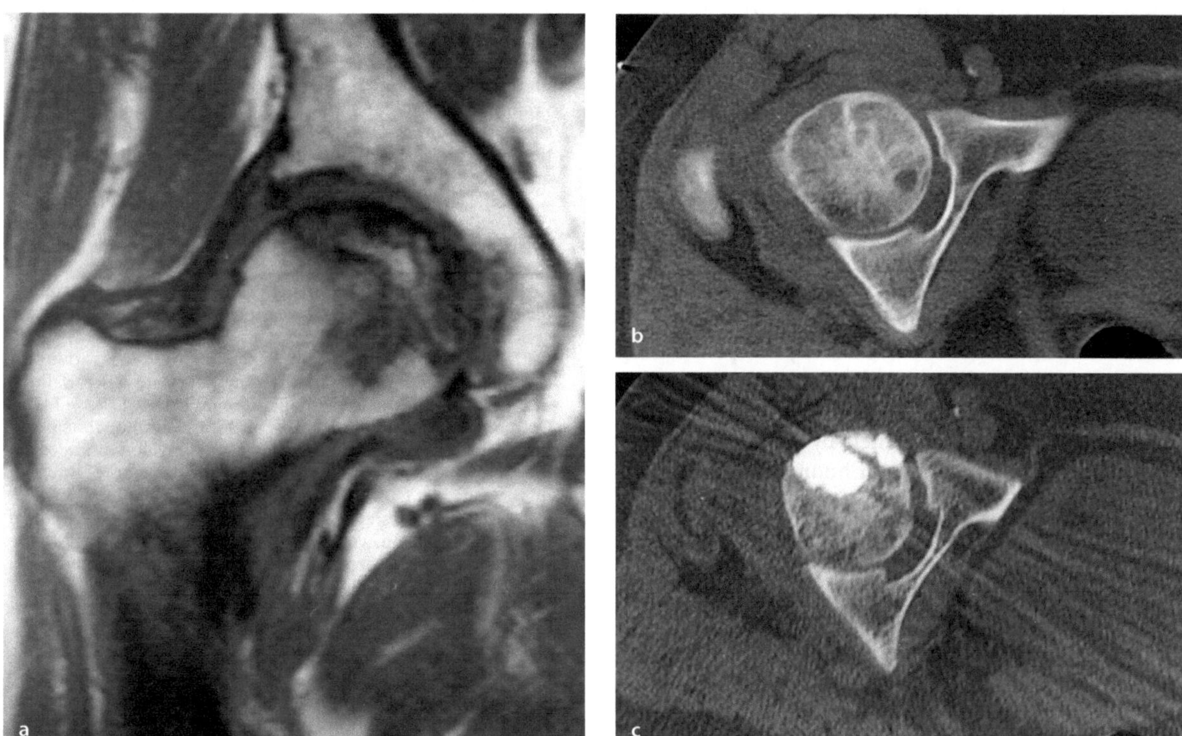

Fig. 15.16 a–c. Aseptic osteonecrosis of a right hip. **a** MRI picture before cementoplasty. **b** CT scan picture before cementoplasty and **c** after cementoplasty

Cement Injection

Cement is injected in the same way as in vertebroplasty. Polymerization time is adapted to needle caliber and lesion size as well as to the thickness of the preserved cortical bone. Cement of more viscous consistency (thick cement) is preferred if the lesion is close to the joint (particularly the acetabular roof). Most authors rotate the femur head during cement injection to limit the thickness of a small cement fragment that may eventually pass through the acetabular cartilage.

Scanography after cement injection assures proper control of successful filling of osteolytic zones (the average quantity of injected cement is 10 to 12 ml), particularly for pelvic bone lesions. Another important purpose of scanography is to look for any possible leakage outside the bone and to quantify it.

If bone biopsy is also required, the concentric tube system described for vertebroplasty can be completely adapted for percutaneous cementation. For deeper locations, such as the pelvis, longer sets are preferred.

Complications, Secondary Effects, and Surveillance

General complications are the same as in vertebroplasty. Complementary material can be found in references: [32, 34, 36, 42, 44]. Local complications are generally represented by cement leakage:

- Leakage in soft tissue occurs in 70% of cases without any evident clinical signs. In other cases, local pain could be due to local inflammatory reactions or compressive effect on a vasculonervous structure. This local pain generally disappears after lidocaine plus prednisolone infiltration;
- Cement leakage into the joints can be responsible for a rapid chondrolytic effect, but this complication is rare. Intra-articular injections of the local anesthetic/cortisone preparation are generally very effective.

Soft tissue hematomas are also reported (1%). They can be avoided if contraindications are respected.

Infections can be minimized by implementing rigorous aseptic conditions and using cement containing an antibiotic.

Secondary effects, represented by possible pain increase during the first couple of hours after the procedure, generally vanish with the administration of anti-inflammatory drugs.

Results

The efficacy of this procedure, subjectively assessed by remission of pain , is quantified by the reduced use of analgesics. Functional results are manifested by re-establishing the standing position and walking. The immobilization and hospitalization period is short, and it must be remembered that these patients generally do not expect to live much longer, and preventing decubitus complications is very important. Analgesia resulting from the procedure can be expected to appear 16 to 72 h thereafter. Percutaneous cementation can be practiced before, during or after the beginning of radiotherapy (which normally shows its effectiveness in pain relief later than cementation, namely, a week or two such treatment). The consolidation effect also appears later, after 2 or 3 months.

Conclusion

Percutaneous cementoplasty remains a palliative therapy in the majority of cases and permits significant amelioration of patient comfort by giving them the possibility of re-establishing their daily activities in a short period of time. Indications should be normally discussed and undertaken in multidisciplinary settings with the participation of pain therapists, oncologists, rheumatologists, surgeons, and radiologists.

References

Vertebroplasty

1. Bascoulergue Y, Duquesnel J, Leclercq R et al (1988) Percutaneous injection of methyl methacrylate in the vertebral body for the treatment of various diseases. Percutaneous vertebroplasty (abstract). Radiology 169:372
2. Centenera LV, Choi S, Hirsch JA (2000) Percutaneous vertebroplasty treats compression fractures. Diagn Imaging (San Franc) 22:147–148, 153
3. Chiras J, Cognard C, Rose M et al (1993) Percutaneous injection of an alcoholic embolizing emulsion as an alternative preoperative embolization for spine tumor. AJNR 14:1113–1117
4. Chiras J, Deramond H (1995) Complications des vertébroplasties. In: Saillant G, Laville C (eds) ƒchecs et complications de la chirurgie du rachis: Chirurgie de reprise. Sauramps Médical, Paris, pp 149–153
5. Cortet B, Cotten A, Deprez X, Deramond H (1994) Vertebroplasty with surgical decompression for the treatment of aggressive vertebral hemangiomas. Rev Rheum 61:14–21
6. Cotten A, Deramond H, Cortet B et al (1996) Preoperative percutaneous injection of methyl methacrylate and N-Butyl cyanoacrylate in vertebral hemangiomas. AJNR 17:137–142
7. Cotten A, Dewartre F, Cortet B et al (1996) Percutaneous vertebroplasty for osteolytic metastases and myeloma: effects of the percentage of lesion filling and the leakage of methylmethacrylate at clinical follow-up. Radiology 200:525–530
8. Debussche-Depriester C, Deramond H, Fardellone P et al (1991) Percutaneous vertebroplasty with acrylic cement in the treatment of osteoporotic vertebral crush fracture syndrome. Neuroradiology 33:149–152
9. Deramond H, Darrasson R, Galibert P (1989) Percutaneous vertebroplasty with acrylic cement in the treatment of aggressive spinal angiomas. Rachi 1:143–153
10. Deramond H, Depriester C, Toussain P (1996) Vertébroplastie et radiologie interventionnelle percutanée dans les métastases osseuses: technique, indications, contre indications. Bull Cancer Radiother 83:277–282

11. Galibert P, Deramond H (1990) La vertébroplastie percutanée comme traitement des angiomes vertébraux et des affections dolorigènes et fragilisantes du rachis. Chirurgie 116:326–335
12. Galibert P, Deramond H, Rosat P, Le gars D (1987) Note préliminaire sur le traitement des angiomes vertébraux par vertébroplastie acrylique percutanée. Neurochirurgie 33:166–168
13. Gangi A, Kastler BA, Dietemann JL (1994) Percutaneous vertebroplasty guided by a combination of CT and fluoroscopy. AJNR Am J Neuroradiol 15:83–86
14. Goltra D (2001) Vertebroplasty for osteoporotic compression fracture: effective treatment for a neglected disease. AJNR Am J Neuroradiol 22:595
15. Grados F, Depriester C, Cayrolle G et al (2000) Long-term observations of vertebral osteoporotic fractures treated by percutaneous vertebroplasty. Rheumatology (Oxf) 39:1410–1414
16. Hardouin P (1998) Place des biomatériaux et des techniques percutanées dans l'arsenal thérapeutique du rhumatologue. Rev Rhum [Ed Fr] 65:120S-121S
17. Heini PF, Walchli B, Berlemann U (2000) Percutaneous transpedicular vertebroplasty with PMMA: operative technique and early results. A prospective study for the treatment of osteoporotic compression fractures. Eur Spine J 9:445–450
18. Heuss JD, Doppman JL, Oldfield EH (1994) Brief report: relief of spinal cord compression from vertebral hemangioma by intra-lesional injection of absolute ethanol. N Engl J Med 331: 508–511
19. Jarvik JG, Deyo RA (2001) Vertebroplasty for osteoporotic compression fracture: effective treatment for a neglected disease. AJNR Am J Neuroradiol 22:594–595
20. Kaemmerlen P, Thiesse P, Jonas P et al (1989) Injection percutanée de ciment dans les vertèbres métastatiques. Presse Méd 18:983–984
21. Kaemmerlen P, Thiesse P, Jonas P et al (1989) Percutaneous injection of orthopedic cement in metastatic vertebral lesions. N Engl J Med 321:121
22. Lapras C, Mottolese C, Deruty R et al (1989) Injection percutanée de méthyl-méthacrylate dans le traitement de l'ostéoporose et l'ostéolyse vertébrale grave (technique de P. Galibert). Ann Chir 43:371–376
23. Levin SA, Perin LA, Hayes D, Hayes WS (2000) An evidence-based evaluation of percutaneous vertebroplasty. Manage Care 9:56–60, 63
24. Martin JB, Jean B, Sugiu K et al (1999) Vertebroplasty: clinical experience and follow-up results. Bone 25:11S-15S
25. Mathis JM, Barr JD, Belkoff SM et al (2001) Percutaneous vertebroplasty: a developing standard of care for vertebral compression fractures. AJNR Am J Neuroradiol 22:373–381
26. Maynard AS, Hensen ME, Schweickert PA et al (2000) Value of bone scan imaging in predicting pain relief from percutaneous vertebroplasty in osteoporotic vertebral fractures. AJNR Am J Neuroradiol 21:1807–1812
27. Murphy KJ, Deramond H (2000) Percutaneous vertebroplasty in benign and malignant disease. Neuroimaging Clin North Am 10:535–545
28. O'Brien JP, Sims JT, Evans AJ (2000) Vertebroplasty in patients with severe vertebral compression fractures: a technical report. AJNR Am J Neuroradiol 21:1555–1558
29. Peh WC, Gilula LA, Zeller D (2001) Percutaneous vertebroplasty: a new technique for treatment of painful compression fractures. Mo Med 98:97–102
30. Weil A, Chiras J, Simon JM et al (1996) Spinal metastases: Indications for and results of percutaneous injection of acrylic surgical cement. Radiology 199:241–247

Cementoplasty

31. Cotten A, Deprez X, Migaud H et al (1995) Malignant acetabular osteolyses: percutaneous injection of acrylic bone cement. Radiology 197:307–310
32. Cotten A, Duquesnoy B (1995) Percutaneous cementoplasty for malignant osteolysis of the acetabulum. Presse Med 24: 1308–1310
33. Cotten A, Bonnel F, Leblond D, Duquesnoy B (1998) Traitement local des ostéolyses malignes. Rev Rhum [Ed Fr] 65:122S-124S
34. Gangi A, Kastler BA, Dietemann JL (1994) Percutaneous vertebroplasty guided by a combination of CT and fluoroscopy. AJNR Am J Neuroradiol 15:83–86
35. Gangi A, Dietemann JL, Schultz A et al (1996) Interventional radiologic procedures with CT guidance in cancer pain management. Radiographics 16:1289–1304, discussion: 1304–1306
36. Gangi A, Guth S, Dietemann JL, Roy C (2001) Interventional musculoskeletal procedures. Radiographics 21:E1
37. Healey JH, Brown HK (2000) Complications of bone metastases. Cancer 88:2940–2951
38. Leclair A, Gangi A, Lacaze F et al (2000) Skeletal Radiol 29:275–278
39. Marcy PY, Palussière J, Magne N et al (2000) Percutaneous cementoplasty for pelvic bone metastasis. Support Care Cancer 8:500–503
40. Mercadante S (1997) Malignant bon pain: pathophysiology and treatment. Pain 69:1–18
41. Schocker JD, Brady LW (1982) Radiation therapy for bone metastasis. Clin Orthop 169:38–43
42. Stark A, Bauer HC (1996) Reconstruction in metastatic destruction of the acetabulum. Support rings and arthroplasty in 12 patients. Acta Orthop Scand 67:435–438
43. Takahashi I, Niibe H, Mitsuhashi N et al (1992) Palliative radiotherapy of bone metastasis. Adv Exp Med Biol 324:277–282
44. Weill A, Kobaiter H, Chiras J (1998) Acetabulum malignancies: technique and impact on pain of percutaneous injection of acrylic surgical cement. Eur Radiol 8:123–129

Aspiration and Lavage of Calcific Shoulder Tendinitis

16

Jean-Michel Lerais, Philippe Sarliève,
Georges Hadjidekov, Cyril Riboud, Bruno Kastler

Introduction and Pathophysiologic Characteristics

Calcific shoulder tendinitis or tondinopathy is a very common painful condition of the shoulder. These deposits are very rare before age 30 and after age 70 [15, 33, 40], but almost 20% of painful shoulders that occur between these ages are due to calcific deposits. They can in fact be found in 7–20% of individuals in this age group, the sex ratio women to men being 2:1. Asymptomatic calcifications are noted in 33–66% of cases, but 15–25% of them are bilateral and symptomatic [2]. Periarticular and soft tissue precipitations in tendons, bursae, ligaments, and capsules cause acute discomfort. Calcium can invade the joint to cause acute arthritis [20].

This disease is called in Europe apatite crystal deposition disease; that substance is the main mineral component of the skeleton [27, 29]. In the past (1965) Welfling et al. termed the condition "multiple calcifying tendinitis disease" [42]; today in the English literature it is called "hydroxyapatite deposition disease" (HADD) [38]. The calcium deposit appears dense, round with clearly defined margins without trabecular and cortical structure.

Symptomatic tendinous calcium deposits are mainly situated in the supraspinatus tendon (80–90%), but can also be found in those of the infraspinatus, subscapularis, and teres minor muscles. Atypical localizations have recently been seen in the bicipital groove (biceps brachialis, pectoralis major) and the deltoid tendon at its proximal insertion (Fig. 16.1) [10–24].

The exact pathogenesis of the apatite crystal formation in these sites is uncertain. Their appearance is considered idiopathic and not a degenerative change and they are assumed to be produced within avascular soft tissues [29]. The tissue hypoxia theory of Uthoff and Sarkar postulates a cyclic course of four stages. First local hypoxia creates a critical zone vulnerable to calcification. Then fibrocartilaginous metaplasia and necrosis replace tissue in this area followed by calcific deposit. A non-invasive resolution by resorption of calcium can be attempted (Fig. 16.2, subacromial bursa). Acute pain can be expected to accompany such an effort, but complete healing can occur (as in Fig. 16.2).

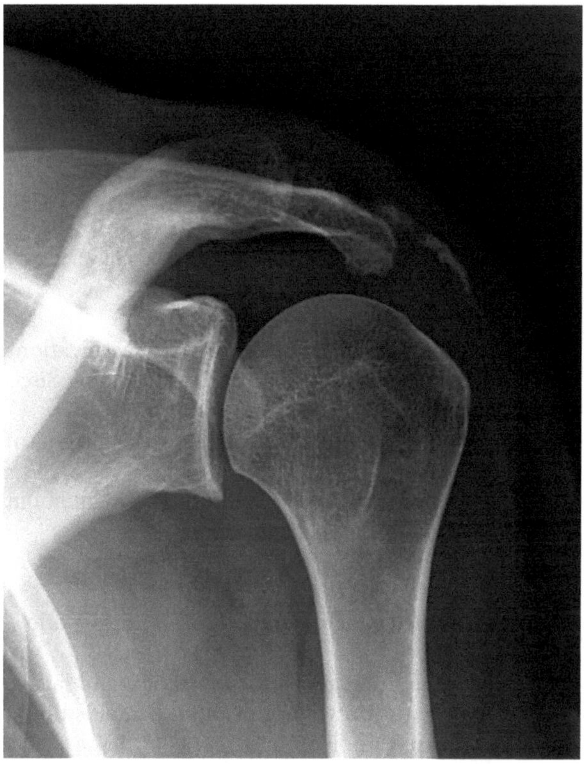

Fig. 16.1. Woman of 48 with chronic pain at night. Apatite calcification in deltoid tendon which is unusually located. A-L is successful while no change in size is seen after a year

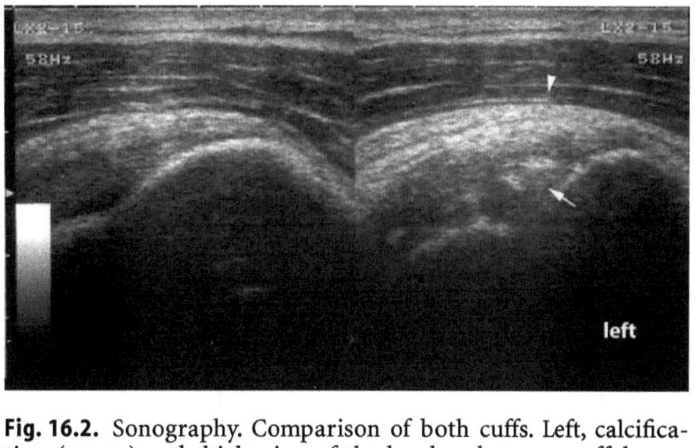

Fig. 16.2. Sonography. Comparison of both cuffs. Left, calcification (*arrow*) and thickening of the borders between cuff, bursa, and deltoid. There is an inflammatory bursa without liquid (*arrowhead*)

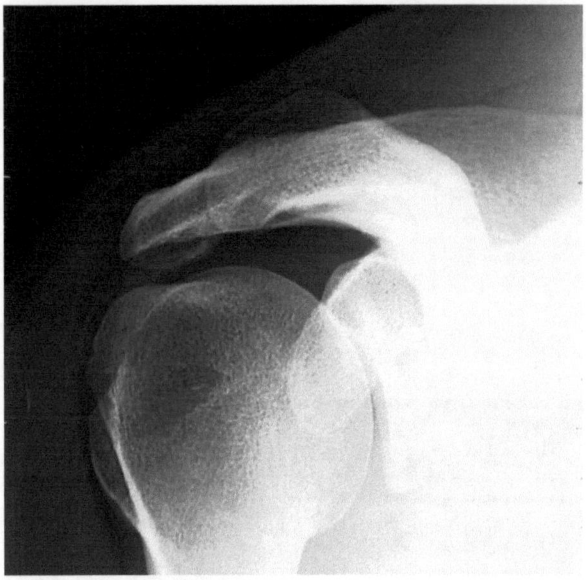

Fig. 16.3. Man of 47 with acute crisis, motion restricted. Calcification with fuzzy contours of the supraspinatus and tendency to evacuate into the subacromial bursa. Aspiration of milky liquid

Several calcific shoulder tendinopathy classifications have been proposed. We prefer the Arthroscopic Society's Mole classification [31]:

- A type; homogeneous with clearly defined margins of calcification
- B type: heterogeneous, polycyclic, or fragmented but with clearly defined calcific margins
- C type: heterogeneous without defined margins of calcification
- D type: calcified attachments to bone (enthesopathy).

A and B type are indications for aspiration and lavage (A-L). C type with fuzzy margins often contains liquid and is easy to aspirate (Fig. 16.3).

Aspiration of D type is not indicated because these calcifications are linear, thin, striated, and degenerative and cannot be aspirated. (Gartner's classification should be noted as being very similar to Mole's [28]).

Anatomy

Calcification is precisely located with X-ray views in different rotations. The supraspinatus tendon is seen with external rotation; those of the supraspinatus and infraspinatus are seen a with neutral position; the. posterior parts of the supraspinatus and infraspinatus tendons (as well those of teres minor and subscapularis) are localized with internal rotation(See Fig. 16.4).

Indications

While apatite calcifications are in most cases asymptomatic, when they cause either an acute inflammatory reaction or chronic and debilitating pain, treatment is indicated [2, 5, 19, 42].

Acute Inflammatory Reaction

Acute and relentless pain limits active and passive motions of the shoulder. The patient may be mildly febrile with inflammatory signs; septic arthritis must be excluded. X-ray is very useful because calcifications can be easily seen [27, 38]. The resorption of the deposit is fast and results in a heterogeneous and fuzzy appearance. Sometimes calcification appears in the subacromial-subdeltoid bursa within 7–21 days [27, 33, 36]. Radiological follow-up is then very useful.

Aspiration of calcified deposits was in the past – Flint (1913), Patterson (1937), then Welfling (1964) – introduced to cure acute crises. The aim is to give prompt and significant pain relief within 21–48 hours, when medical treatment is ineffective after 48–72 hours. According to our experience, only 10 to 20 % of cases require treatment in the acute phase.

There is no study in the literature about the exact place of A-L for the acute inflammatory crisis.

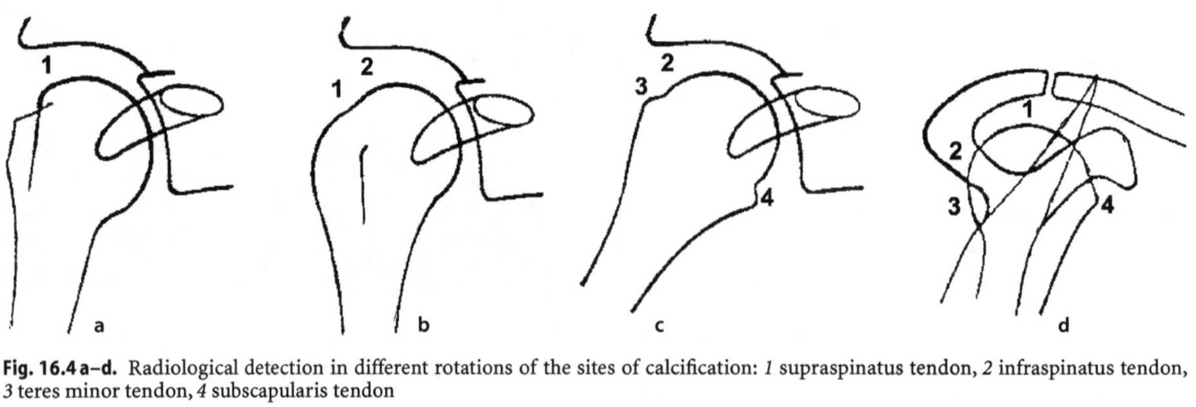

Fig. 16.4 a–d. Radiological detection in different rotations of the sites of calcification: *1* supraspinatus tendon, *2* infraspinatus tendon, *3* teres minor tendon, *4* subscapularis tendon

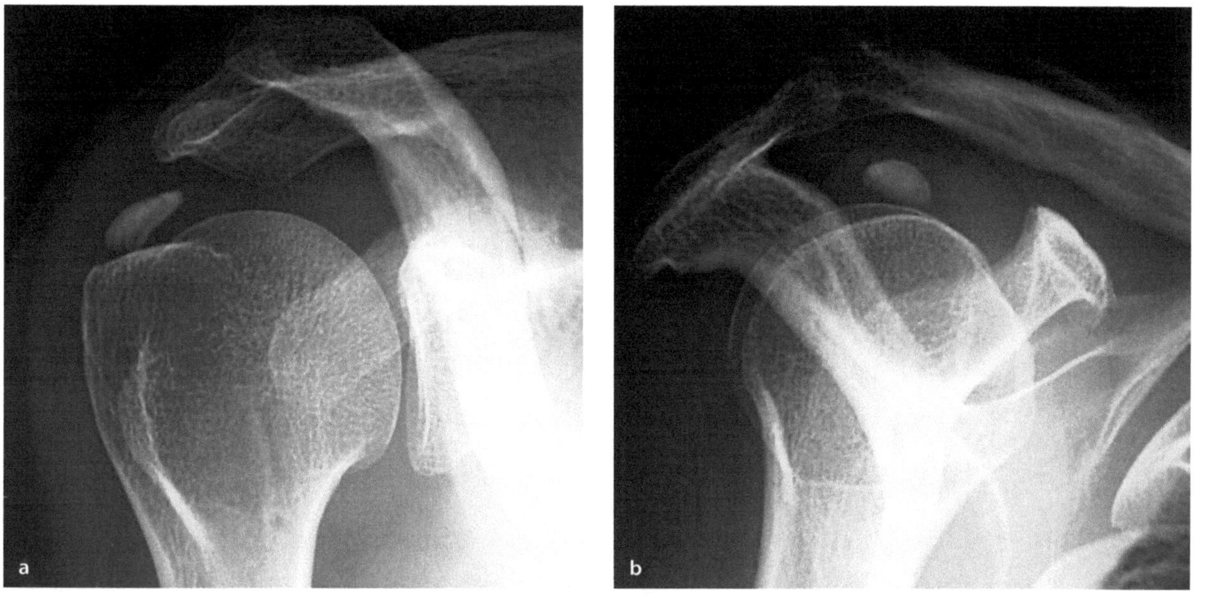

Fig. 16.5 a, b. woman of 38. Chronic night pain. Large A type calcification of the supraspinatus tendon

Chronic Pain

In almost 80–90% of the cases A-L is indicated for chronic shoulder pain of more than 3 month's duration [12, 32]. Clinical tests are made to check that the tendon is symptomatic and to exclude an impingement syndrome, which can lead to failure of the treatment in almost 25% of the cases [34]. The impingement reduces motion in certain types of movement with a painful ache, but without night pain [35].

But this distinction is often difficult because the calcification itself causes what might be called an impingement syndrome. Lavage of the subacromial bursa associated with the calcification relieves the pain temporarily [33].

Besides not being a degenerative calcification, apatite calcification doesn't involve a rotator cuff tear [2, 5, 42], although other authors believe it does and must be systematically looked for [22, 23]. Because the technique establishes the distinction, we always use static and dynamic US study (according to JL Brasseur [8]) rather than the sometimes confusing MRI.

The number, size, contours, superficial or deep situation of the calcifications are noted as well as location in the tendon. All these items will be compared with X-ray plain films. A calcification larger than 5 mm in diameter with size and shape show no change on successive standard films is a good indication for treatment [35].

Sometimes sonography shows a bursa with thick echogenic walls (greater than 2 mm). This indicates an inflammatory bursa (Fig. 16.2) for which lavage is beneficial.

If there is liquid in the subacromial bursa it is important to look for liquid in the sheath surrounding the biceps brachialis tendon, for its presence here as well as in the bursa signifies a complete rotator cuff tear [8].

For some, a partial tear of the deep surface of the supraspinatus tendon doesn't contraindicate A-L, nor does glenohumeral arthritis [1]. We, however, don't think A-L is a good treatment in such cases. According to Farin loss of echogenic shadow behind a calcification indicates that it is rather soft [17]. But apatite calcifications don't actually have an echogenic shadow, even when they are large. It is impossible to know their consistency in advance.

Solid indications for A-L are in summary:

- Age 55 or below
- Chronic night pain for 2–3 years
- Range of motion not restricted
- Calcification types A B more than 1.5 mm in diameter of the supra- or infraspinatus tendon(Figs. 16.5–16.7)
- Sonography shows no complete tear.

In case many calcifications exist, these further criteria may help select the one most requiring treatment:

- Clinical and sonographic evidence with pain during the sonographic procedure
- Larger calcification
- Tendon edema (Figs. 16.8, 16.9) [1, 35].

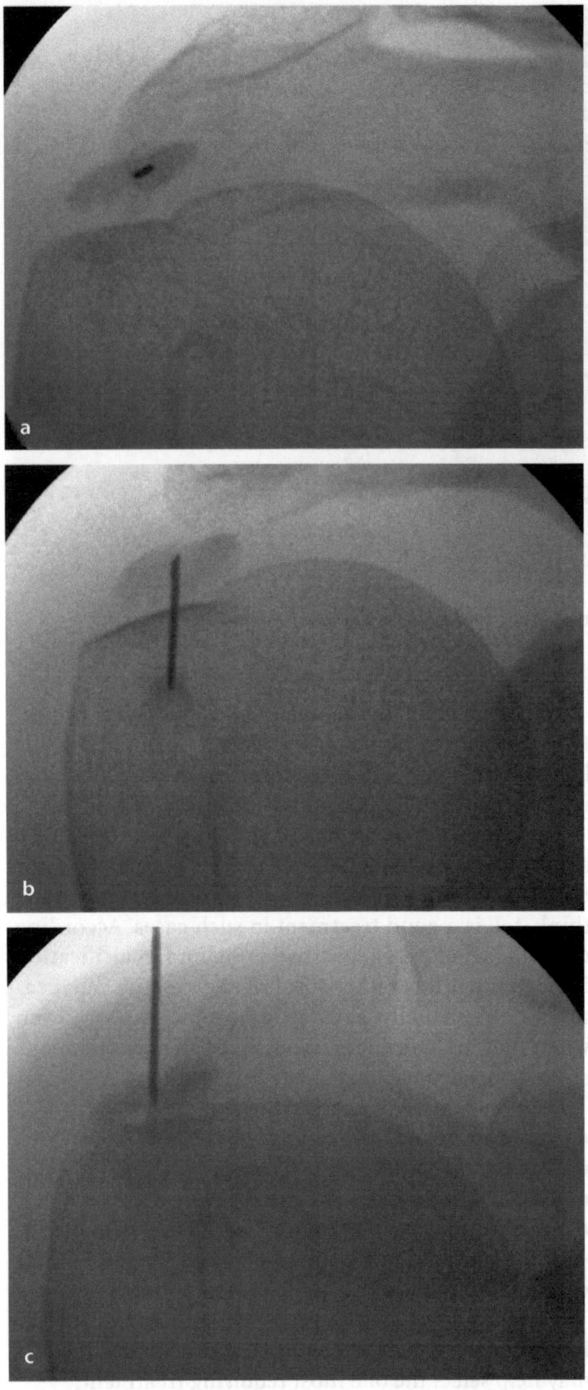

Fig. 16.6 a–c. Same patient, aspiration, fluoroscopic procedure. If correctly placed the needle tip will remain within the calcification when the X-ray beam is tilted in maximal cephalad and caudal directions

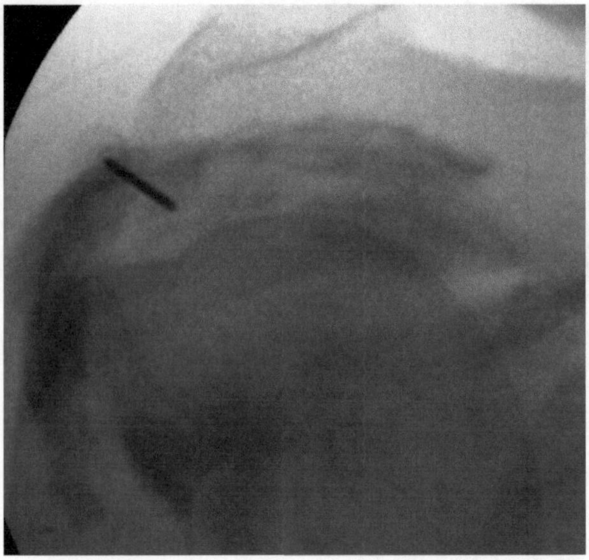

Fig. 16.7. Same patient, bursography after lavage. Calcification is no longer visible

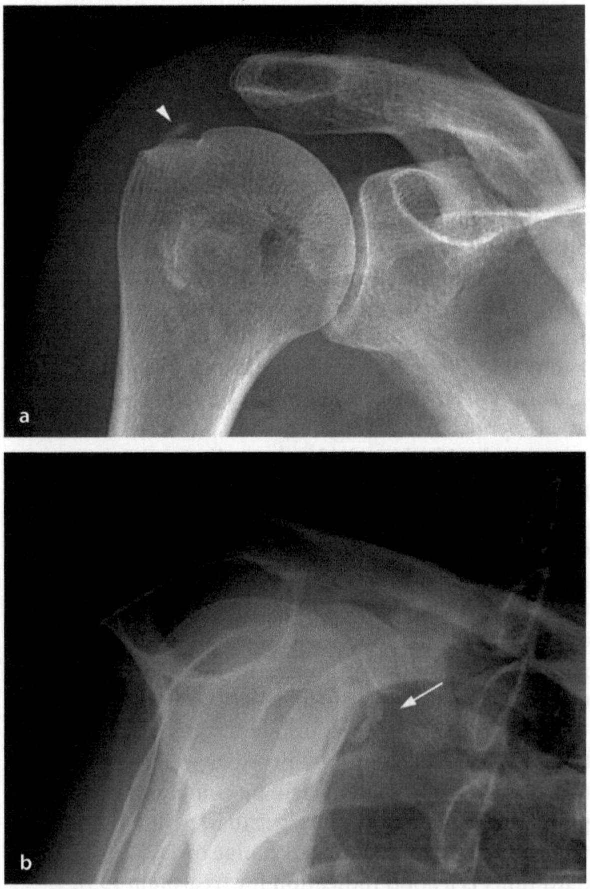

Fig. 16.8 a, b. Man of 38, chronic night pain. There are several calcifications, the smallest, A type is situated in the supraspinatus (*arrowhead*). The largest, B type is in the subscapularis (*arrow*). However, clinical tests and sonography show that the one located in the supraspinatus tendon was painful. Aspiration is successful

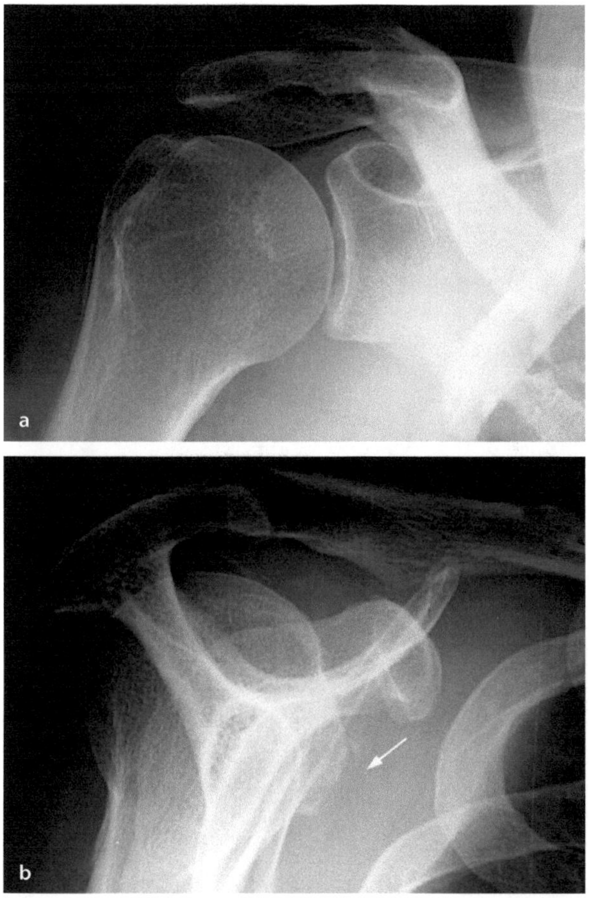

Fig. 16.9 a, b. Same case; Follow-up 2 years after treatment. Supraspinatus calcification has disappeared, subscapularis calcification has decreased in size and is asymptomatic

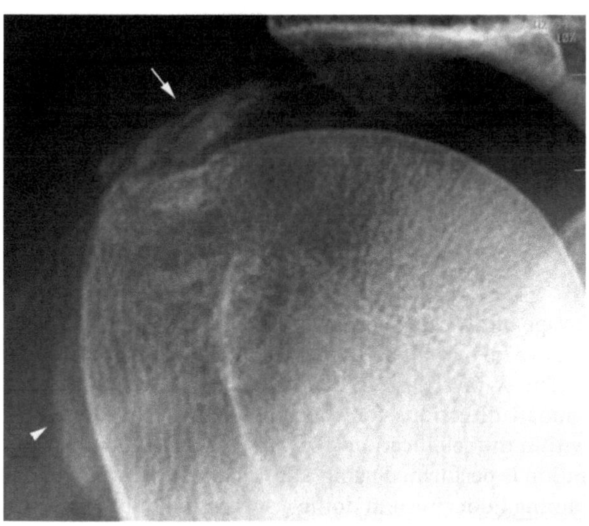

Fig. 16.10. Woman of 36, chronic pain. Large, B type calcification of the supraspinatus tendon (*arrow*). Calcification of the subacromial bursa (*arrowhead*)

Contraindications

Idiopathic Adhesive Capsulitis

Also called "frozen shoulder syndrome," this is characterized by insidious progressive restriction of passive motions. The average incidence of the condition in the general population is 2–3 % [3] but it is more frequent in diabetes mellitus. Passive external rotation is specifically restricted. X-rays and CT scan are normal. At an early stage MRI shows post-gadolinium enhancement of the joint capsule and synovial membrane in the rotator space and in the axillary recess (subscapularis bursa, coracohumeral ligament). Bone marrow edema of the humeral head is also seen. This pattern seems to be specific for inflammation and increased skin temperature [33]. Later on in the disease process, there is no more inflammation or synovial abnormality but only fibrosis and capsulitis, appearing like Dupuytren's contracture on arthroscopy [9, 43]. In most cases adhesive capsulitis is idiopathic, affecting post-menopausal women and diabetics (36% of the latter) [9]. Arthrography is the only means of making the diagnosis. It usually shows a reduced articular capacity (less than 10 ml), although sometimes the volume is almost normal and the diagnosis is difficult. Reflex sympathetic dystrophy (algodystrophy) and adhesive capsulitis are very similar and it is no use lavaging and aspirating calcifications in such cases because the stiffness doesn't change. Distension arthrography must be undertaken [33].

Associated Rotator Cuff Tear

This is uncommon, but when it does occur, only arthroscopic or open surgery are useful [23]. Thus, rotator cuff tear must be ruled out before A-L is attempted. In our experience, if a young woman is afflicted with a calcification and sonography is normal we don't use another imaging method. But if A-L doesn't give a good result we have in the past proceeded with CT scan-arthrography because sonography might be in error regarding the diagnosis of partial tear of the tendon [13].

Coagulopathies

A-L with milder antithrombotic agents such as aspirin is allowed [30], but antivitamin K agents must be stopped 3 days before the procedure, and treatment with heparin used as a temporary replacement [30]. In accord with Thumbo et al. [40] and Gorgona et al. [21] we think it possible to make intra-articular and periarticular punctures even if the INR is over 4–5 without complications. Only a slight articular hemorrhage has been described, before the puncture [21]. If the patient is under heparin or low-molecular-weight heparin (HBPM), the morning injection is not given and A-L is performed just before the other injection with an interval of 12 hours when the drug's activity is very low [26].

C and D Type Calcifications

These are degenerative, linear, granular calcifications within the tendons and entheses. They can neither be aspirated nor disintegrated. A lavage of the subacromial bursa may be considered, however.

Technique

Materials and Methods

Forty-nine shoulders of 40 consecutive patients (30 women, 10 men) with chronic (35) or acute (5) shoulder pain were treated. Deposits were situated in the supraspinatus (36) or infraspinatus tendon (4), larger than 5 mm in 15, smaller in 25, but all larger than 1.5 mm in diameter. Thirty-eight patients were improved, with (12) or without (26) disappearance of the calcification. Continued presence of deposits has not been systematically followed.

Clinical and X-ray Diagnosis

The most important selection criteria have been worsening of pain at night and isometric tests such as the Jobe test.

Plain film diagnostic views have included antero-posterior, internal, neutral, and external rotations, and a subacromial lateral Lamy view.

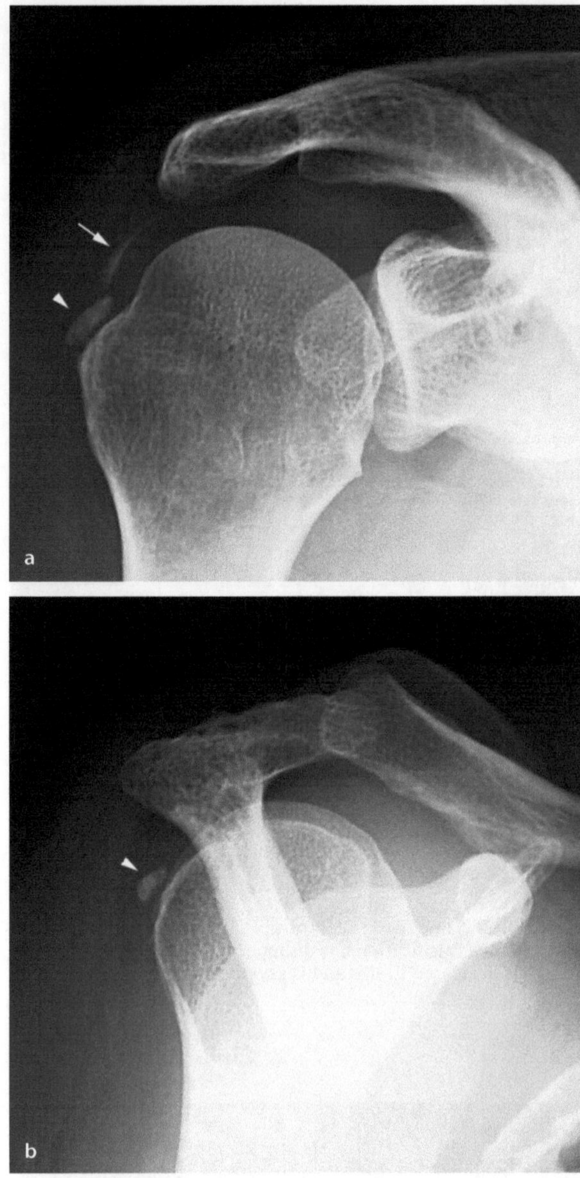

Fig. 16.11 a, b. Woman of 35, chronic pain. Infraspinatus tendon A type calcification. Internal and profile views show the calcium deposit (*arrowhead*). Thin calcification of the subacromial bursa (*arrow*)

Needle Placement

A direct antero-posterior approach under fluoroscopic guidance is used with the patient is in supine position, even if the calcification is behind the great tuberosity (Figs. 16.11, 16.12) [12, 32, 35]. A US-guided technique has also been described using 22 or 25 gauge needles [1, 16, 18]. With X-ray beam centered vertically, aseptic conditions obligatory, a 20 or 21 gauge needle is inserted to the center of the calcification. We don't use bigger needles (e.g., 14–18 gauge) because of concern for tendon rupture upon repeated puncture [1, 33]. We don't use simultaneous placement of two needles in the tendon for calcification lavage because of lack of better results even with large calcifications [11]. We use 15–20 ml or more of lidocaïne, 0.5% or 1%, for local anesthetic lavage of the calcification and bursa. A syringe of 1.5 ml cortivazol or 1 ml bethamethasone is locally injected.

The X-ray beam is tilted in maximal cephalad and caudad directions for checking that the needle tip is within the calcification (Figs. 16.6, 16.12). Calcium aspiration is performed using a 20 cc Luer-lock syringe containing lidocaine and doing a succession of propulsions and suctions with the syringe piston. The goal is to fragment the granulomatous calcific deposit and thus facilitate its resorption.

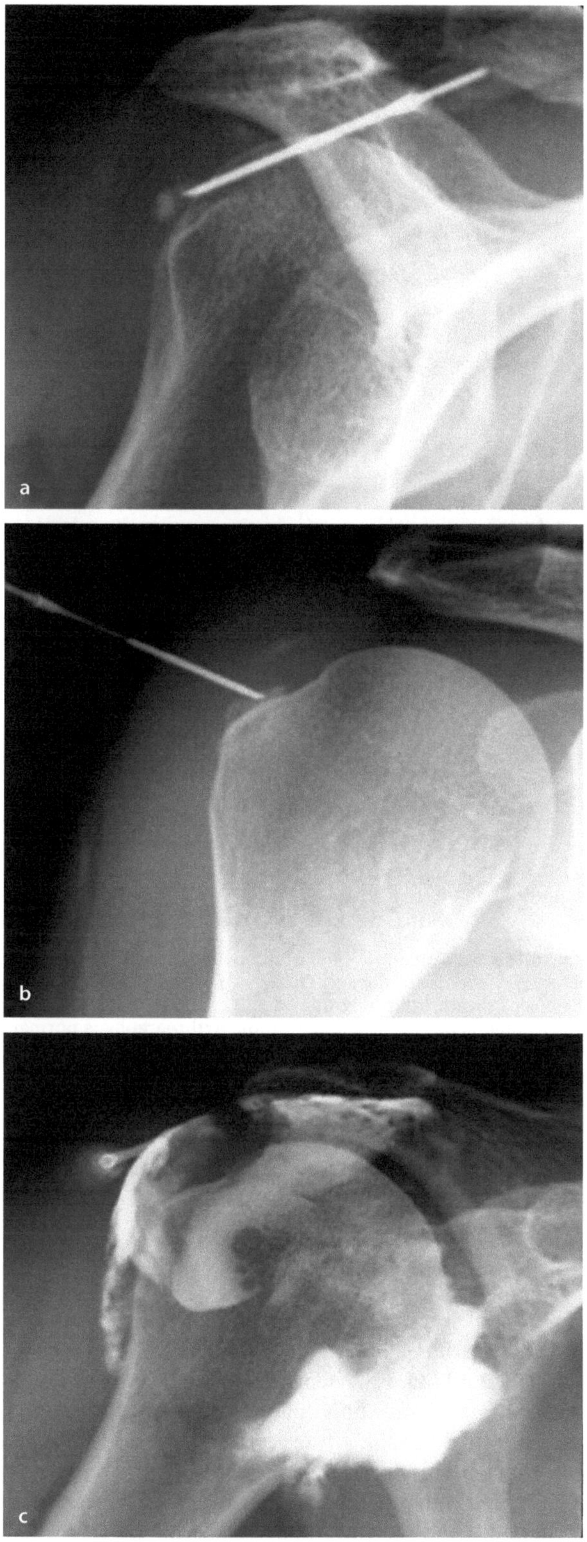

Fig. 16.12 a–c. Same patient. **a** Direct anterior approach although the calcification is posterior. **b** Lateral stereotaxic views. **c** Bursography

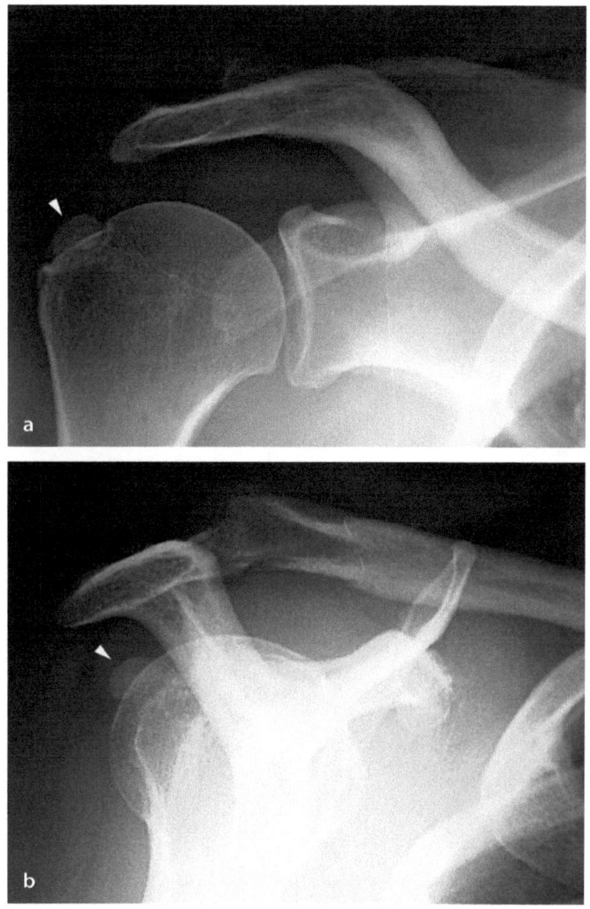

Fig. 16.13 a, b. Woman of 54, chronic pain. Infraspinatus A type large calcification (*arrowhead*). Erosion of the great tuberosity

Sometimes aspirated calcium appears in the syringe as a white cloudy milk. More often the calcification has a hard consistency and no calcium can be aspirated. Grinding and washing the calcific deposit in order to obtaining a decrease of its radiological density, or a hole within it, accelerates the process of spontaneous resorption (Figs. 16.13, 16.14) [35].

Half of the corticosteroid is injected within and around the calcification. Aspiration of large amounts of calcium and secondary resorption of calcification on plain films were found to be significantly associated with good clinical results [32, 34].It is not essential to remove the calcium deposit entirely. But it is important to open the calcium-containing cavity, create a communication with the bursa, and wash the inflammatory proteins [35].

Lavage of the bursa with lidocaïne ends the procedure. The needle is withdrawn and easily placed into the subacromial bursa, which is more superficial. Then, after making a bursography, the second half of the corticosteroid is injected into the bursa (Figs. 16.11–16.15).

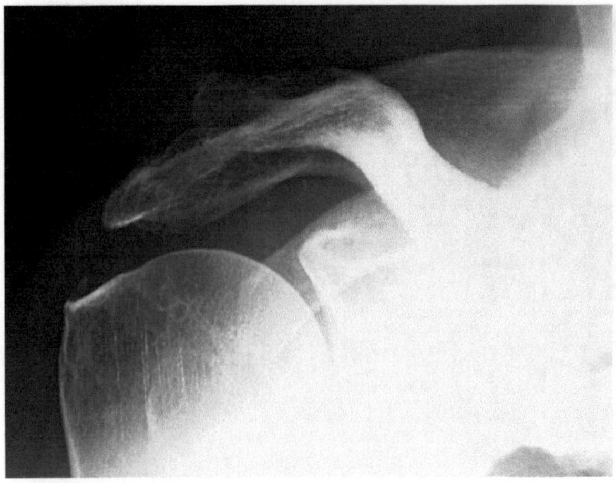

Fig. 16.14. Same patient. Follow-up at 3 months. The calcification has disappeared. Good clinical result

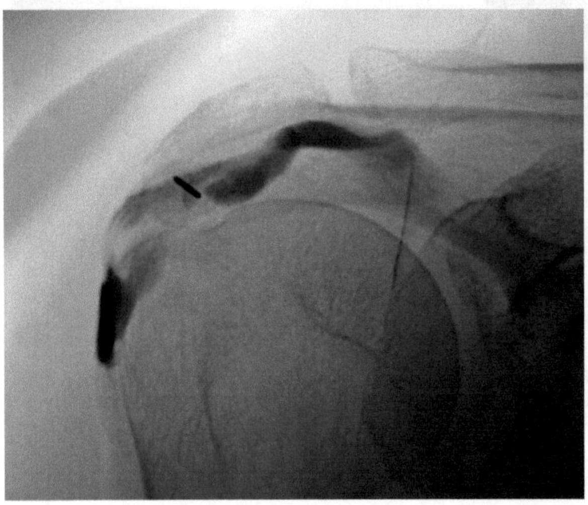

Fig. 16.15. Bursography

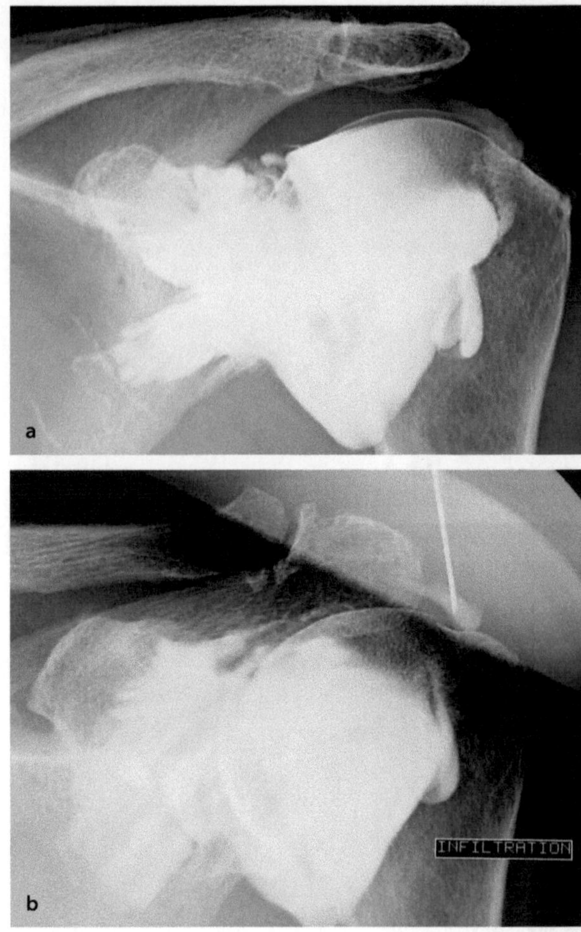

Fig. 16.16 a, b. Woman of 69, chronic pain. Exhaustive check-up before A-L because of the age. There is an excess of liquid around the biceps sheath, but sonography doesn't show a rotator cuff tear. Supraspinatus B type large calcification. Arthrography is normal. A-L in the same session, good clinical result

Follow-up

In one third of cases a painful reaction follows the procedure [4, 18, 34] caused by resorption of the calcification. This is managed with local application of ice, prescription of antalgics and non steroidal anti-inflammatory agents. It lasts rarely more than 2–4 days, more often 24 hours [11, 35]. In most cases, patients are immediately improved with lidocaine, and later the pain disappears, first at night then during the day.

The shoulder should be kept at rest for at least 2 days; we have found that a bandage or orthopedic device is not necessary for this. We take additional plain X-rays only if the patient is not improved. If a second session is required we make use of CT arthrography or MRI (Fig. 16.16).

Complications

Septic Risk

The risk of infection is no greater than for any other articular, periarticular, or foraminal injections (reportedly 1:77,300) [25, 39]. Aseptic protocol includes use of a surgical mask and only one passage of the needle through the skin [25]. While reports of septic complications have been effectively nonexistent in the literature, special care must be taken with those at high risk such as diabetics and immunosuppressed patients. Of course the skin should be scrubbed as free from contamination as possible, but puncture through the skin is not the only mechanism of sepsis. Oral corticosteroids can cause immunosuppression and thus increase the risk of hematogenic infection. In the study of David-Chausse

59 of 1,080 septic arthritis cases occurred during oral corticotherapy and 11 when immunosuppressors were given, all 70 without local injection [14].

Exacerbation of pain occurs in about one third of the patients and usually means resorption of calcium deposit (for treatment see above).

Secondary Rotator Cuff Tear

There is theoretical risk of perforation of the rotator cuff. This risk is directly correlated with needle diameter, and so the tendency is to decrease the size of the needles. We use 21 gauge (as also advocated by Brasseur [7]). Others use 22 gauge or even 25 gauge if the calcification is quite small [1].

Only one patient in our experience has incurred a full thickness (thin; 2 mm) tear, and it was not clear that this was a result of the procedure, quite possibly having been already present. One should not hesitate to investigate shoulders of patients who show no improvement with CT arthrography or MRI.

Side Effects

Some vague discomforts have been described that are difficult to ascribe to A-L. The procedure is generally well tolerated and painless.

Results

Pain relief appears at the end of the first week in 60–70% of cases, is maximized during the second week [11], and after a month the results can be considered as established. No increase of pain has been noted. A second session can be tried after 4 to 6 weeks (or even earlier on the 15th day) if the improvement is considered unsatisfactory.

If the calcification has disappeared, it exceptionally comes back in situ. But about 20% of patients will have recurrence of pain within two years because calcification has not disappeared but persisted. They are candidates for repeat aspiration and lavage.

Long term results judged good to excellent were achieved in 66% to 90% of cases, while 6% were unchanged [1, 11, 18, 32, 35, 37].

Comparison Between A-L and Arthroscopic Excision

See Table 16.1. Arthroscopy does not provide a useful approach for completely removing calcification [1, 12], although opening the calcium-containing cavity facilitates its resorption. But reduction in size and density of calcification is a good indicator of successful treatment, which occurs in 56% of cases [18, 35]. This frequency is superior to its spontaneous disappearance (5.4% after 3 years, Bosworth [5], 30% after 4 years Noel [33])

The technique of A-L is easy, less painful than arthroscopic resection, and the adhesive capsulitis rate is the same [6].

The cost of aspiration and lavage is lower and general anesthesia is not needed.

Associated techniques are possible at arthroscopy (synovectomy, acromioplasty, resection of coraco-acromial ligament) but they are rarely useful if the indications were clearly established [4].

Conclusion

When the calcium crystal holds out against medical treatment and becomes chronic A-L may be attempted. It is a safe technique with a low rate of complications, and morbidity is almost nil. Two sessions are sufficient. Healing or significant clinical improvement is noted in 75% of cases at 5 years follow-up. Fluoroscopic guidance, which even with newer improvements involves a

Table 16.1. Comparison between A-L and arthroscopy

	A-L	Arthroscopy
Good clinical results	70–90% at 12 months	Up to 90% at 12 months
Calcification's disappearance	50%	Up to 80%
Failures	6% at 5 years	5% at 1 year
Guidance	Fluoroscopy or sonography	Fluoroscopy or sonography
Irradiation	+	0
Pain after the procedure	A few days	A few weeks
Complications	Adhesive capsulitis : 1–3 %	Adhesive capsulitis : 2%
Cost	+	+++
Anesthesia	local	general

certain radiation exposure, may be replaced by sonography. Ultrasonography is accurate for depict and localizing calcification even though the internal structure and density of calcium crystals can't be seen.

The long term results of aspiration and lavage and arthroscopy are the same but aspiration and lavage is the easier route to take.

References

1. Aina R, Cardinal E, Bureau N et al (2001) Calcific shoulder tendinitis: treatment with modified US-guided fine-needle technique. Radiology 2:455–461
2. Amor B, Cherot A, Delbarre F (1977) Le rhumatisme à hydroxyapatite (la maladie des calcifications tendineuses multiples). Rev Rhum 44:301–316
3. Anton HA (1993) Frozen shoulder. Can Fam Physician 39: 1773–1777
4. Bard H, Vigneron AM (2000) Traitements physiques externes des tendinopathies calcifiantes. In: de Seze †, Ryckewaert A, Kahn MF et al (eds) L'Actualité rhumatologique. Elsevier, Paris, pp 437–449
5. Bosworth BM (1941) Calcium deposits in the shoulder and subacromial bursitis. A survey of 122 shoulders. JAMA 116: 2477–2482
6. Boyer T (1993) Traitement arthroscopique des calcifications de l'épaule. In: de Sèze, Ryckewaert A, Kahn MF et al (eds) L'Actualité rhumatologique 1993. Expansion Scientifique Française, Paris, pp 311–318
7. Brasseur JL (1997) Note technique: ponction des calcifications de l'épaule. Sixième Journée d'Imagerie Ostéo-Articulaire de la Pitié-Salpétrière. Paris, 10–11 oct 1997
8. Brasseur JL, Tardieu M (1999) Échographie du système locomoteur. In: Blery M (ed) Collection d'Imagerie radiologique. Masson, Paris
9. Bunker TD, Anthony PP (1995) The pathology of frozen shoulder: a Dupuytren like disease. J Bone Joint Surg 77:677–683
10. Chadwick CJ (1989) Tendinitis of the pectoralis major insertion with humeral lesions. J Bone Joint Surg 71:816–818
11. Chevrière A, Carlier RY, Feydy A et al (2000) Ponction-rétrospective de 50 périarthrites traitées. J Radiol 81:971–974
12. Comfort TH, Arafiles RP (1978) Barbotage of the shoulder with image intensified fluoroscopic control of needle placement for calcific tendonitis. Clin Orth Rel Res 135:171–178
13. Dardel P, Jacob D, Lerais JM et al (2002) Analyse comparée échographie-IRM dans les ruptures de la coiffe des rotateurs. GETROA, Paris, 21 oct 2002: JFR
14. David-Chaussé J, Dehais J, Boyer M et al (1981) Les infections articulaires chez l'adulte. Atteintes périphériques et vertébrales à germes banals et bacilles tuberculeux. Rev Rhum 48:69–76
15. Dryll A, Bardin TH (1989) Rôle pathogène des microcristaux d'apatite. Press Méd 18:564–565
16. Farin PU (1996) Consistency of rotator cuff calcifications. Observations on plain radiograph, sonography, computed tomography and at needle treatment. Invest Radiol 31:300–304
17. Farin PU, Jaroma H, Soimakallio S (1995) Rotator cuff calcifications: treatment with US-guided technique. Radiology 195: 841–843
18. Farin PU, Rasanen H, Jaroma H, Harju A (1996) Rotator cuff calcifications treatment with ultrasound-guided percutaneous needle aspiration and lavage. Skeletal Radiol 25:551–554
19. Flint J (1913) Acute traumatic subdeltoid bursitis. A new and simple treatment. JAMA 19:1224–1225
20. Fritz P, Bravo, Bardin TH (1998) Maladie des dépôts extra-articulaires d'apatite. In: Laredo JD (ed) Imagerie ostéo-articulaire. Pathologie générale. Flammarion, Médecine-Sciences, Paris, pp 531–536
21. Gorgona M, Waterman J (1998) Arthritis and Rheum 41 [Suppl]:S234
22. Hsu HC, Wu JJ, Jim YF et al (1994) Calcific tendonitis and rotator cuff tearing: a clinical and radiographic study. J Shoulder Elbow Surg 3:159–164
23. Jim YF, Hsu HC, Chang CY et al (1993) Cœxistence of calcific tendonitis and rotator cuff tear: an arthrographic study. Skeletal Radiol 22:183–185
24. Kraemer EJ, El-Khoury GY (2000) Atypical calcific tendinitis with cortical erosions. Skeletal Radiol 29:690–696
25. Lavie F, Rozenberg S, Bourgeois P (2002) Complications sévères au décours d'infiltrations rachidiennes de corticoïdes. In: de Seze †, Ryckewaert A, Kahn et al (eds) L'actualite rhumatologique. Elsevier, Paris, pp 293–303
26. Lemaire V, Charbonnier B, Gruel Y et al (2002) Antiagrégants, anticoagulants et infiltrations: comment faire? Rev Rhum 69:8–11
27. Liote F, Fritz P (1997) Rhumatisme apatitique, aspects particuliers. Ann Radiol 40:56–60
28. Loew M, Daecke W, Kusnierczak D et al (1999) Shock wave therapy is effective for chronic calcifying tendonitis of the shoulder. J Bone Joint Surg 81B:863–867
29. Malghem J, Vandeberg B, Lecouvet F et al (2002) Arthropathies microcristallines. In: Imagerie du pied et de la cheville. Sauramps Médical, GETROA, pp 221–237
30. Mejjad O, Favre S (1997) Anticoagulants et anti-agrégants plaquettaires: l'infiltration est-elle possible et comment? Lettre Rhumatol 237:12–13
31. Mole D, Kempf JF, Gleyze P et al (1993) Société Française d'Arthroscopie. Résultats du traitement arthroscopique des tendinopathies non rompues de la coiffe des rotateurs. Rev Chir Orthop 79:532–541
32. Moutounet J, Chevrot A, Godefroy D et al (1984) Ponction infiltration radioguidée dans le traitement des périarthrites calcifiantes rebelles d'épaule. J Radiol 65:569–572
33. Noël E (1997) Le traitement des tendinopathies calcifiantes et de la rétraction capsulaire de l'épaule. Rev Rhum 705–715
34. Normandin C, Seban E, Laredo JD et al (1988) Aspiration of tendinous calcific deposits. In: Bard M, Laredo JD (eds) Interventionnal radiology in bone and joints. Springer, Berlin Heidelberg New York, pp 270–285
35. Parlier-Cuau C, Champsaur P, Nizard R et al (1998) Percutaneous treatments of painful shoulder. Radiol Clin North Am 36:589–596
36. Patterson RL (1937) Treatment of acute bursitis by needle irrigation. J Bone Joint Surg 19:993
37. Pfister J, Gerber H (1994) Treatment of calcific humero-scapular periarthropathy using needle irrigation of the shoulder: retrospective study. Z Orthop Ihre Grenzgeb 132:300–305
38. Resnick D (1995) Calcium hydroxyapatite crystal deposition disease. In: Resnick D, Niwayama G (eds) Diagnosis of bone and joint disorders, 3rd edn. Saunders, New York, pp 1615–1648
39. Seror P, Pluvinage P, Lecocq d'Andre F et al (1999) Frequency of sepsis after local corticosteroid injection. Rheumatology 38:1272–1274
40. Thumboo J, O'Duffy JD (1998) A prospective study of the safety of joint and soft tissue aspirations and injections in patients taking warfarin sodium. Arthritis Rheum 41:736–739
41. Uhthoff HK, Sarkar K (1989) Calcifying tendinitis. Clin Rheumatol 3:567–581
42. Welfling J, Kahn MF, Desroy M et al (1965) Les calcifications de l'épaule. La maladie des calcifications tendineuses multiples. Rev Rhum 325–333
43. Wiley AM (1991) Arthroscopic appearance of frozen shoulder. Arthroscopy 7:138–143

Other Analgesic Bone Procedures

17

Bruno Kastler, Hatem Boulahdour,
Jean-Michel Lerais, Philippe Sarlieve,
Marie Jacamon, Annie Pousse, Michel Parmentier,
Fabrice-Guy Barral, Benoît de Billy,
Christophe Clair, Jean-Pierre Cercueil, Denis Krause

Treatment of Bone Tumors

Bruno Kastler, Hatem Boulahdour, Jean-Michel Lerais, Marie Jacomon, Annie Pousse, Michel Parmentier, Fabrice-Guy Barral

Secondary lesions are the most frequently encountered bone tumors. These are metastases mainly (80%) from cancer of the breast, lung, or prostate. Classic therapeutic procedures for such bone invasion include chemotherapy, radiotherapy, and more rarely surgery. These methods and even major analgesics are often ineffective against the pain they bring, mechanisms for which include, among others, compression of nerve endings, pathological fractures, and chemical releases such as bradykinin, prostaglandins, substance P and histamine.

Tumoral Alcoholization

Absolute alcohol is injected in various analgesic procedures and in particular in the neurolyses described in this book. The early percutaneous treatments under CT guidance for analgesic purposes that we proposed under CT-guidance over ten years ago required injections of absolute alcohol into the tumor with good results in terms of pain relief (Fig. 17.1) [10, 11]. Alcohol is not very costly and can be injected with flexible 20 or 22 gauge spinal-type needles. It is not however possible to treat condensed bony forms in which alcohol doesn't spread homogeneously.

The quantity of alcohol and number of needles inserted into the tumor depend on its size (see Fig. 17.1). The procedure is often very painful, particularly in the case of bone tumors and must be carried out under general anesthesia (or major sedation). Prior to the injection of alcohol into the tumor, an injection of a mixture of lidocaine and/or ropivacaine and contrast medium (hyperdense) is administered for the dual purpose of diminishing the pain of alcoholization and anticipating the possible spread within the tumor. It should, however, be remembered that unlike an anesthetic–contrast mixture, alcohol is not only hydro- but also liposoluble. It is thus not possible to treat tumors adjacent to nerves, particularly motor nerves, with alcohol. Moreover, repeated CT slices must be acquired to monitor diffusion (hypodensity within the tumor) as the alcohol is instilled, the slightest undesirable diffusion requiring the needle(s) to be repositioned and/or the intervention discontinued.

In the case of tumors in contact with or having invaded the sympathetic system (paravertebral), sympatholysis slightly above the lesion can be carried out at the same time. The same is true in the case of costal localization where it is possible to carry out neurolysis of the pertinent intercostal nerve(s).

RF Tumor Ablation

Due to these uncertainties of alcoholization (diffusion problems, risk of reaching nerves), radiofrequency ablation is clearly our current preference for bone tumor treatment. Dry electrode radiofrequency (RF Radionics (Burlington, MA, USA) 3FG with a voluntarily restricted ablation volume) is used routinely in many cases, some of which are described in this work, e.g., thoracic sympatholysis, intercostal neurolysis.

To obtain a larger, ovoid lesion of a controlled size, different techniques are used: "umbrella" electrodes (Rita, Fremont, CA, USA; Boston Scientific, Natick, MA, USA), internal circulation electrodes (Radionics, Valleylab (Boulder, CO, USA), Celon (Teltow, Germany), and external perfusion electrodes [Berchtold (Tuttlinger, Germany)]. For tumor ablation, particularly in bone, we recommend internal circulation straight-needle devices [13], because umbrella devices cannot be properly opened within bone lesions. External perfusion electrodes raise the same issues as alcoholization (non-homogenous diffusion in the tumor, risk of damaging nerves) [12, 13, 14] (Figs. 17.2–17.4).

Moreover, two electrodes are necessary for the current to circulate: one electrically insulated electrode whose tip is bare (active conduction exposed tip) and a second electrode which is either:

- A neutral plate on the patient's skin (principle of monopolar RF)

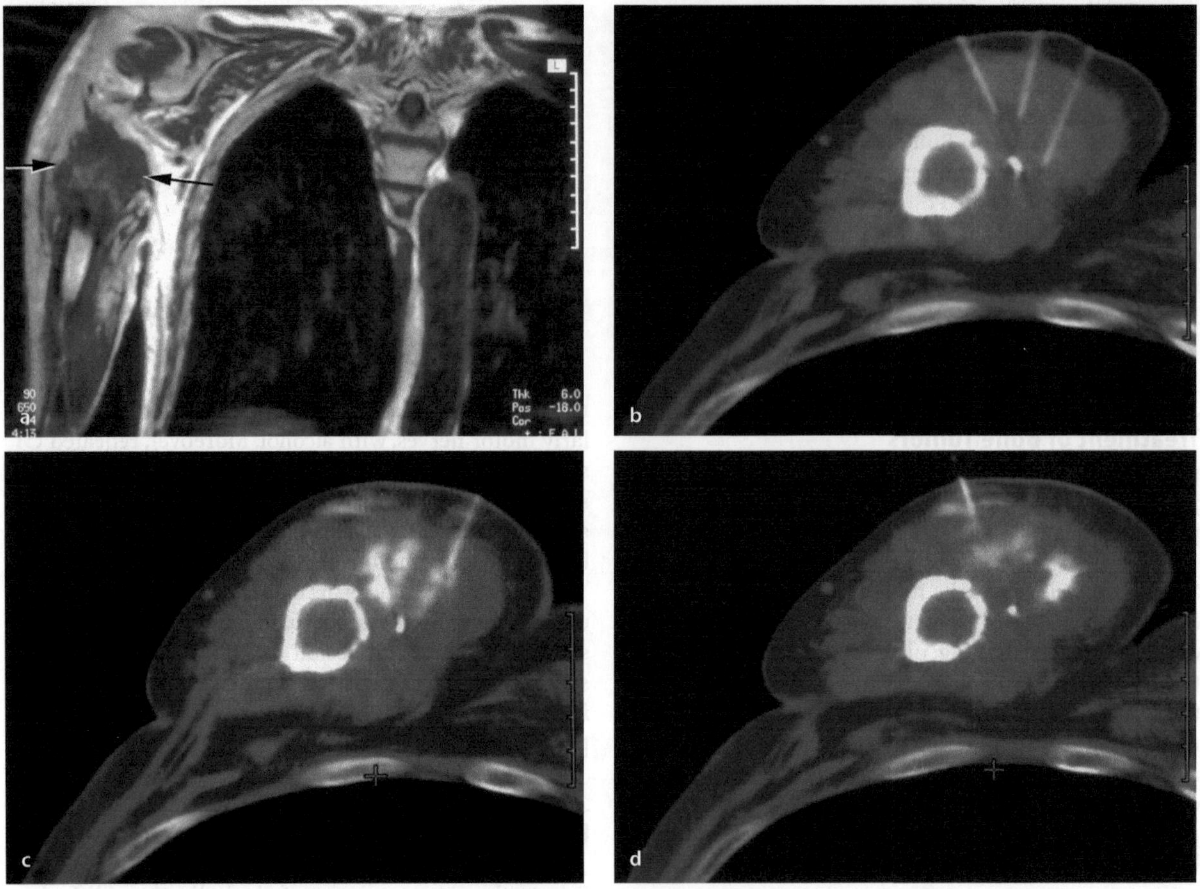

Fig. 17.1a–d. Extremely painful humeral metastasis (*arrows*) from lung cancer. **a** MRI axial slice at T1. **b** Insertion of three needles into the mass. **c** Injection of anesthetic-contrast mixture. **d** Instillation of alcohol. Pain relief within 24 hours of 50%. We currently treat this type of lesion by radiofrequency

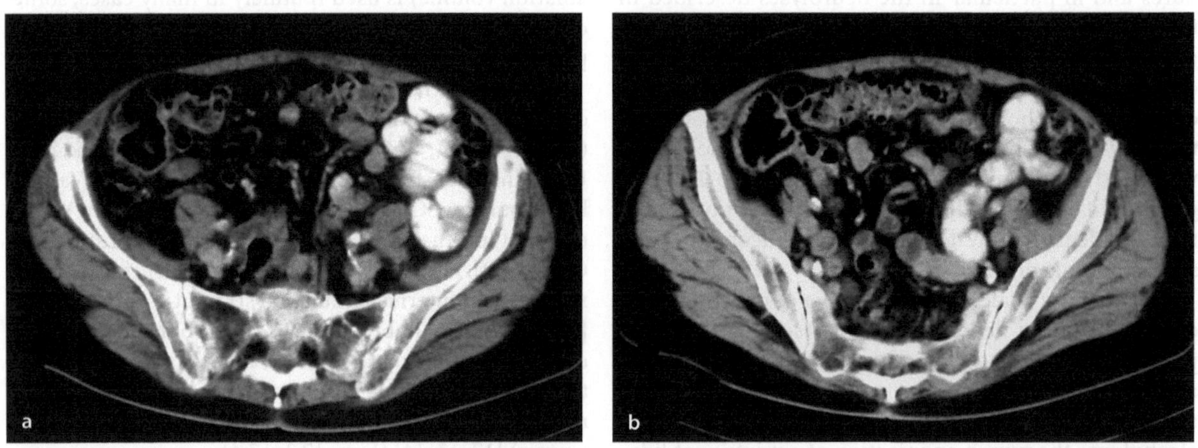

Fig. 17.2a–h. A 70-year-old bed-ridden patient, shriveled right leg, with very painful metastatic regions from breast cancer qualified for L3 irradiation. **a, b** An exam carried out 7 months earlier showed no lesion. **c, d** The two regions (*arrows*) are treated in a single session, **e** the first 2.7 cm in diameter at the level of the anterosuperior ischial spine with a single needle, and **f** the second 5.6 cm in diameter at the level of the iliac wing with a cluster needle (3 needles). Application of RF current (Radionics) for 12 and 25 minutes respectively). **g** A tissue vaporization effect (bubbles) appears within the mass. **h** Infiltration of lidocaine and cortivazol is carried out at the end of the procedure along on the path (*arrow*) of the iliohypograstric and ilioinguinal nerves (see Chap. 14; electrode *arrowhead*). Invasion of the nerves by the smaller metastases probably partly explains the inguinal radiation. The next day the patient sat and walked without pain and left the palliative care unit in 3 days

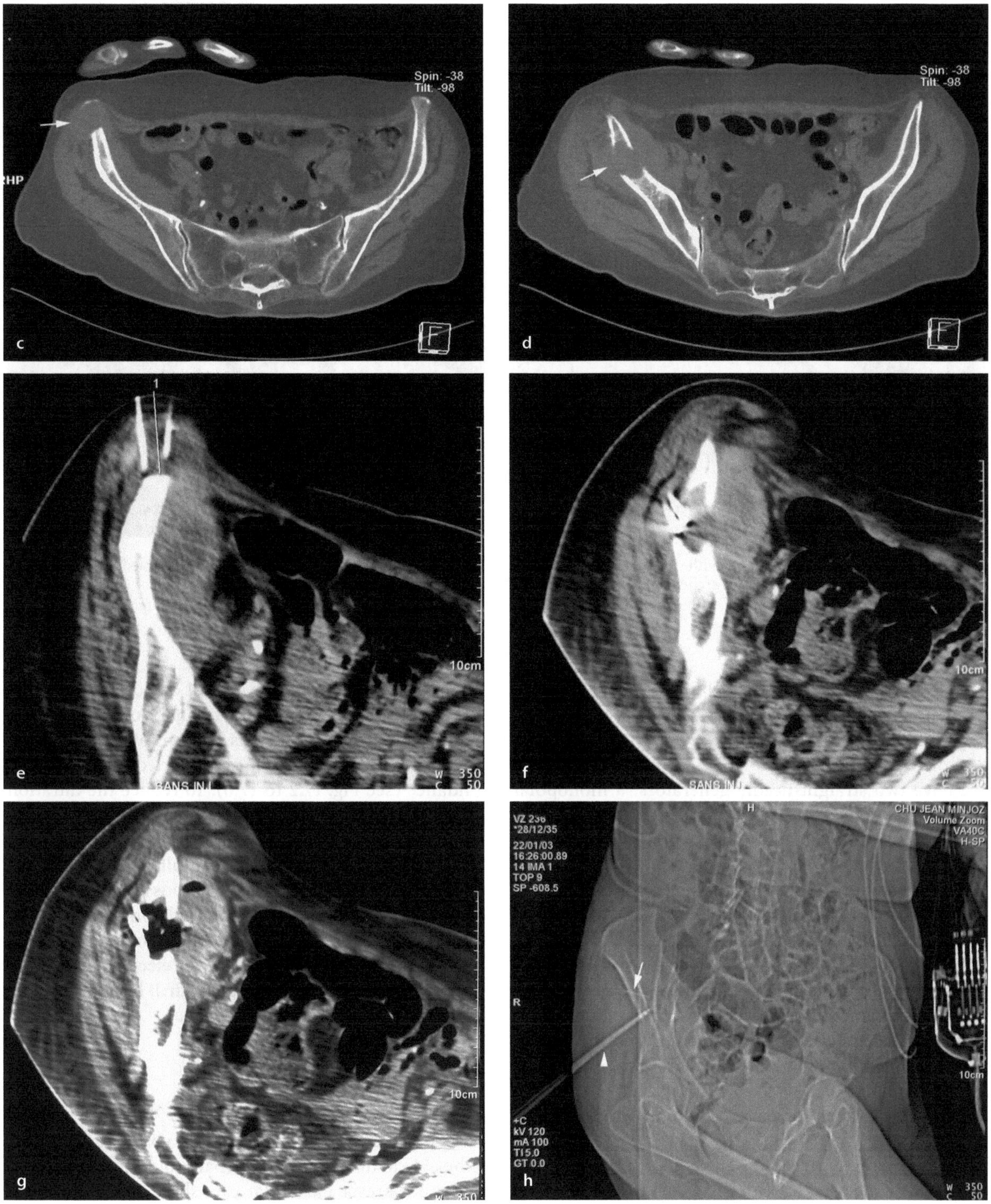

Fig. 17.2 a–h. *(Continued)*

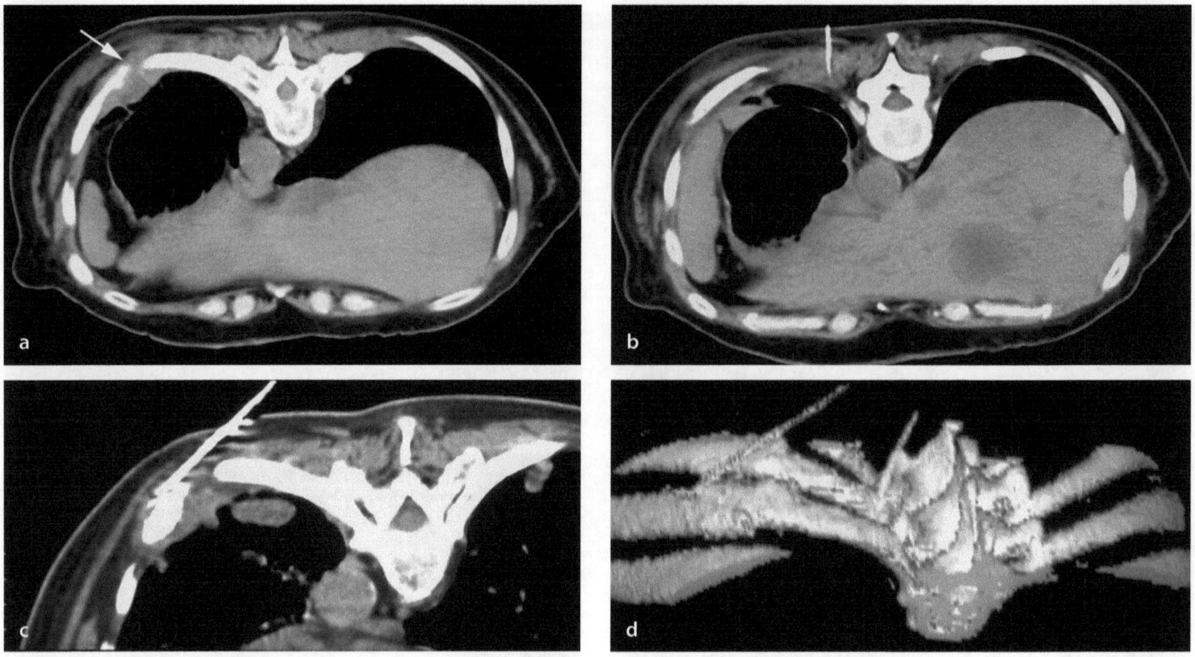

Fig. 17.3. **a** Sixty-year-old patient with metastases (from the breast) located in the posterior costal arches of the 7th and 8th ribs (*arrow*). **c** The lesion is treated by RF with a simple bipolar needle (Celon) and **b** an infiltration was also performed. **d** A 3D reconstruction shows the two needles on target

- A second conductive zone within the same needle insulated from the first electrode (more recent principle of bipolar RF).

We have two straight-needle generators: a monopolar system (Radionics) and more recently a bipolar system (Celon; internal circulation application with two electrodes at its tip).

The advantages of the bipolar approach compared to the classic monopolar system are multiple:

- No need for a neutral plate on skin (no risk of burning)
- Energy concentrated between two electrodes (better control over the lesion's size and less risk of damaging peripheral motor nerves)
- More efficient (effective for larger lesions, with possibility of multipolar treatment with two, even three needles)
- Possibility of treating patients with pacemakers.

We are currently treating all bone tumor lesions, particularly metastases. with this generator and results in terms of pain relief have been very good [13, 14].

Indications

The lesions we treat must be accessible by a safe percutaneous route, be no more 5 to 6 cm in diameter (or more if the effect intended is analgesic and not aimed at tumor eradication), and be at least one or two centimeters from a nerve structure (spinal cord, peripheral nerve). The usual precautions in terms of blood clotting are taken, and the procedure is carried out under CT guidance (see Fig. 17.2 to 17.6). To reduce the duration of the procedure, tumors over 3.5 cm can be treated by one electrode, or by two or three for multipolar effect. This protocol also holds true for multiple lesions (up to three lesions at a time). It is fully possible, apart from drilling problems, to treat condensed bony lesions without any difficulty. To perforate long bone path or thick cortical bone it is handy to use an electrical drill (see Chapter 15) or the Laredo-Hamze drill biopsy set (Cardinal Health Inomed Toulon-France).

Technique and Results

The procedure is carried out under conscious sedation to be able to detect any abnormal projected pain, paresthesia or paresis. Particular care should be taken when treating vertebral locations where it is mandatory to avoid any harm to neural structures (spinal cord or motor nerve roots). After subcutaneous anesthesia, a 22 gauge needle is inserted into the center of the tumor; it anesthetizes the path and the tumoral zone using a ropivacaine (70%) – lidocain mixture. It is left in place to easily guide the electrode needle down to the target using the tutor technique (see Chap. 3). Sharply bending

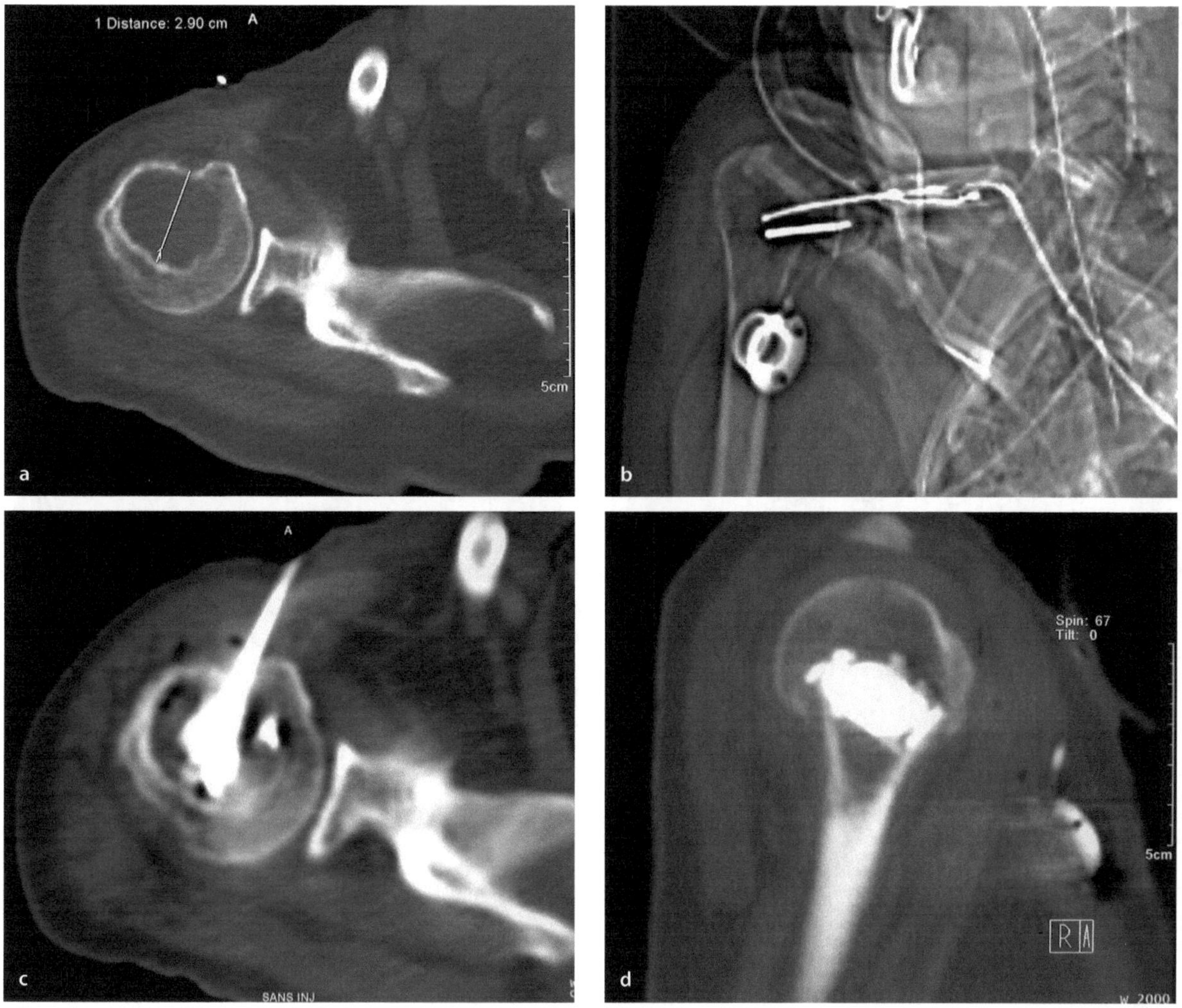

Fig. 17.4a–d. Humeral lytic metastasis of a lung cancer. **a** MRI with sagittal slices at T1. **b** Insertion of two bipolar needles (Celon), one of them coaxial with an 11 gauge (Cook) biopsy needle (after needle mandrel removal); retrieval of biopsy needle trocar until its tip is no longer in contact with the conducting tip (active proximal electrode). RF current applied for 15 minutes. **c, d** Needle removed and cement inject through to consolidate pathological fracture

the portion of the anesthesia needle that remains above the skin makes it easier to insert the electrode needle in beside it, its plastic end no longer a hindrance. Once the electrode is in position, cooling circulation (40 ml/min) is begun before application of the RF current. The current is maintained for 8 to 45 minutes depending on the size of the lesion (2 to 8 cm, respectively). At the end of this time the perfusion is ceased (causing a significant temperature rise) and the needle is carefully removed, thermocoagulating and sterilizing the insertion path and minimizing the risks of neoplastic insemination. The analgesic effect is immediate and often spectacular (the positive response rate was over 80% for our series [12, 14]). Patients found relief for between 1 to 12 months (sternal metastases), with an average of 2–3 months. Pelvic lesions responded particularly well [13, 14]. CT control scans performed up to three months later revealed that some lesions did not increase in size (anticarcinogenic potential). If pain and/or tumor recurs, the procedure can be repeated.

For weight-bearing bones including vertebrae, RF can be completed with cementoplasty ad/or vertebroplasty [13, 14]. making it possible to thermocoagulate the bone. And RF performed before cementoplasty and/or vertebroplasty makes it possible to sterilize the lesion before consolidation which is of interest particularly in unique locations. Indeed a drawback of performing cementoplasty (or vertebroplasty) solely is that during the cement injection at the pasty phase (often under pressure), there is a potential risk of dissemination of malignant cells either locally or by the hematogenous spread (vertebrae often harbor hyper-

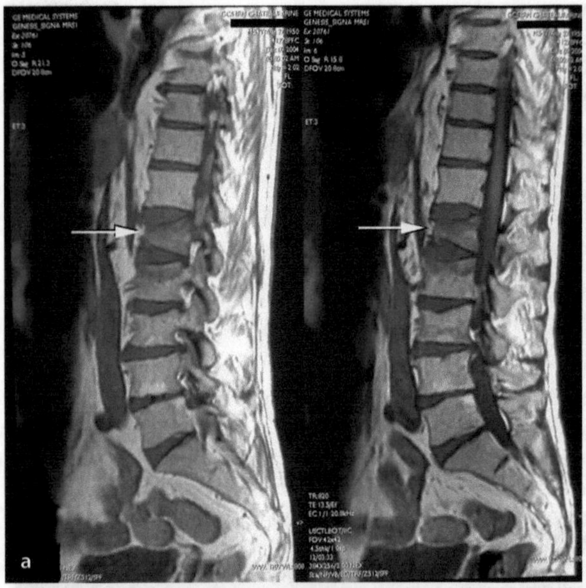

Fig. 17.5a–d. Vertebral metastasis (L1) of a lung cancer with painful fracture compression. **a** Sagittal T1 MRI slices. **b** First insertion of a 11 gauge (Cook) biopsy needle in L1 vertebra by transpedicular access; removal of needle mandrel and then insertion of a bipolar needle (Celon) coaxial through biopsy needle trocar to target; removal of needle trocar until its tip is no longer in contact with the conducting tip (proximal electrode). Removal of radiofrequency needle. The tip of the biopsy needle is reinserted at the junction of the anterior and middle third of the vertebral body; **c** injection of acrylic cement under CT guidance. **d** Frontal view

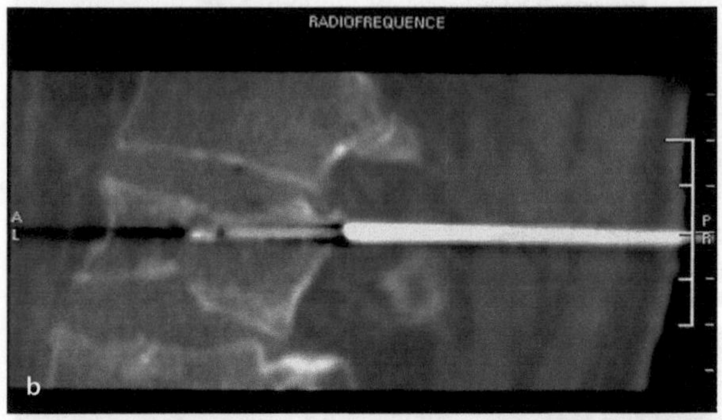

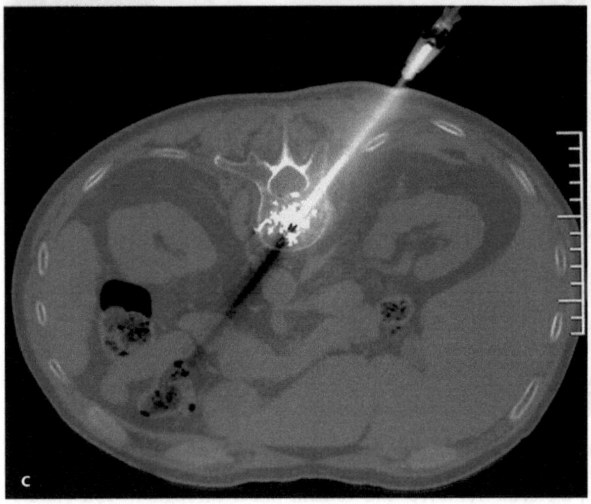

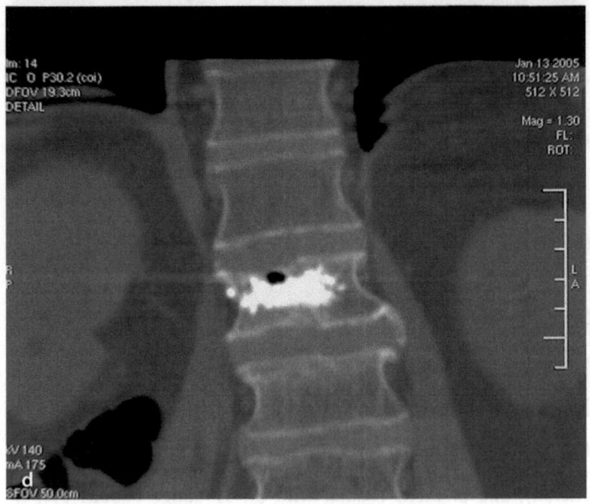

vascularized lesions). This is important particularly in single accessible metastatic locations. The fact that these techniques can be carried out during the same procedure is of course an advantage of their combination. However special care has to be taken to avoid contact of needle electrode with biopsy needle trocar (for further explanation see Figs. 17.5, 17.6). For these bone RF procedures the patient is observed for one night and usually discharged the following day.

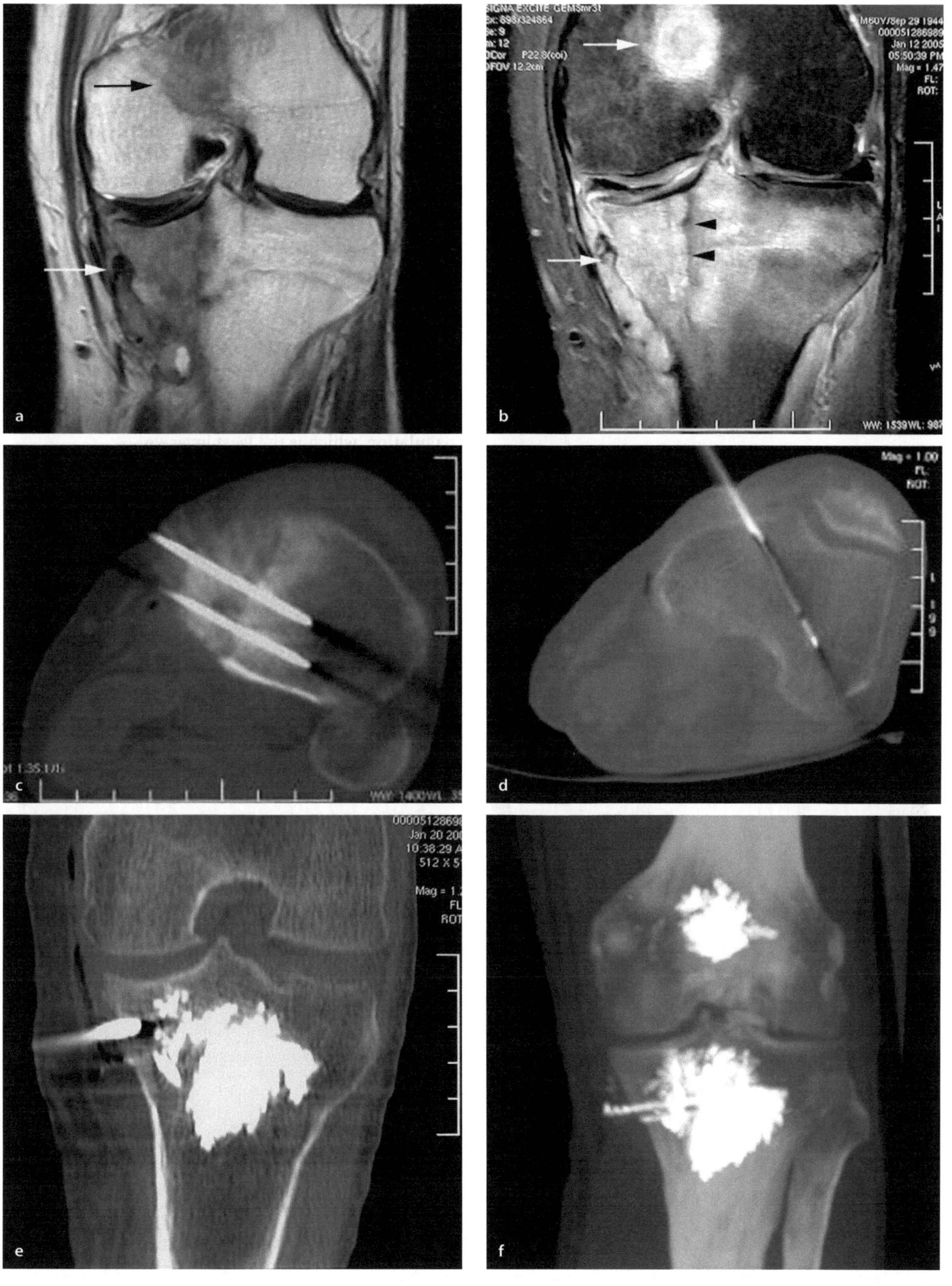

Fig. 17.6 a–f. Fifty-four-year-old patient, metastatic melanoma; wheel-chair bound, impossible to bear weight on lower left limb. Metastasis of inferior extremity of femur and superior extremity of tibia (*arrows*), with clearly visible pathological fracture (*arrow heads*) on frontal slices on views **a** T1 and **b** T2. **c** Bipolar radiofrequency (Celon) treatment is carried out with two needles in the tibial lesion and **d** one needle in the femoral lesion, followed **e, f** by acrylic glue injection. The patient walked pain free the same evening

CT-Guidance Therapy of Osteoid Osteoma

Bruno Kastler, Philippe Sarlieve, Christophe Clair, Benoît de Billy, Fabrice-Guy Barral

Diagnosis

Osteoid osteoma is a benign osteoblastic tumor occurring in young people, often accompanied by severe pain at night, and having a good response to salicylic acid. The diagnosis often requires scintigraphy. The size, physical appearance, and exact position of the nidus are indicated by a CT or possibly an MRI scan. The radiological picture is often sufficient for diagnosis. When doubt exists, a biopsy should be carried out.

Technique

Less and less invasive treatments under CT guidance of this benign tumor can be offered as an alternative to surgery (including the percutaneous, resection discussed here [21, 30, 32]), namely alcoholization or thermocoagulation by RF or laser [23, 24, 25, 35]. The full destruction or excision of the nidus (75% located in the tibia or femur) is necessary for total recovery.

The lesions treated must be accessible by a safe percutaneous path and for RF be at least one to two centimeters from a nerve structure (spinal cord, spinal column, peripheral nerve). The usual precautions in terms of clotting must be observed. The procedures are carried out usually under general anesthesia (particularly in children) and followed step by step under CT guidance. We currently prefer radiofrequency thermocoagulation, which is the least invasive.

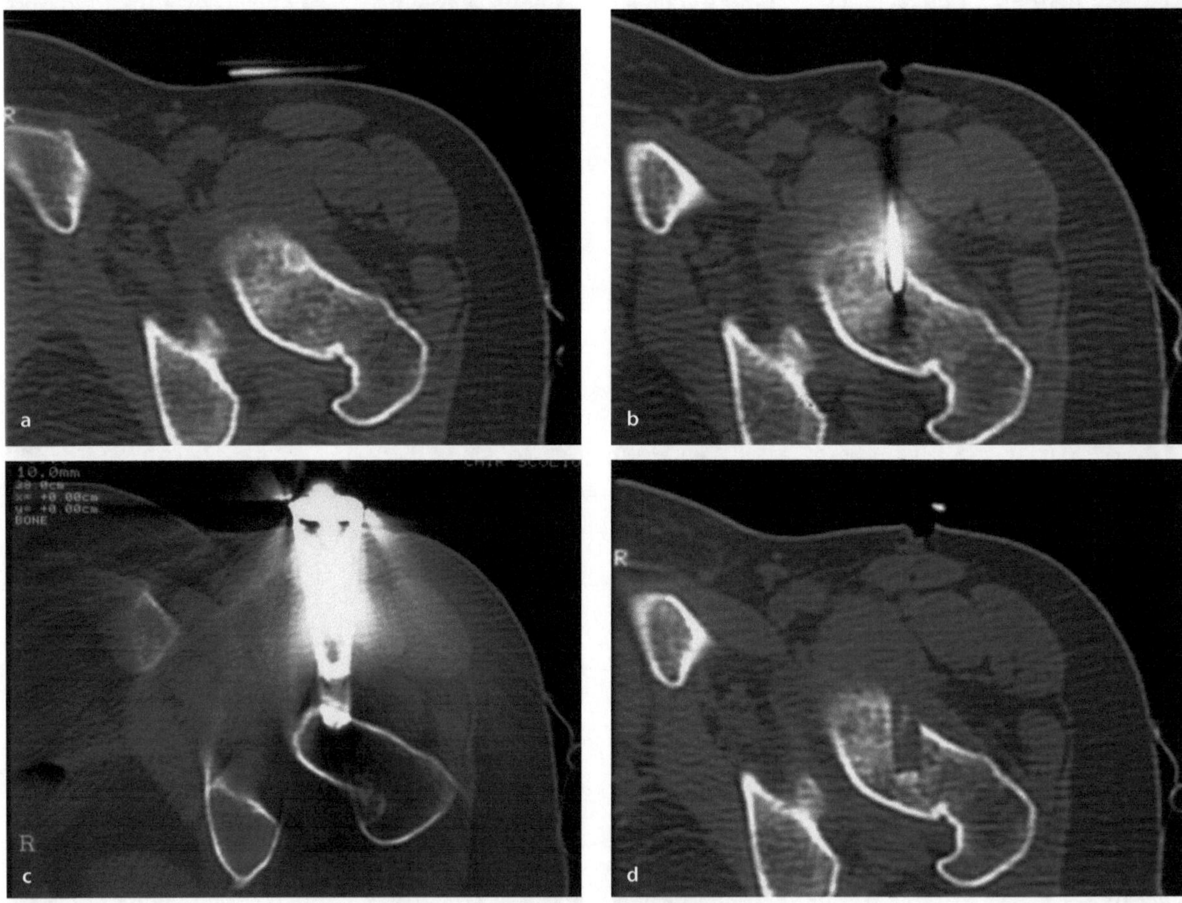

Fig. 17.7 a–d. Osteoid osteoma of the neck of the femur. **a** Anterior approach after cutaneous location. **b** Positioning of the guide mandrel and **c** the trephine (c). **d** View after excision

Percutaneous Resection

The technique calls upon the Kohler set: after subcutaneous anesthesia, a Kirschner wire is positioned in the nidus under CT-guidance to locate the trephine (7 to 10 mm external diameter) using a mandrel (Figs. 17.7, 17.8). After drilling a pilot bore in the bone, monitored by one or several CT slices, all the necrotic tissue is removed (for histological analysis). A CT scan verifies the quality of the ablation. Limited or partial resections (thin trephine) can benefit from another drill or possibly complementary sclerosis by alcoholization.

The complications reported of this method are cutaneous burns at the point of entrance, resulting from the heat produced by the high rotating speed of the trephine (which can be prevented by the use of a sheath around the trephine), muscle hematoma, fractures of long bones (when fragile), osteitis.

For most locations, particularly as in small bones, vertebra, and joints, radiofrequency thermocoagulation is a less invasive alternative.

RF Treatment

After subcutaneous anesthesia, first a 22 gauge needle is inserted into the center of the tumor. This ensures that the path is anesthetized and enables, using the tutor technique (see Chap. 3), the easy guidance of the biopsy needle (14 gauge 10 cm) into the heart of the nidus (using a mallet if necessary; see Fig. 17.9). In the case of any diagnostic doubt, a coaxial biopsy should be carried out. The mandrel is then removed, maintaining the needle trocar anchored in the bone. The 16 gauge 15 cm bipolar electrode (Celon) is coaxially inserted through the biopsy needle into the nidus and held in place. The biopsy needle trocar must now be carefully removed until its tip is no longer in contact with the conducting tip i.e. the proximal electrode of the bipolar needle (at least 1 cm or more) to prevent any conduction of current along the biopsy needle; it must be thus kept away from the proximal electrode during the entire RF process (see Fig. 17.8). After establishing cooling circulation (40 ml/min), RF current can be started and maintained for between 6 and 15 minutes (temperature can reach 80–90°). After this, the perfusion is stopped and the needle is rapidly removed in order to thermocoagulate the insertion path. Patients feel pain relief soon after the procedure is over. Radiofrequency for this purpose is used as a routine technique at present in our department with excellent results.

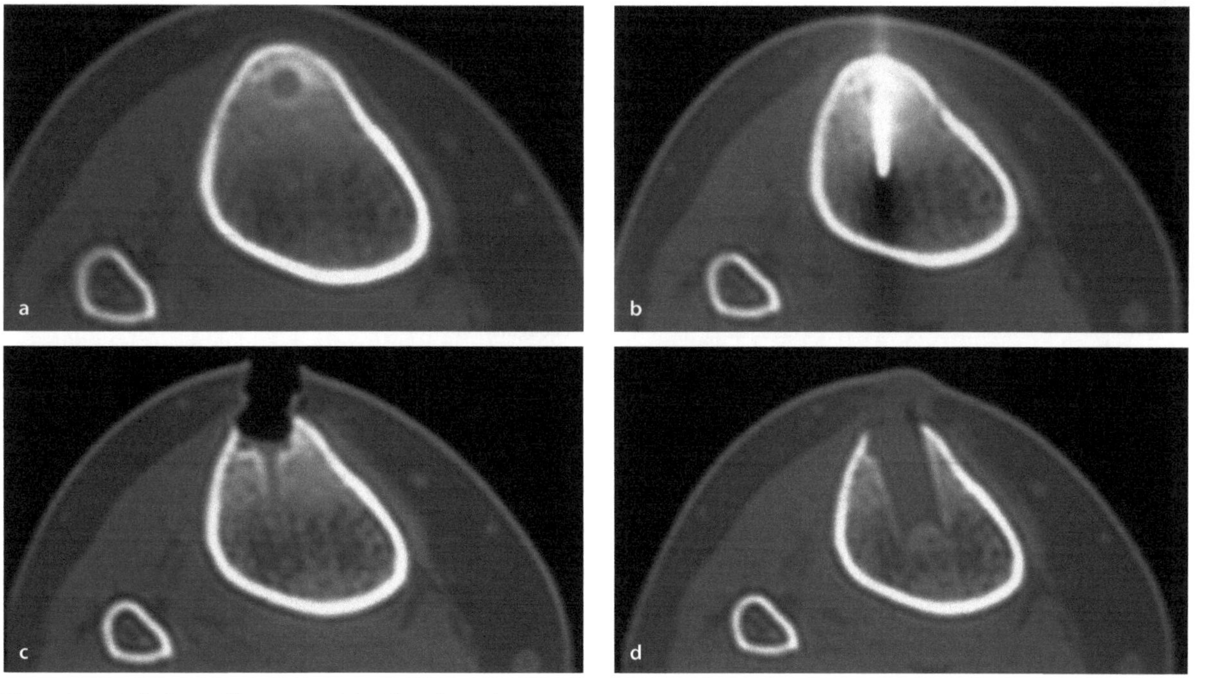

Fig. 17.8. **a** Typical osteoid osteoma with nidus of the tibial crest. **b** Positioning of the guide mandrel; **c** excision limited during first drill with trephine, **d** completed by a second drill

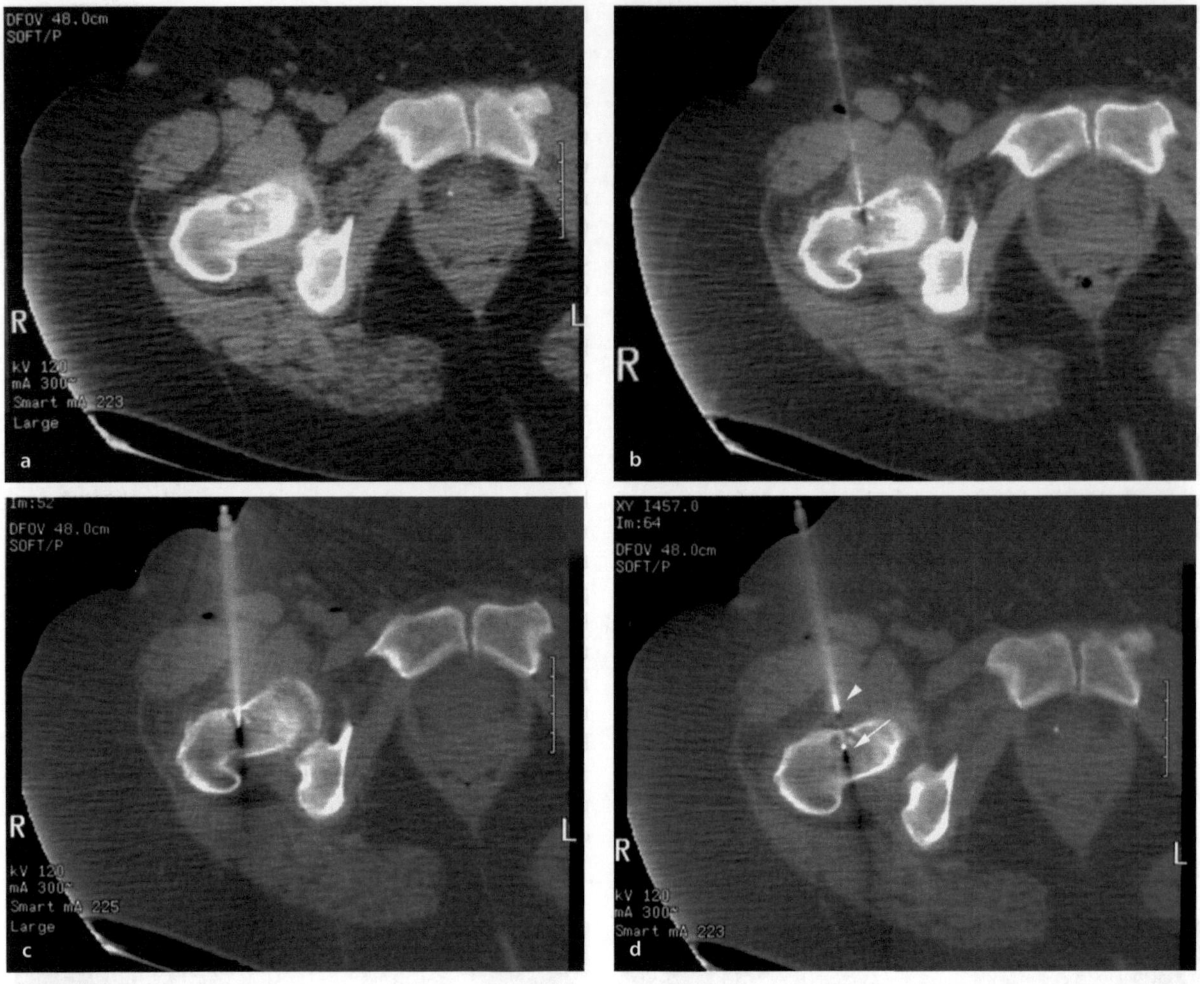

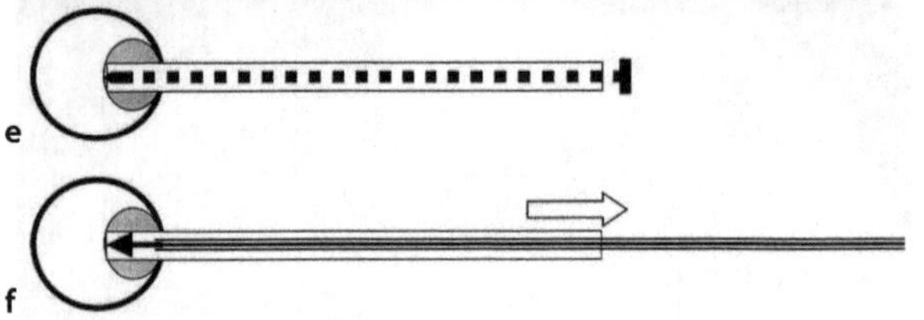

Fig. 17.9. **a** Osteoid osteoma of the neck of the femur; **b** anterior approach and path of a 22 gauge spinal needle used for anesthesia and left in position. **c, d** Positioning of the 11 gauge 10 cm biopsy needle (mandrel and trocar) whose tip penetrates the nidus (a biopsy can be performed if necessary). **e** Removal of mandrel (*dotted line*) and **f** introduction of the bipolar needle coaxial with the trocar to target. **g** Retrieval of biopsy needle trocar until its tip is no longer in contact with the conducting proximal electrode. The RF needle is held in place by the lesion (*arrow* in **d**) for thermocoagulation

Embolization of Bone Metastases in Kidney Cancer

Jean-Michel Lerais, Jean-Pierre Cercueil, Denis Krause, Bruno Kastler

Introduction

Embolization acts by reducing the pressure of renal cancer metastases to bone on the periosteum which is richly innervated. It creates a bone and cell necrosis, reduces the edema and vascular stasis.

Bone metastases occur in 30–45% of renal cancer cases [7], in which case the average survival time is five months [8]. These bone metastases affect primarily the spine (dorsal and lumbar) then the pelvic bone and the femur. Kidney cancer is the fourth greatest source of spinal metastases (after breast, prostate, and lung cancer). Bone metastasis can also be located on the limbs (distal to the knee and elbow 6–10%) as well as intracortically and subperiostally [3, 8, 19].

Bone metastases reveal the cancer in 60–70% of cases; they can be isolated but are more frequently multiple.

Pain is their principal syndrom. They are often lytic and can destroy the cortical bone, often taking on a pseudosarcomatous or pseudoangiomatous appearance with neovascularization and arteriovenous shunts [25, 30]. Bone metastases are hypervascularized (as is the primary tumor) in 65–75% of cases.

Extreme pain, lack of chemosensitivity, and neurological risk can result in a decision to attempt the arterial embolization technique, particularly when the bone metastasis is singular. It may also be performed preoperatively to facilitate tumor removal [1, 7].

Technique

Catheterization

Position of a 5F or 6F valve introducer in the femoral or humeral artery. For atheromatous patients with winding arteries, a long guiding (40 cm) introducer is often useful. Highly stable Simmons 1, 2 or "sidewinder" catheters or a Cobra 2 (Cardeon, Cupertino, CA, USA) with a distal tip are used. Hydrophilic guides make highly selective stable anti-reflux catheterization possible. Coaxial 3F micro-catheters (Terumo, Tokyo; Tracker, Target, Boston Scientific) are often very useful. Arterial cartography must be excellent in order to identify small radicular medullary arteries stemming from lumbar (above L3), intercostal (mainly T4 to T9), intestinal, renal, or gonad arteries. Embolization of arteries in the buttock is avoided because of risk of cutaneous or muscular necrosis [5].

Embolization Materials

Non-resorbable embolic materials are used for both proximal and distal sites.

Distal embolization

Inert Particles

- Polyvinyl or polyvinyl alcohol sponge (Ivalon, Ultra-Ivalon, Ivalon Inc., San Diego).
- Deformable acrylic polymer gelatin impregnated microspheres (Embosphere; Biosphere, Rockland, MA, USA) prevent aggregation in the catheter. The particles are calibrated from 1 to 100μ and diluted in contrast media, diameters below 300μ passing through coaxial micro-catheters. They enable excellent distal occlusion [2].

Liquid Agents

- Cyanoacrylate (Histoacryl; Sutherland Medical, Oakleigh, Victoria, Australia) is a biological adhesive that polymerizes on contact with the blood in less than a second [26]. It is diluted in an oil contrast media [Lipiodol Ultrafluid (LUF); E-Z-EM Canada, Montreal] at a ratio of 1:3, 1:4, or 1:5 and injected in coaxial micro-catheters opacified with LUF to avoid polymerization in the catheter [2, 5]. Cyanoacrylate is capable of occluding large vessels (Fig. 17.10).
- Alcohol (96% ethanol) is less often used. It leads to severe, often very painful tissue necrosis; it dilutes very rapidly in the blood which limits risk in the case of reflux into the aorta, yet still can result in hemolysis [26]. Its use in the spine is restricted by the risk of intracanalar diffusion.

Proximal Embolization

Metallic coils (Gianturco-Anderson-Wallace): these are tiny bits of steel to which fibers of wool or Dacron are added to facilitate thrombosis. The caliber of the coils must be adapted to that of the catheters. They result in proximal occlusion, similar to a surgical ligature, that complement the use of particles (Fig. 17.11) [2, 15, 26].

Efficacy

Embolization is considered effective when arteriography reveals that less than 25% of the tumoral volume is opacified and pre-operative loss of blood is no more than 150–300 ml [4, 5]. Seventy-five percent of patients lose between 450–1,500 ml of blood during surgery [5, 34].

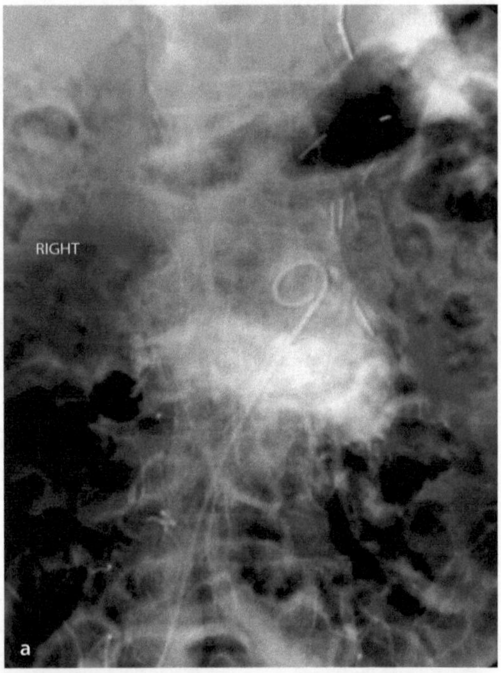

Fig. 17.10 a–d. Sixty-nine-year-old patient, left kidney operation in 1996. In 1997 metastasis of left femur and L3 operated and irradiated. **a** Aortography frontal view and selective catheterization of left and right lumbar arteries L3, showing **b** hypervascularization and **c** tumoral blush. Embolization by Embospheres (300–500 μ; two bottles) and (500–700 μ; 1 bottle). Flow remained rapid. Completed with Histoacryl and Lipiodol Ultrafluid: disappearance of tumoral blush. **d** View after embolization: the left L3 artery remains opaque, thrombosed by the glue and lipiodol

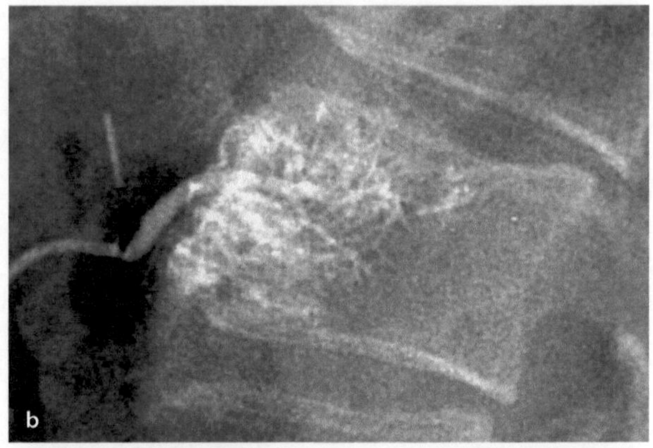

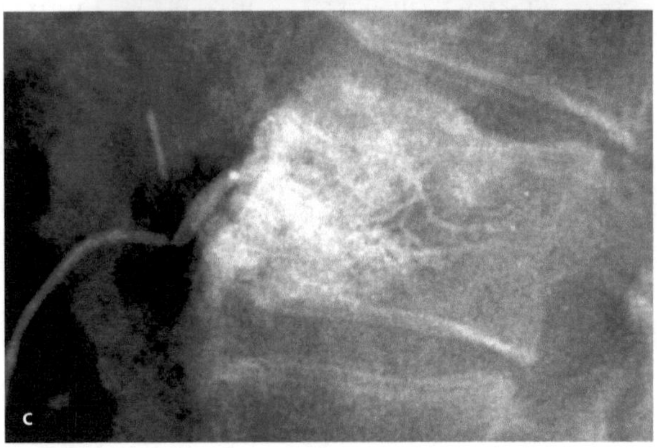

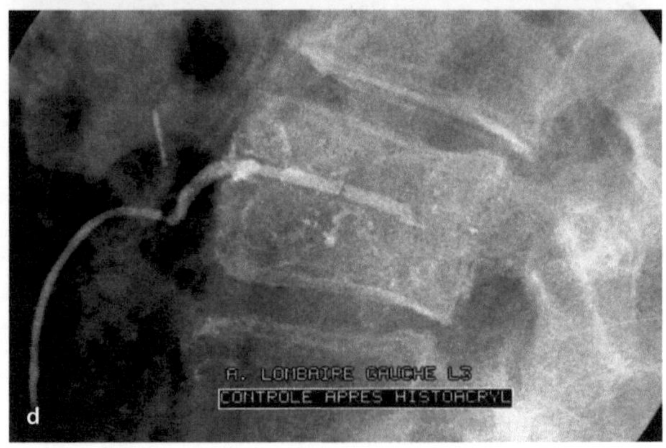

Results

As stated earlier, embolization acts to reduce tumoral pressure on the periosteum, which is richly innervated, by creating a bone and cell necrosis, reduces the edema and cell necrosis. Osteoblastic activity with bone regrowth has been observed around the tumor (Fig. 17.12) [1, 27] in a percentage varying from 0 to 4% of cases depending on the author [33, 36]. Blood loss during ensuing surgery is reduced, enabling pathological fractures to heal normally [1, 5]. Surgery must be carried out within three days after embolization to reduce the risk of revascularization [5, 15].

The size of the bone metastasis is reduced in 80–100% of cases [5, 33, 36]. CT scans show hypodense central necrosis 4 to 9 months after embolization.

Pain disappears in 75–100% of cases; improvement begins within 12 hours and lasts for 2 to 9 months [1, 5, 7, 33, 36]. For optimal pain relief Yilmaz advocates repeating the embolization up to three times [6].

Material is becoming standard, but the type in current use that is chosen has little effect on the benefit obtained, which can be significant if embolization is total [30].

A post-embolization syndrome is constant, which includes pain in the embolized region and abdomen, nausea, and moderate fever. It does not last more than 1 to 5 days; the pain responds well to usual analgesics and the fever to non-steroidal anti-inflammatories.

Survival after embolization is usually between 17 and 37 months, depending on whether it is purely palliative or preoperative, with an average time of 28 months [5, 16, 22].

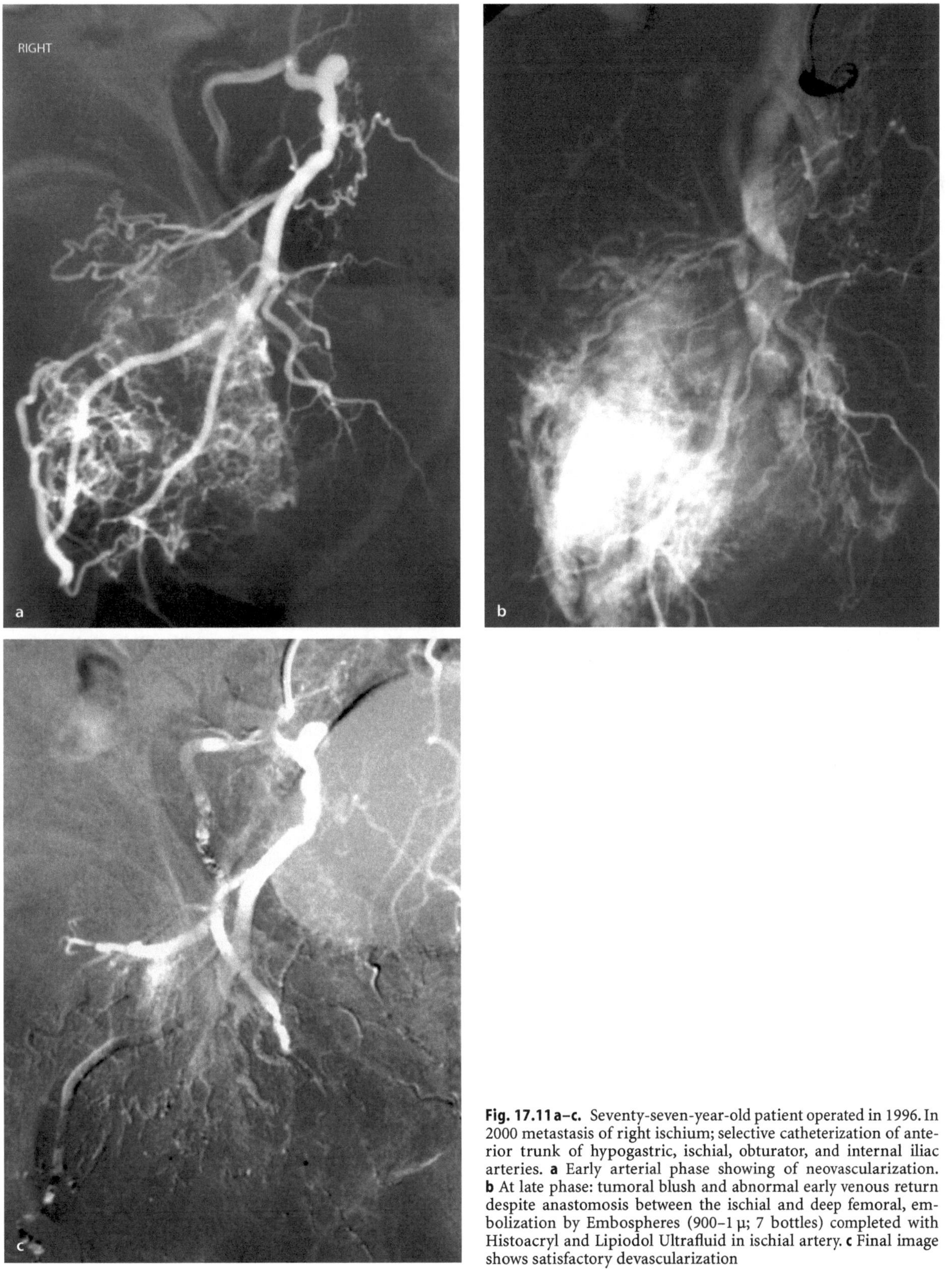

Fig. 17.11 a–c. Seventy-seven-year-old patient operated in 1996. In 2000 metastasis of right ischium; selective catheterization of anterior trunk of hypogastric, ischial, obturator, and internal iliac arteries. **a** Early arterial phase showing of neovascularization. **b** At late phase: tumoral blush and abnormal early venous return despite anastomosis between the ischial and deep femoral, embolization by Embospheres (900–1 μ; 7 bottles) completed with Histoacryl and Lipiodol Ultrafluid in ischial artery. **c** Final image shows satisfactory devascularization

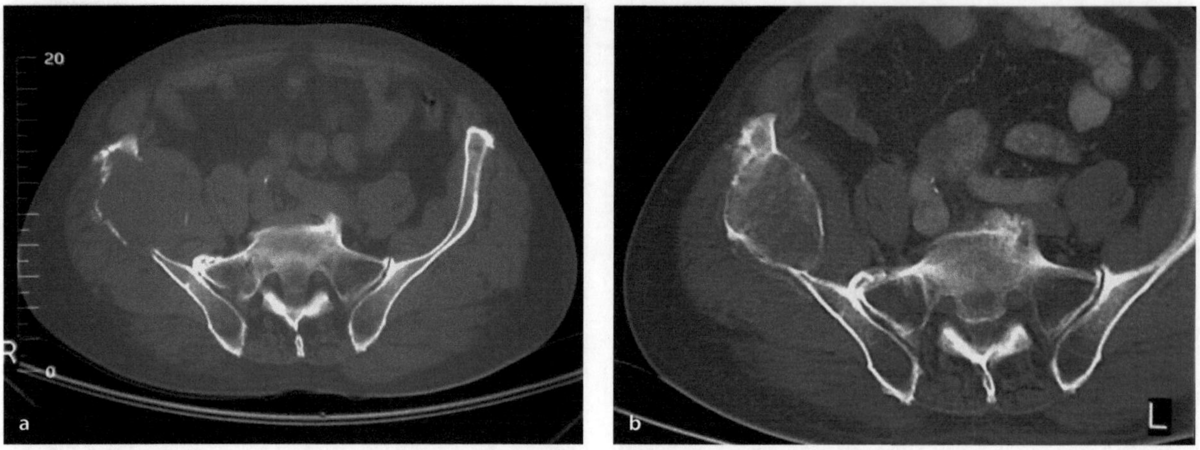

Fig. 17.12a, b. Seventy-five-year-old patient. Cancer of right kidney with surgery in 1995). **a** In 1998 metastasis of right ilium treated by embolization with Embospheres and Histoacryl and radiotherapy. **b** Follow-up films in 2000 shows cortical reconstruction almost complete, and analgesic effect was good

Complications

Paresis or sometimes even paralysis of foot muscles sometimes occurs after embolization of lumbar internal iliac arteries due to involvement of radicular arteries and perivascular plexi (5–33%). This complication is usually temporary but can be permanent [5, 7, 15, 20, 33] and is most often seen following the use of ethanol [15].

While this complication has been regarded as a risk germane to the procedure, other reported mishaps can be considered accidents, and include:

- Mesenteric infarction after ileal occlusion
- Hypertension from thrombosis of the adrenal artery
- Lung emboli in connection with a tumor-caused arteriovenous shunt
- Partial necrosis of skin of a lower limb 8 days after alcohol embolization[1, 15].

The rate of "accidental" complications has been found not to exceed 2% in a large series [5].

Conclusion

Taken as stand-alone therapy or performed as a preoperative measure, embolization of bone metastases is an interesting procedure for use in severely painful hypervascularized metastases. Best results are achieved in its facilitative pre-op role, but it also increases patients' pain-free survival. It can also be used following massive doses of radiotherapy administered for purely palliative purposes.

References

1. Barton PP, Waneck RE, Karnel FJ, Ritschi P, Kramer J, Lechner GL (1996) Embolization of bone metastases. JVIR 7:81–88
2. Baudrillard JC, Lerais JM, Auquier F, Toubas O, Lacour P (1986) Les différents matériels d'embolisations et agents pharmacologiques utilisés en radiologie vasculaire interventionnelle. Feuillets Radiol 26:125–135
3. Bouvier M, Lejeune E, Bonvoisin B, Biron P (1982) Les métastases osseuse distales du membre supérieur. Ann Radiol 25:359–362
4. Bowers TA, Murray JA, Charnsangavej C, Soo CS, Chuang VP, Wallace S (1982) Bone metastases from renal carcinoma: the preoperative use of transcatheter arterial occlusion. J Bone Joint Surg 64:749–754
5. Cercueil JP, Holtzmann P, Ravel A, Boyer L, Krause D (1997) Embolisation rénale: technique et indications. Radiol J Cepur 7:24–30
6. Chiras J, Gaston A, Gaveau T, Sellier N, Marsault C, Bories J (1983) Embolisation préopératoire en pathologie rachidienne. à propos de 21 cas. J Radiol 64:397–403
7. Chuang VP, Wallace S, Swanson D, Zornoza J, Handel SF, Schwarten DA, Murray J (1979) Arterial occlusion in the management of pain from metastatic renal carcinoma. Radiology 133:611–614
8. Conroy T, Malissard L, Dartois D, Luporsi E, Stines J, Chardot C (1988) Histoire naturelle et évolution des métastases osseuses. à propos de 429 observations. Bull Cancer 75:845–857
9. Gangi A, Dietemann JL, Gasser B et al (1997) Interstitial laser photocoagulation of osteoid osteomas with use of CT guidance. Radiology 203:843–848
10. Gangi A, Kastler B, Klinkert A, Dietemann JL (1994) Injection of alcohol into bone metastases under CT guidance. J Comput Assist Tomogr 18:932–935
11. Gangi A, Kastler B, Quoix E et al (1992) Traitement palliatif des métastases osseuses par alcoolisation (article à caractère didactique). Feuillets Radiol 32:117–119
12. Kastler B (2004) Radiofrequency treatment in the management of pain in bone metastasis with straight needles. Scientific session Radiological Society of North America, 90th scientific assembly and annual meeting. Chicago, 28 Nov – 3 Dec 2004. Radiology [Suppl]

13. Kastler B (2005) Radiofrequency combined with cementoplasty under CT-guidance in the management of pain in bone metastasis. Scientific session European congress of Radiology Vienna March 2005. European Radiology [Suppl]
14. Kastler B, Boulahdour H, Barral F-G (2005) Pain management in bone metastasis of pulmonary origin: New interventional and metabolic techniques. Rev Mal Respir 22:8594–85100
15. Gellad Fe, Sadato N, Numaduchi Y, Levine A (1990) Vascular metastatic lesions of the spine: preoperative embolization. Radiology 176:683–686
16. Hare W, Lond F, Holland C (1983) Paresis following internal iliac artery embolization. Radiology 146:47–51
17. Hoey MF, Mullier PM, Lee DA, Kastler B (1997) Needle ablation of the liver using radiofrequency energy and interstitial saline infusion. Scientific exhibit. Radiological Society of North America, 83th scientific assembly and annual meeting, Chicago, 30 Nov - 5 Dec 1997. Radiology [Suppl] 205:705
18. Hoffel JC (2001) Percutaneous excision of osteoid osteoma. Radiology 218:302–303
19. Jardé O, Frigent F, Obry C, Murat JL, de Moegen J, Vives P (1986) Les métastases osseuses des doigts. à propos de 3 observations. Revue de la littérature. J Radiol 67:621–624
20. Keller FS, Rösch J, Bird CB (1983) Percutaneous embolization of bony pelvic neoplasms with tissue adhesive. Radiology 147: 21–27
21. Kohler R, Mazoyer JF, Besse JL, Bascoulergue Y (1990) Treatment of osteoid osteoma with percutaneous resection under CT control. A report of 5 cases. Rev Chir Orthop Reparatr Appar Mot 76:284–287
22. Munk PL, Torregiani G, Legiehn G, Morris DC, Ho SGF (2001) Palliative treatment of metastatic bone pain by embolization. Clin Radiol 56:339
23. Osti OL, Sebben R (1998) High frequency radiowave ablation of osteoid osteoma in the lumbar spine. Eur Spine J 7:422–425
24. Rosenthal DI, Springfield D, Alexander A, Rosenberg AE (1992) Ablation of osteoid osteomas with percutaneously placed electrode: a new procedure. Radiology 183:29–33
25. Rosenthal DI, Springfield D, Gebhart MC et al (1995) Osteoid osteomas: percutaneous radiofrequency ablation. Radiology 197:451–454
26. Rossi C, Ricci S, Boriani S, Biagini R, Ruggieri P, de Cristfaro R, Roversi RA, Khalkhali I (1990) Percutaneous transcatheter arterial embolization of bone and soft tissue tumors. Skeletal Radiol 19:555–560
27. Rowe DM, Becker GJ, Rabe ER, Holden RW, Richmond BD, Wass JL, Sequeira FW (1984) Osseous metastases from renal cell carcinoma: embolization and surgery for restoration of function. Radiology 150:673–676
28. Sanhaji L, Gharbaoui IS, Hassani Re et al (1996) Un nouveau traitement de l'ostéome ostéoide: la sclérose percutanée à l'éthanol sous guidage scanographique. J Radiol 77:37–40
29. Sans N, Morena-Maupome H, Galy-Fourcade D et al (1999) Résection percutanée sous contrôle TDM des ostéomes ostéoides. J Radiol 80:457–465
30. Stepanek E, Josph S, Campbell P, Porte M (1999) Embolization of a limb metastasis in renal cell carcinoma as a palliative treatment of bone pain. Clin Radiol 54:855–857
31. Towbin R, Kaye R, Meza Mp et al (1995) Osteoid osteoma: excision using a CT-guided coaxial technique. AJR 197:451–454
32. Trèves R, Legoff JJ, Doyon D, Chasle G, Arnaud M, Jacob P, Burki F, Desproges-Gotteron R (1984) L'embolisation thérapeutique ou embolisation palliative à visée antalgique des métastases osseuses d'origine rénale. Rev Rhum 51:1–5
33. Varma J, Huben RP, Wajsman Z, Pontes JE (1984) Therapeutic embolization of pelvic metastases of renal cell carcinoma. J Urol 131:647–649
34. Wallace S, Granmayeh M, de Santos LA et al (1979) Arterial occlusion of pelvic bone tumors. Cancer 43:322–328
35. Woertler K, Vestring T, Boettner F et al (2001) Osteoid osteoma: CT-guided percutaneous radiofrequency ablation and follow up in 47 patients. J Vasc Interv Radiol 12:717–722
36. Yilmaz S, Sindel T, Culeci E (2002) Repeated palliative embolization of renal cell carcinoma. Clin Radiol 57:319–320

Fractures of the Pelvic Girdle: CT-guided Percutaneous Fixation

Patrick Eude, Ghislaine Eude, Fernand De Peretti

18

Introduction

The pelvic girdle is a resistant ring-shaped bony structure upon which the high-intensity mechanical stress of major trauma often generates two, three, or even four fractures or disruptions. Such injuries are inherently unstable, leading to secondary displacements that may jeopardize standing and walking. This kind of injury can also remain persistently painful, even after consolidation seems to be achieved.

Open surgical fixation is a solution that allows reduction and stabilization of displaced fractures. This is, however, a difficult, complex measure and thus mostly restricted to displaced lesions.

Fractures with little displacement are treated conservatively with bed rest for 3 to 6 weeks; a continuous traction device is frequently used for both longer and shorter periods than this. But this treatment may lead to the well known cutaneous, vascular, and/or visceral complications of a prolonged bed stay.

Percutaneous fixation aims to stabilize fractures by driving screws across the fracture, utilizing very accurate CT guidance and only a small skin opening. This method allows a quick resumption of ambulation and a hospital stay limited to a few days.

Reminders

Anatomic Basis

It is necessary to focus on the essential part played by the posterior ligamentous structures in the stability of the sacroiliac complex. Consolidation of these injuries depends upon ensuring the stability primarily of disrupted posterior, but also of anterior musculoskeletal elements.

The relationship between the ring of bone and the pelvic contents explains the frequency of associated visceral and vascular wounds. It is also a reason to avoid endopelvic intrusion while driving pins and screws.

An acetabular approach requires look-out for the femoral vessels and nerve anteriorly and the sciatic nerve posteriorly. These elements are clearly visible on CT slices and can therefore be avoided. Because of the position of the sciatic nerve, the posterior approach is, however, dangerous.

Classifications

Several classifications have been published of traumatic lesions of the pelvic ring and acetabulum. Some are according to the direction of the traumatic vector [12], others to the mechanism of injury [18, 26]. Those we present below are more descriptive and widely used. Each classification describes elementary fracture lines followed by complex associations of (mostly unstable) fractures and disruptions.

Pelvic Ring Injuries (Tile)

Good reference articles for this and the next two subsections are those of Pennal, Tile, Denis, Letournel and associates. [4, 5, 6, 25].

A-type injuries are stable lesions, either because there is no disruption of the posterior arch (A1) or because there is a nondisplaced posterior fracture (A2). Since the ligamentous structures are preserved, the lesion is stable.

B-type injuries result from a lateral stress vector in external rotation (B1), or when there is internal rotation with anterior impact, ipsilateral (B2) or contralateral (B3). B1 is also called "open book injury" and includes two subgroups according to the amount of symphysis pubis disruption (± 25 mm).

Another specific injury involves internal rotation on one side and external rotation on the other ("bucket handle injury") due to asymmetric compression of the pelvis, such occurs when wheels of a vehicle roll over a body from one side to the other.

Sacrum (Denis)

Neurological consequences of pelvic trauma are frequently due to sacral fractures, and so this classification is based on the correlation between anatomic features and neurological involvement.

Fewer than 6% of vertical fractures of the ala, lateral to the foramina (type 1), are accompanied by neurological signs (usually referable to L5).

Vertical fractures through the sacral foramina (type 2, called "postage-stamp") entail neurological signs in 28%, usually of S1 and S2, seldom L5.

Fractures of the sacral canal (type 3) are often comminuted and nearly 57% come with neurological signs.

Acetabulum (Letournel)

Elementary fracture lines (including transverse lines) affect the posterior wall, posterior column, anterior wall, and anterior column of the acetabulum.

Complex fractures represent an association between at least two elementary lines:

- T-shaped fractures
- Transverse fractures also involving the posterior wall
- Posterior transverse fractures also involving the anterior wall or column
- Posterior column plus posterior wall fractures (frequently associated with hip dislocation)
- Anterior and posterior column fractures.

And still more complex associations can be seen.

Indications

The choices of percutaneous technique and specific procedure are made in coordination between radiologists and surgeons, the advice of the anesthetists of course is needed.

Time Limits

In most traumatic injuries of pelvic bones, associated visceral and vascular lesions are to be feared, but their clinical manifestations can be initially obscure and delayed. Exhaustive investigation is therefore mandatory before undertaking a percutaneous procedure [9, 16]. Moreover, the prone position can favor hemodynamic destabilization of such lesions. This is a reason why it is often considered safer to wait at least two days before performing a screw fixation, especially using a posterior or posterolateral approach.

On the other hand, a prolonged supine position should be avoided, since it allows bedsores or other usual complications to appear. Early stabilization can also prevent a consolidation in a faulty position that requires surgical correction.

The optimal period to operate thus seems to range from to 3 days to 3 weeks.

Injury Type

Posterior Arch Fractures

Type-C injuries due to a longitudinal (cephalocaudal) stress vector, whether iliac or sacral, can be treated percutaneously if the displacement is smaller than 15 mm and after installing an efficient continuous traction device. Highly displaced fractures that need a tricky reduction have to be treated by open surgery.

Transverse injuries (B-type) and sacroiliac disruptions should first undergo external reduction, kept steady with a large adhesive strip applied anteriorly, after which the patient can be positioned properly for the procedure. The percutaneous incursion is then directed to stabilizing the posterior uni- or bilateral lesion. If an anterior lesion is associated, it should be fixed only if it threatens acetabular stability.

"Open Book" Fractures

"Open book" fractures represent an excellent example of associated surgical and radiological treatment. An open reduction of the pubic gap can allow one to look for a possible vascular or visceral wound (of the bladder, for instance) and then to perform an accurate internal plate fixation [15]. Posterior fixation. especially in bilateral injuries, should be performed a few days later and lead to a really strong setting that will allow early ambulation (Fig. 18.1).

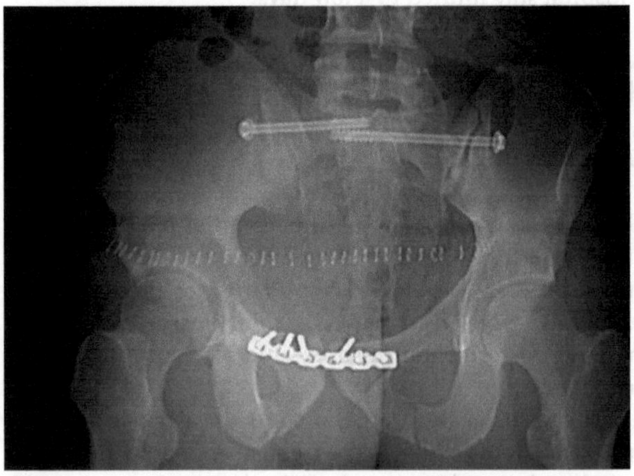

Fig. 18.1. "Open book" fracture. Open reduction and internal fixation of a pubic disruption using plate and screws. Later percutaneous fixation of a bilateral sacroiliac disruption

Percutaneous Solutions

Percutaneous solutions have been more recently proposed for acetabular fractures that are more complex and require a highly accurate reduction to prevent osteoarthritis. Delayed displacement, which would only occur in unstable injuries, can be avoided by screw fixation [22]. Such a procedure is to be considered after applying a traction device efficient enough to reveal even a slightly displaced fracture. The main indications are (1) frontal or sagittal fractures reaching from the acetabular roof across the iliac wing, (2) posterior fractures with threat of hip dislocation, and (3) fractures of the upper part of the anterior column.

For posterior injuries, a percutaneous approach may prevent periarticular ossifications from delayed occurrence, which would then require weighty treatment (radiation therapy or surgery) [2].

"Non Indications"

Injuries considered stable do not require fixation as long as they do not jeopardize the stability of the pelvic girdle.

Such is the case for fragmented fractures (A1 type of Tile), notably of the ilium. For A2 fractures, considered stable, the need for percutaneous fixation can be discussed. The main advantage of this solution is quick eradication of pain and early ambulation. This option can be used for patients at high risk for the complications of long bed rest [11,22].

Isolated fractures of the pubic rami need no special treatment. When associated with a posterior injury, however, screw fixation of this one will help in stabilizing the whole. Similarly, a fracture line of the anterior column running ahead of the weight-bearing zone of the acetabulum should not be operated.

An excessive delay required by a shaky state or by the more urgent management of other pathology (e.g., neurological problem, infection) renders percutaneous fixation a useless gesture since the fracture will become stable on its own after 3 to 4 weeks and because any undesirable callus or pseudarthrosis will be correctable only by an open and generally difficult surgical procedure.

Further Considerations and Contraindications

The type and the degree of displacement is the essential point in decision-making. Vertical shear fractures most often require an open reduction and internal fixation, especially if the displacement is larger than 15 mm.

Comminuted fractures of the sacrum accompanied with neurological signs, especially when a spinal lesion is associated, must be investigated, decompressed, and fixed by open surgery.

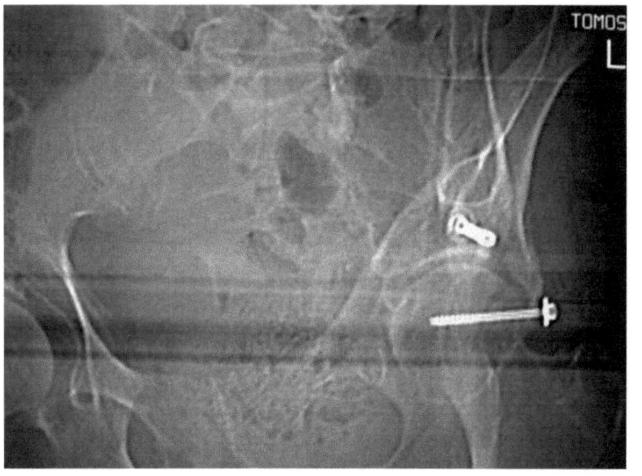

Fig. 18.2. Fixation of a comminuted acetabular fracture in a 96-year-old man who fell. He could sit in his armchair the day after operation, i.e., 3 days after accident

Comminuted fractures of the acetabulum, especially when there is a gap between the fragments, must be operated to restore a correct anatomical configuration. In certain cases however, an additional percutaneous fixation of some fragments can avoid a second open approach. An intra-articular fragment most often requires quick removal through an opening. On the other hand, in some cases when stabilization is more important than the quality of reduction (e.g., in old age), a less traumatic percutaneous intervention allows the patient to sit and even stand quickly (Fig. 18.2).

The overall conditions of the injured person does not always allow him or her to maintain the required position, in particular the prone position that is mostly used in the posterior approach (sacroiliac joint and posterior column). Damage from skin and other soft-tissue trauma can rule out the procedure if situated obstructively, and can also prevent access for spinal anesthesia. When the delay before intervention becomes too long for any reason, and the patient remains bedridden, the advent of bedsores requires abstention.

The Procedure

Preliminaries

Upon admission of the patient a traction device should be applied as soon as the vital parameters allow. A dislocation of the femoral head is reduced as soon as possible.

The initial radiological evaluation limits itself mostly to the frontal and oblique views, because it is now known that the essential diagnostic step is a CT scan of the whole pelvis with multiplanar and sometimes 3D reconstructions. Often accompanying this exam may be one or more contrast-aided series investigating vascular and visceral elements. If an abdominopelvic CT scan is immediately performed (for instance in case of total body screening), flat X-rays are redundant.

In unstable vascular situations, a pelvic clamp is set, then an angiographic exploration, possibly followed by therapeutic embolization, may be performed. This represents no contraindication for a later fixation that can be done as soon as the hemodynamic state of the patient is normalized.

Protocol and Technique

The CT room is thoroughly cleaned and disinfected just before the intervention. When possible, the anesthesia is prepared in a room close to the CT. Access is restricted to those whose presence is necessary, in sterile surgical garb. Rigorous asepsis is mandatory throughout the procedure.

The patient is settled in a comfortable position on the CT table and metallic marks are emplaced on the skin (usually spinal needles). A CT scan is executed in slices, 5 mm thick for the sacroiliac joint and 3 mm for the acetabulum. Indelible marks are made where the implants are to be introduced prior to disinfecting and dressing the skin. A transparent sterile veil is affixed to the skin and CT gantry as a separation from personnel.

Appropriate surgical hardware is arranged on one or two dressed tables. The procedure is generally led by a radiologist and a surgeon or by two radiologists. If the latter, a surgeon has to be on close call in case of an emergency.

A skin incision of about 1 cm is performed and followed by careful dissection down to contact with bone. A guide pin is then hammered a few millimeters into the bone. The position of the pin is monitored by some slices of the same thickness as for the initial CT. When the proper position is confirmed, the pin is advanced with a drill (pneumatic or electric) until its extremity can be seen beyond the fracture line. The length of the screw can then be exactly measured with the CT calipers. We use cannulated self-drilling and self-tapping screws, preferably in titanium, which can be seen tolerably well on MRI examination. For posterior arch fixation, screws of 7 to 8 mm in diameter are chosen, with a length from 60 to 140 mm according to the orientation. For the acetabulum, we use screws from 4 to 6 mm in diameter, and the tip of the screw has to run 2 to 3 mm beyond the opposite cortex. Injuries of the posterior arch are ideally fixed by two screws positioned in two different planes and in different directions. A better result is obtained when the shank of the screw lies immediately adjacent to bone cortex and the tip is situated beyond the median line. Only when the screw is in exactly the right place and correctly tightened can the pin be removed.

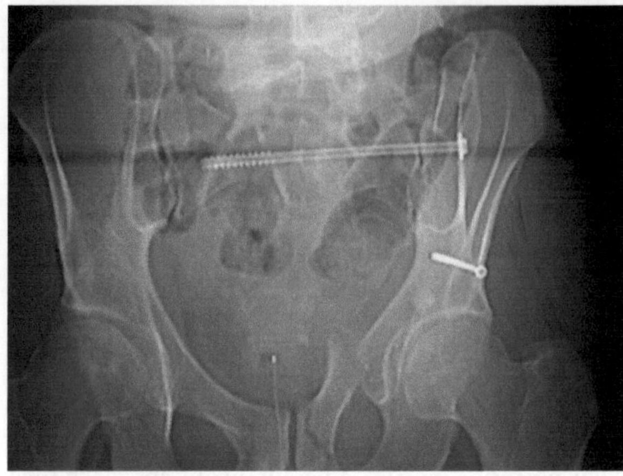

Fig. 18.3. Fractures of left sacrum and acetabulum fixed during the same operation

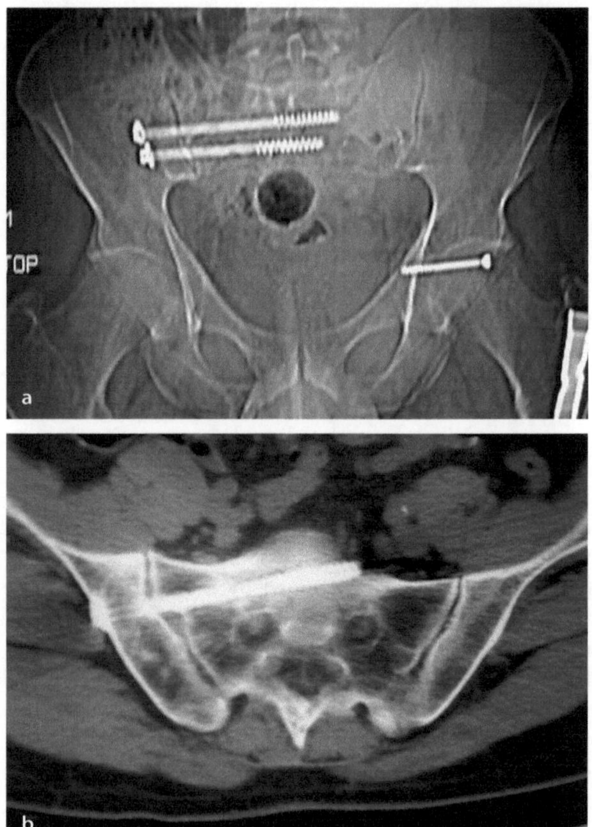

Fig. 18.4a, b. Right sacroiliac disruption associated to a fracture of the left acetabulum. **a** Single procedure fixation. **b** View of sacroiliac fusion after 10 months

Ipsilateral or contralateral associated injuries can be treated at the same time (Figs. 18.3, 18.4). In case of

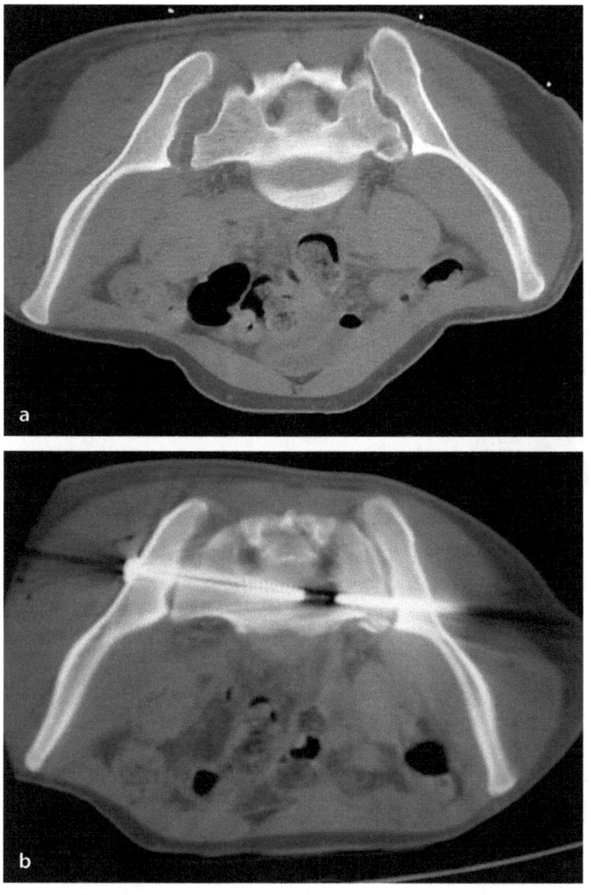

Fig. 18.5. **a** Right sacroiliac disruption and fracture of left ala of sacrum. **b** Bilateral fixation in a single procedure

bilateral lesions, two operators can act simultaneously (Fig. 18.5).

The cutaneous breach is closed by one or two stitches, with or without deep reinforcement. It is sometimes possible to introduce two screws through a single 1.5 to 2 cm opening. It is not necessary to use drains because the bleeding is usually less than 25 ml.

A final CT of the whole pelvis is obtained, the scout view being used as a control radiograph. Reconstructions can complete the iconography. The patient, after a short stay in a recovery room, is put back to bed. Standing is most often possible the next morning.

Surveillance, Complications

The various published series, as well as our personal experience (75 cases) at the Saint Roch Hospital in Nice and H. Mondor Hospital in Aurillac, confirm this technique as one with very few complications.

Vascular, nervous, and visceral injuries are avoided by a prudent approach. A careful preoperative study of the trajectory, especially for structures at risk, and the taking of control slices during the procedure assure minimal risks. Thus far, no patient of ours has had to undergo a blood transfusion as a result of the percutaneous procedure.

In our experience with sacral procedures, no screw has threatened a nervous or vascular structure because of a breach of the foramen. One screw placed in S1 via an obliquely ascending route was seen to have its tip in the L5-S1 disk, but without any clinical consequence.

No case of postoperative infection has thus far occurred. We have injected a single dose of a first generation cephalosporin at the beginning of each procedure, but other use of antibiotics has only been for problems such as open fractures or visceral wounds.

During the initial postoperative phase, the patient must refrain from weight bearing on the operated side. Within this period a thromboembolic accident is prevented by a systematic prescription of low molecular weight heparin (LMWH). Painkiller is injected with an automatic syringe on demand; it is rarely needed for more than 48 hours.

We have had no case of secondary displacement or failure of the implants. The traction device was most often removed at the end of the procedure (thus taking advantage of the spinal anesthesia). In one case of fixation of a complex acetabular fracture and one case of comminuted fracture of the femur, traction was maintained for two weeks.

A visit to the radiologist and surgeon is scheduled for 45 and 90 days post-procedure, then ideally after 6 months, the last two being preceded by CT examination. We have to give notice that several of our patients who incurred accidents while on holiday came from other regions or even from foreign countries, and thus have escaped our follow-up.

Results

Immediate

The acute painful phase did not exceed 48 hours in 87% of the cases, allowing for quick removal of venous access for the less seriously wounded patients.

Sitting then standing with help was successful the following morning in 90% of the cases. The exceptions were those with associated injuries of the spine or lower limbs.

The patient could be discharged from hospital when able to ambulate with crutches or equivalent device, most often within 3 to 5 days. In some cases delay occurred while the rehabilitation department sought accommodation for the patient. More often the patient was sent back home if there were no steps to climb and if help was available, rehabilitation to proceed on an outpatient basis.

A perfect compression of the fracture was not always achieved because of the interposition of small fragments, in particular in fractures of the iliac wing, but strong consolidation was finally obtained. The result was radiologically satisfactory according to Jacob's criteria [13] in 83% of the cases.

Delayed

Jobs were resumed after 3 months and normal preoperative job activity was achieved in about 6 months. The resumption of sport and leisure activities also began in 3 months. The persistence of daily pain after one year is described in 15% of the cases, mostly after sacroiliac injuries, and in 12% occasionally during efforts (the average quotation being 3 on a pain scale of 10 maximum). Less than 7% of the patients, however, admit being disappointed by the result.

The cautious indication for fixation of vertical shear injuries allowed us not to find significant lower limb length discrepancy. One patient had a 2 cm shortening due to a fracture of the femur with faulty healing.

In one man a comminuted injury of the sacroiliac joint turned into pseudarthrosis that required a further conventional open fixation. He was a severely multitraumatized patient we received at the beginning of our series, who could be operated only after one month, a situation that can be now practically judged a bad indication. A delay longer than three weeks is now considered a contraindication to percutaneous screwing.

It will probably be necessary to accumulate experience over a longer period to be able to foresee the frequency of osteoarthritic degeneration of the sacroiliac joint, and most especially of the acetabulum, and to estimate the influence that the screw and its position might have on such degeneration and on possible hip replacement.

Discussion

The functional (nonsurgical) treatment of unstable injuries, at first recommended, was found to be unsatisfactory. Letournel's development of open surgery demonstrated that the posterior fixation is essential for these lesions [6]. The technological improvements in medical imaging and in data processing, as well as the development of mini-invasive techniques, served to increase the importance of percutaneous methods for screw insertion under CT scan guidance and thus include them in the field of interventional radiology.

The prone position is preferred for percutaneous treatment of fractures of the posterior arch [14, 15] and for the posterior approach of acetabulum [16]. The lateral (Fig. 18.6) or oblique decubitus (Fig. 18.7) allows

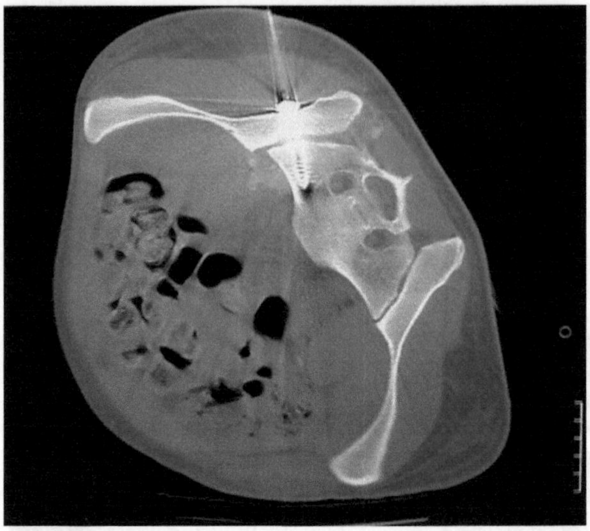

Fig. 18.6. Fracture-disruption of right sacroiliac joint. Fixation in lateral decubitus position

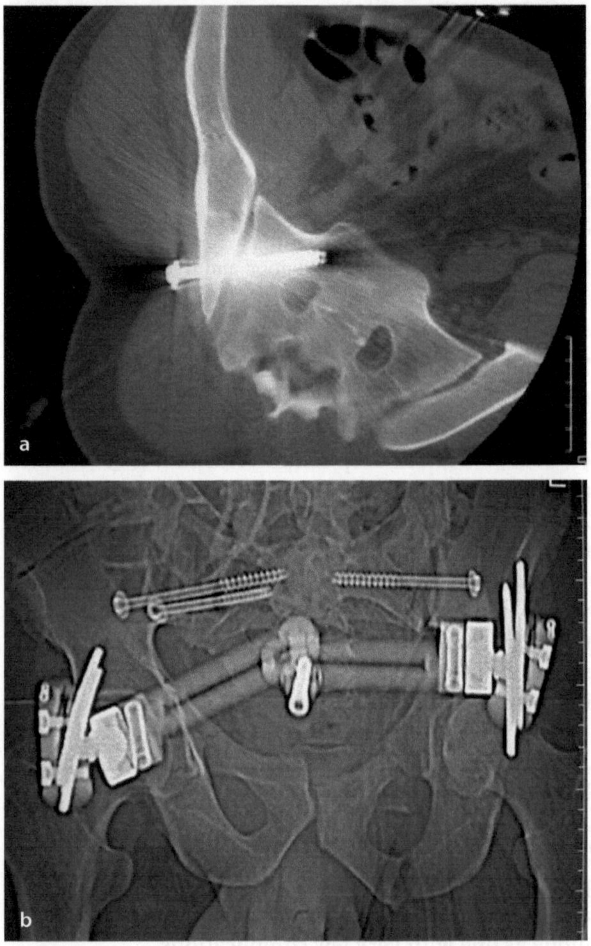

Fig. 18.7a, b. Bilateral sacroiliac disruption with symphysis pubis disruption and left obturator foramen fracture; reduction with external fixation. **a** View during procedure in oblique decubitus. **b** Final view

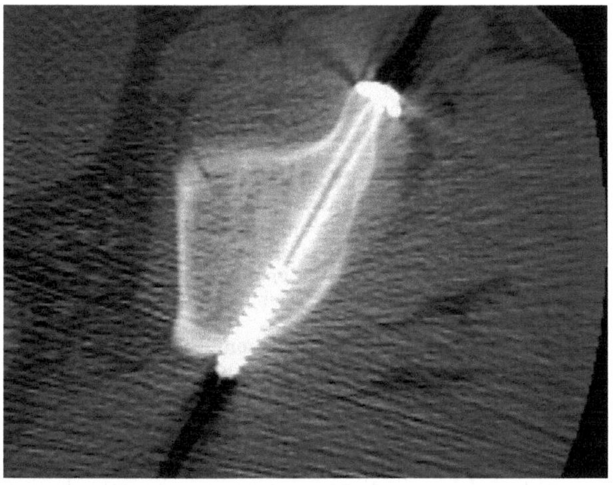

Fig. 18.8. Fracture of the anterior column of left acetabulum. Fixation by the "Corsican Cape" technique

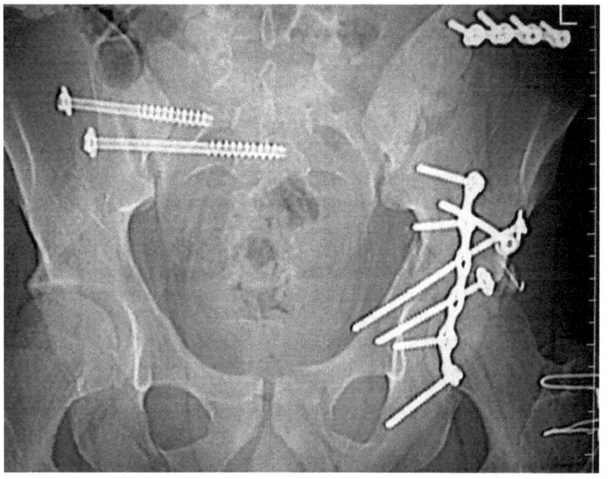

Fig. 18.9. Open reduction and internal fixation of left femur, acetabulum, and iliac wing. Postage-stamp fracture of the right part of sacrum. Percutaneous fixation by two screws one week later

a combined approach, notably in associated injuries of the sacroiliac joint and acetabulum [17]. The supine position is used for the anterior approach to the acetabulum and iliac wing.

In considering the CT slice running through the acetabular roof, one notices it is very like the outlines of the island of Corsica, leading to an easy characterization of the intended approach. The insertion of anteroposterior screw(s) following the longitudinal axis of the acetabulum, used for the fixation of verticofrontal fractures, has thus become Corsican Cape approach [18] (Fig. 18.8).

Utilizing only fluoroscopy for fixation is dangerous [19, 20]. The CT scan is incomparably more precise. The value of a combined technique, fluoroCT, has yet to be adequately determined, and computer-guided navigation is under development [21, 22].

The creation of appropriate technical devices should in the future allow performance of the procedures under permanent traction, and thus widen the indications to a larger number of C-type injuries. The realization of associated procedures, open surgery and percutaneous screw insertion, should improve treatment of some complex fractures, especially of the acetabulum. A delay is necessary of just 2 or 3 days between the two interventions (Fig. 18.9).

The introduction of mobile CT into the interventional radiology room – or even the operating room – is conceivable in trauma centers, which would release the main CT scan for scheduled and emergency examinations.

Conclusion

This "mini-invasive" approach of the traumatic injuries of the pelvic girdle is manifestly promising. This can be demonstrated by noting that, while only a few articles were published during the first years, more and more teams are now interested [23, 24]. The prospects for further development are intriguing.

The development of simulation techniques and of virtual imaging, in which certain teams are already interested, should quickly improve the accuracy (already noticeable) of these interventions.

The considerable shortening of the hospital stay [25, 26] and the small rate of complications add major human and economic arguments to the attractive technical aspect of this therapeutic strategy, based on close cooperation and confidence between surgeons and radiologists.

References

1. Huittinen VM, Slatis P (1972) Fractures of the pelvis: trauma mechanism, type of injury and principles of treatment. Acta Chir Scand 138:563–569
2. Monfort J, Le Neel JC (1973) Les disjonctions récentes de la symphyse pubienne. Indications thérapeutiques à partir de 50 cas. Ann Chir 27:601–608
3. Young JWR, Burgess AR, Brumback RJ, Poka A (1986) Pelvic fractures: value of plain-radiography in early assessment and management. Radiology 160:445–451
4. Tile M, Pennal GF (1980) Pelvic disruption: principles of management. Clin Orthop 151:56–64
5. Denis F, Davis S, Comfort T (1988) Sacral fractures, an important problem. Clin Orthop 227:160–179
6. Letournel E (1980) Acetabulum fractures: classification and management. Clin Orthop 151:81–106

7. Gill K, Bucholz R (1984) The role of CT-scanning in the evaluation of major pelvic fractures. J Bone Joint Surg 66(A):34–39
8. Kellam JF, Messer A (1994) Evaluation of the role of coronal, sagittal and axial CT scan reconstructions for the imaging of acetabular fractures. Clin Orthop 305:152–159
9. Judet R, Judet J (1965) Etude critique du traitement chirurgical de 20 observations de disjonction traumatique de la symphyse pubienne. Presse Méd 73:1787–1792
10. Spencer R (1989) Acetabular fractures in older patients. J Bone Joint Surg 71(B):774–776
11. Burd TA, Lowry KJ, Anglen JO (2001) Indomethacin compared with localized irradiation for the prevention of heterotopic ossification following surgical treatment of acetabular fractures. J Bone Joint Surg 83A(12):1783–1788
12. Helfet DL, Borrelli J, DiPasquale T, Sanders R (1992) Stabilization of acetabular fractures in elderly patients. J Bone Joint Surg 74:753–765
13. Jacob AL, Messmer P (1997) Posterior pelvic ring fractures: closed reduction and percutaneous CT-guided sacroiliac screw fixation. Cardiovasc Intervent Radiol 20:285–294
14. Ebraheim NA, Rusin J (1987) Percutaneous computed tomography stabilization of pelvic fractures: preliminary report. J Orthop Trauma 1:197–204
15. Nelson DW, Duwelius PJ (1991) CT-guided fixation of sacral fractures and sacroiliac joint disruptions. Radiology 180:527–532
16. Gay S, Sistrom C (1992) Percutaneous screw fixation of acetabular fractures with CT guidance: preliminary result of a new technique. Am J Radiol 158:819–822
17. Eude P, Damon F, Eude G et al (2000) Ostéosynthèse percutanée des fractures du bassin sous contrôle tomodensitométrique. J Radiol 81:63–68
18. Eude P, Trojani C, Eude G, Piche S, Aboulker C, de Peretti F (2002) Percutaneous screw fixation of acetabular fractures under computed tomography guidance. Semin Intervent Radiol 19:257–264
19. Templeman D, Schmidt A (1996) Proximity of ilio-sacral screws to neurovascular structures after internal fixation. Clin Orthop 329:194–198
20. Goldberg BA, Lindsey RW, Foglar C, Hedrick TD, Miclau T, Hadad JL (1998) Imaging assessment of sacroiliac screw placement relative to the neuroforamen. Spine 23:585–589
21. Brown GA, Willis MC, Firoozbakhsh K, Barmada A, Tessman CL, Montgomery A (2000) Computed tomography image-guided surgery in complex acetabular fractures. Clin Orthop 370:219–226
22. Jacob AL, Suhm N, Kaim A, Regazzoni P, Steinbrich W, Messmer P (2000) Coronal acetabular fractures: the anterior approach in computed tomography-navigated minimally invasive percutaneous fixation. Cardiovasc Intervent Radiol 23: 327–331
23. Starr AJ, Jones AL, Reinert CM, Borer DS (2001) Preliminary results and complications following limited open reduction and percutaneous screw fixation of displaced fractures of the acetabulum. Injury 32:45–50
24. Crowl AC, Kahler DM (2002) Closed reduction and percutaneous fixation of anterior column acetabular fractures. Comput Aided Surg 7:169–178
25. Pennal GF, Davidson J, Garside H, Plewes J (1980) Results of treatment of acetabular fractures. Clin Orthop 151:115–123
26. Nordin JY (1990) Fractures de l'anneau pelvien. Conférences d'Enseignement de la SOFCOT. Expansion Scientifique Française

Interventional Magnetic Resonance Imaging in Pain Therapy

Principles and Clinical Application

19

Philippe L. Pereira, Jan Fritz, Claus D. Claussen, Bruno Kastler

Introduction and Overview

Back in 1952, Bloch (in Stanford) and Purcell (in Harvard) received the Nobel Prize in physics for "their development of new methods for nuclear magnetic precision measurements and discoveries in connection therewith." Five decades later magnetic resonance occupies a central place in natural science and has evolved into an essential tool in diagnostic radiology. The development of different acquisition techniques as well as the development of different configured MR scanners contributed to the impressive development of medical MR imaging over the last several years. And in interventional radiology, MR imaging has begun to play a more and more important role. Interventional MR imaging is a methodology whereby MR imaging is used to guide therapeutic procedures.

MR imaging offers unique features that make it suitable for interventional purposes:

- Excellent tissue contrast of T1- and T2-weighted MR sequences with or without fat suppression techniques
- Multiplanar imaging capabilities that allow virtually three-dimensional visualization of MR-compatible interventional instruments, thus enabling the exact delineation in difficult anatomic areas during procedures
- Adequate temporal and spatial resolution necessary to perform interventions
- No exposure of patients and interventional radiologists to ionizing radiation
- Identification of vascular structures without the need of contrast agents.

And finally more sophisticated features available in high-field MR scanners (field strength 0.5 Tesla):

- Measurement of different physiological information such as diffusion, perfusion, and quantification of flow
- Temperature monitoring, which is an essential feature in MR imaging-guided percutaneous thermal ablation – by using radiofrequency (RF) or laser – for the control of heat distribution

In addition to the introduction of open configured MR scanners, the development of MR-compatible interventional devices has introduced new diagnostic and therapeutic possibilities for interventional radiologists and surgeons. Dedicated MR scanners help to improve patient safety during interventional MR imaging, reduce the invasiveness of certain surgical procedures, and enable minimally invasive interventions.

Owing to technological progress, it has been made possible to adapt essential interventional hardware such as equipment for anesthesia and technical instruments, including RF devices and therapeutical laser systems, for use in an MR environment. This MR-compatible hardware can be safely handled inside an MR unit, and does not undergo stress or heating in a magnetic field.

The ability of preprocedural MR imaging with high tissue contrast provides the interventionalist with exclusive information for evaluation of the region of interest (ROI), and for planning a procedure. The required spatial and temporal resolution of MR images necessary for MR-imaging guidance can be achieved with fast gradient echo MR sequences at virtually all field strengths (from 0.2 to 1.5 Tesla). Although real-time imaging as obtained in X-ray fluoroscopy is difficult to achieve in MR imaging, today practically all MR systems permit near real-time imaging by image updates within seconds. On one hand, this feature allows excellent navigation and position control of interventional devices in difficult anatomic areas; on the other hand, in combination with physiologic tissue information, it offers unique monitoring capabilities for therapeutic procedures, in particular for thermal ablations or local injections.

With the technical improvement and the absence of ionizing radiation of MR imaging guidance, virtually any intervention can be performed. For a large number of interventions, e.g., MR imaging-guided biopsies, interventional MR imaging has successfully run the gamut of feasibility studies [1]. Nevertheless, the application of interventional MR imaging in pain therapy still remains very limited. The same applies to microsurgical MR imaging-guided spine interventions [2] and to joint infiltrations [3]. To ensure best therapeutic results in pain therapy, an interdisciplinary approach that includes radiologists, anesthetists, surgeons, nurses, and technicians has proved to be essential.

In summary, interventional MR imaging offers unique characteristics in the localization of anatomic and pathologic structures, allowing imaging-guided placement and navigation of interventional devices and enabling direct process monitoring of specific therapies.

The Interventional MR Armamentarium

Even though interventional MR imaging is only at its beginning, it is not precipitous to state that rarely has a medical technique benefited so much from technical developments. This progress is mainly related to the sufficient access to the patient provided by an MR scanner, specially designed for interventional purposes, and to the MR-imaging compatibility of interventional devices and equipment used both inside and outside the magnetic field.

General Considerations and Prerequisites

Following the same principles as applicable to diagnostic MR imaging, interventional MR imaging likewise relies upon the crucial role played by the strength of the static magnetic field (B_0) of an MR scanner. In general, the lower the strength of the magnetic field, the longer the acquisition time. Moreover, with low-field MR scanners the quality of fast imaging and artifacts, such as might be necessary for targeting interventional MR-compatible devices, often remains poor. This drawback is due to the reduced susceptibility, which depends on the homogeneity of B_0. In this context, new possibilities are offered by the introduction of a new generation of interventional high-field MR scanners with a short magnet and a large bore (Magnetom Espree, Siemens, Erlangen, Germany). With this new concept the former compromise between patient access, image quality, and duration of image acquisition is rendered unnecessary;. interventional high field MR scanners allow the use of fast and functional MR imaging without marked restrictions to patient access.

A prerequisite for fast MR imaging with sufficient image quality is a gradient of at least 15 mTesla/m or higher, and a gradient switch time of at least 900 ms. Dedicated interventional open MR scanners are equipped with MR-compatible in-room liquid crystal (LCD) monitors that allow the interventionalist to remain close to the patient. In-room monitoring is particularly useful for direct MR imaging navigation during the placement of interventional devices. A chair that provides an ergonomic position for the interventionalist during the procedure, a flexible optical fiber lamp, and a double pedal for optional device control have proved to be useful interventional equipment.

Moreover, there are sophisticated navigation systems (Siemens, and Marconi, Coventry, UK) that assist the determination of skin entry points and the corresponding optimal slice orientation for interventional MR imaging guidance. The spatial orientation and position of interventional instruments are detected with an optical lasers system (Polaris, Northern DIGITAL, Waterloo, Ontario, Canada for Siemens) that provides continuous information on the position of the device in relation to the system.

Configurations and Designs

To perform interventional MR imaging. unrestricted access to the patient is indispensable. In contrast to the limited patient access of conventional closed MR scanners, various new designs that have been introduced permit interventional access even as scanning proceeds.

The new group includes open-bore MR systems (Magnetom Espree, Siemens, 1.5 Tesla) providing patient access similar to a CT scanner and a still prototypical interventional MR scanner offering unrestricted 360-degree patient access (Fonar-360°-MRI, 0.6-Tesla, Fonar Corporation, Melville, NY, USA). The following list represents an overview of proven and promising concepts, with differences in field strength, configuration, and patient access:

- Low-field MR scanner (0.2 Tesla) generally has horizontally oriented magnets resembling a c-arm (Figs. 19.1, 19.2) with a vertically oriented static magnetic field (Magnetom Concerto, Siemens; Panorama 0.23 T, Philips Medical Systems, Eindhoven, The Netherlands).
- The first open mid-field MR scanner (0.5 Tesla) consisted of two vertically oriented magnets resembling a "Double-Doughnut" and a horizontally oriented static magnetic field (Signa SP, General Electric Medical Systems, Waukesha, WI; Fig. 19.3). New generation mid-field MR scanners, however, also have the c-arm design enabling horizontal patient access (Panorama 0.6T, Philips).
- Additional open high-field MR scanners (1.0 T) suitable for interventional purposes were recently introduced to the market. One new concept is based on a short cylindrical open-bore magnet with a horizontally oriented static magnetic field (Magnetom Espree, 1.5 T, Siemens). Other concepts are based on known designs with horizontal patient access (Panorama 1.0 T, Philips).

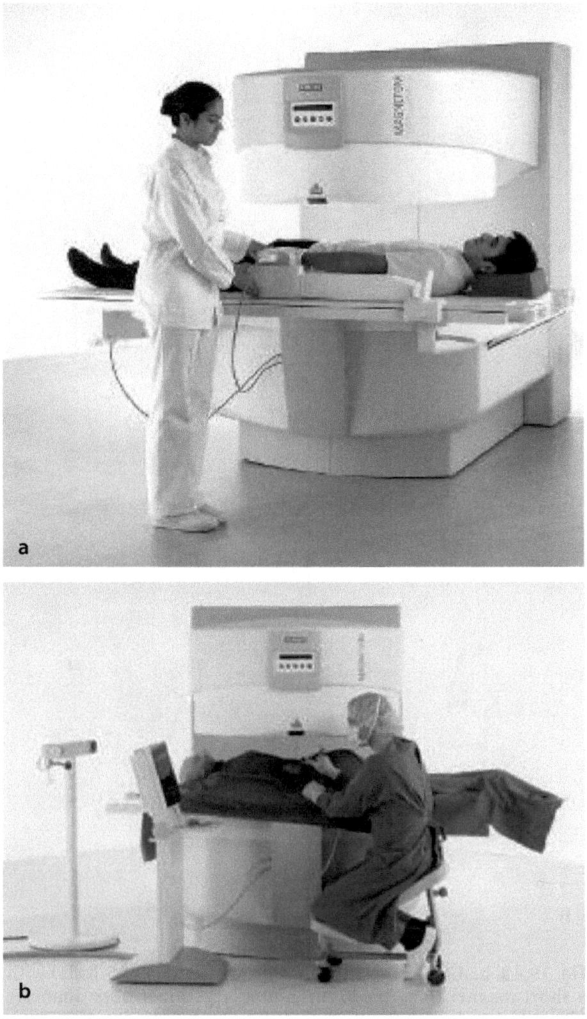

Fig. 19.1. **a** Open low field MR scanner in "C" configuration (Magnetom Concerto, Siemens) enabling comfortable patient positioning and horizontal patient access during interventional procedures, with enough space for proper sterile covering. **b** Interventional scenario with sterile covered puncture site. The in-room monitor provides the interventionalist real-time MR images for navigation and control

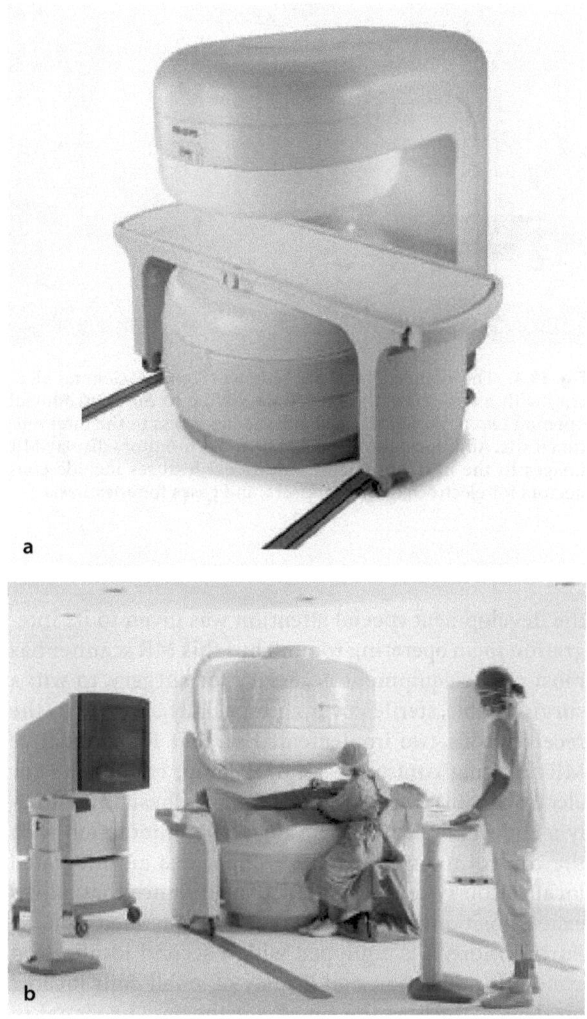

Fig. 19.2. **a** Open low field MR scanner in "C" configuration (Panorama 0.23T, Philips Medical Systems, Eindhoven, The Netherlands). The image shows the c-arm shaped design. **b** The image shows an interventional MR imaging scenario. Useful additional equipments are an MR-compatible in-room monitor for navigation and real-time action control as well as an additional workstation panel

Interventional Low-field MR Scanners

The permanent magnet in an open low field MR system (0.2 Tesla) has in general a "C" shape (Figs. 19.1, 19.2). The magnetic field is oriented vertically between the upper and lower poles. This design allows a horizontal patient access of approximately 280 degrees. The field of view allows interventional and diagnostic MR imaging. The ring-shaped flexible receiver coils (Fig. 19.5) placed around the patient can be shifted very easily in order to gain access to the puncture site. The coils can be easily covered sterilely. A close placement of the coil to the puncture site is desirable in order to achieve a high signal-to-noise ratio and best imaging quality.

Interventional Mid-field MR Scanners

The first open mid-field MR scanner was developed by engineers of General Electric (Signa SP, General Electric) [4] (Fig. 19.3). The prototype of this system was installed at Brigham and Women's Hospital, Boston, MA, USA, in 1994. This MR scanner consists of a superconducting 0.5-Tesla magnet with imaging capacities close to those of standard MR scanners. The central vertical opening allows the interventionalist continuous patient access during procedures. This type of configuration allows virtually unlimited patient access. The difference between this MR scanner and other superconducting MR systems is the absence of a cooling system. During

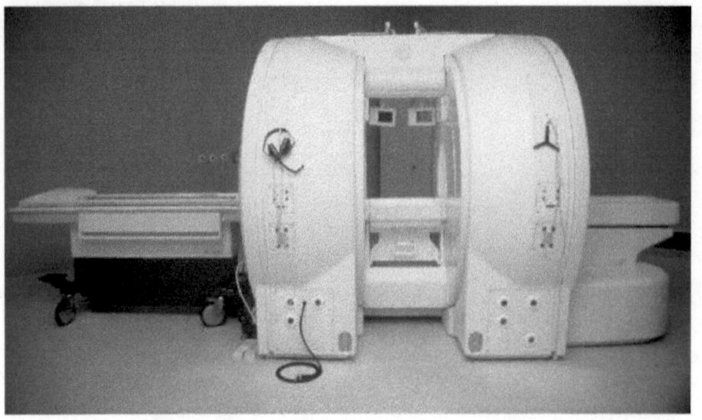

Fig. 19.3. The "double donut" MR scanner (Signa SP, General Electric) with a field strength of 0.5 Tesla. Owing to the ventrodorsal opening two physicians have simultaneous access to the interventional site. Additional implemented in-room monitors display MR images to the interventionalist. Additional features include connectors for electrocoagulation, lasers, and gases for anesthesia

the development special attention was given to its integration in an operating room. Thus this MR scanner has most of the equipment necessary for surgery, to wit: a surgical table, sterile covering especially adapted to the receiver coils, two implemented screens for interactive MR imaging control, a surgical lamp, connectors for electrocoagulation, equipment for anesthesia, and finally a communication system for verbal interaction with the control room . This MR scanner has an integrated localization system for interactive guidance that allows exact positioning of instruments in defined spaces. Furthermore, it is equipped with a second localization system for detection and display of small coils located on devices such as the tip of a catheter. The signal of such a coil delivers the exact position of the catheter and can be used to continuously adjust the level of the MR images of the catheter (active tracking). Owing to these two systems and to the field strength, it is possible to perform MR imaging with a frequency of 20 frames per second, i.e., near real-time imaging (MR fluoroscopy) of good quality. On the integrated in-room monitors the movement of the instrument can be seen virtually as with conventional X-ray fluoroscopy.

Since this concept has turned out to be extremely expensive, the design of present interventional mid-field MR scanners has changed toward horizontal access MR scanners as known from the low-field MR scanners.

Owing to the field strength, these MR scanners again allow performance of MR imaging with a frequency of 20 frames per second, providing near real-time visualization on the integrated in-room monitors in the manner of conventional X-ray fluoroscopy.

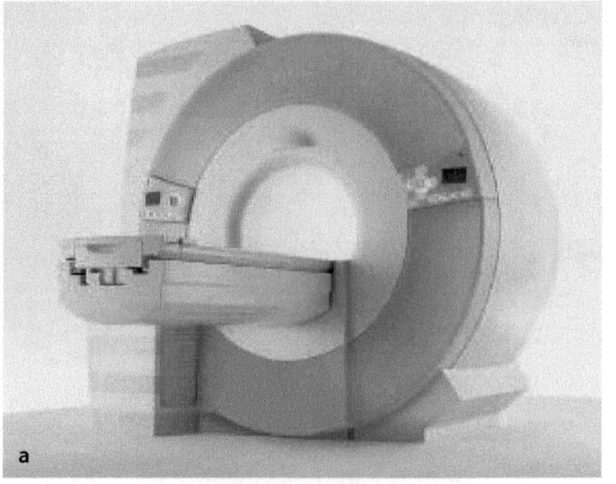

a

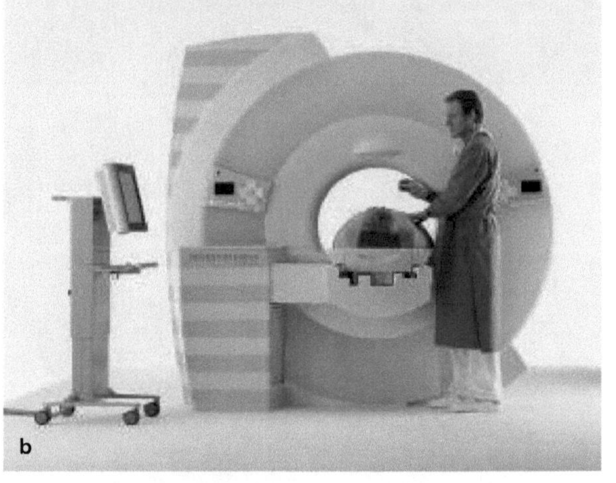

b

Fig. 19.4 a, b. Ultracompact high-field MR scanner (1.5 Tesla) with a short magnet (length 120 cm) and a large inner bore diameter (70 cm) enabling patient access for interventional purposes. **a** Apart from the patient access **b** similar to CT-guided interventions, the high-field technology enables MR fluoroscopy for device guidance and interactive real-time imaging as well as process monitoring using acquisition techniques such as diffusion and perfusion imaging and functional magnetic resonance imaging of the highest quality during interventions

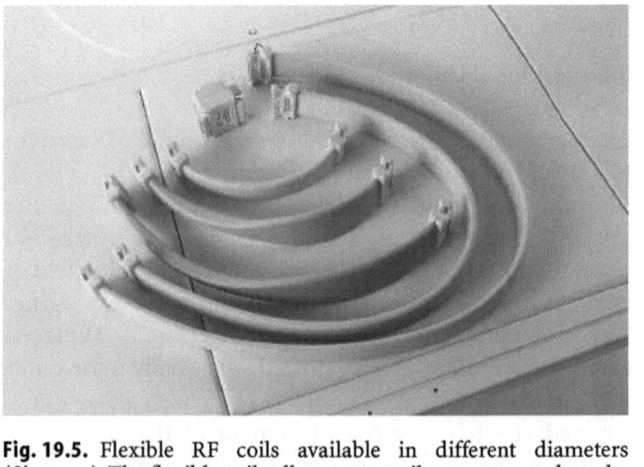

Fig. 19.5. Flexible RF coils available in different diameters (Siemens). The flexible coils allow easy sterile coverage and can be shifted during the intervention in order to facilitate sufficient access to the puncture site.

Interventional High-field MR Scanners

Apart from the open design with horizontal patient access, the latest development in interventional high-field MR imaging is a short closed open-bore MR scanner (Magnetom Espree, Siemens) with a design similar to a CT scanner (Fig. 19.4). The system consists of a 1.2 m short 1.5-Tesla magnet with an inner diameter (bore) of 70 cm. This promising concept might set new standards for interventional MR imaging in accessibility, flexibility, performance, and comfort.

The use of true high-field MR scanners for interventional MR imaging makes it possible to take advantage of high quality MR images without the previously described limitations of an open low-field MR systems. These systems combine features of interventional MR imaging such as MR fluoroscopy for device guidance and interactive real time imaging. as well as process monitoring during interventions using new acquisition techniques such as diffusion and perfusion imaging and functional magnetic resonance imaging of the highest quality.

Safety Issues and Patient Monitoring

The MR Environment and MR Compatibility

The magnetic field, the RF pulses, and the gradients contribute to the special conditions that characterize the environment of an MR scanner. All materials brought into the magnetic field (steel, titanium, plastic, nickel alloy, aluminum, and tungsten, or polymerized composites) cause image distortion of various degree. This phenomenon is based on the magnetic susceptibility of and among different materials. The interactions result in artifacts that can vary from less than one millimeter to a complete distortion of the image.

Ferromagnetic materials most severely influence magnetic fields and MR imaging. In general, conventional steel instruments are composites with a high proportion of ferromagnetic material that cause large artifacts and make MR images uninterpretable (Fig. 19.6). For this reason, "MR compatibility" primarily concerns non-ferromagnetic materials.

When using ferromagnetic equipment or devices in a magnetic field, three types of interactions (inductions) are especially important:

- Artifacts that severely compromise image quality
- Magnetic traction forces
- Heating of instruments to cause burns.

However, with the growing range of application of interventional MR imaging the definition of MR compatibility has moved beyond the simple concept of magnetism related to the nature of the instrument. Beside the question of how the selected material will influence the MR signal other factors also have become important, including magnetic field strength, the behavior of instruments with different angulations to the magnetic field, and the type and parameters of MR sequences used for interventional MR imaging. For example, certain instruments known as MR-compatible may become invisible in a position parallel to the orientation of the magnetic field. On the other hand, large bore needles (>14 gauge) produce disquieting artifacts when oriented perpendicular to the direction of the static magnetic field. To a lesser degree, the frequency, the bandwidth, the read-out direction, and the time of echo (TE) are additional factors that have the potential to influence the MR signal.

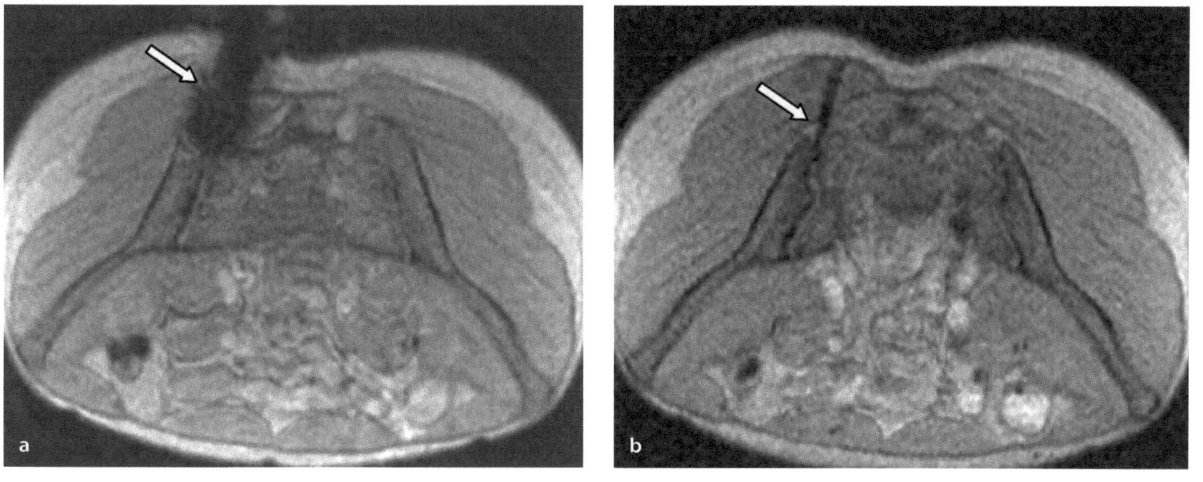

Fig. 19.6 a, b. MR-imaging-guided steroid infiltration of the sacroiliac joints in a patient with sacroiliitis due to seronegative spondylarthropathy. Comparison of MR imaging visualization of **a** a conventional therapy needle (*white arrow*) and **b** a MR-compatible therapy needle specially design for MR-imaging-guided interventions (*white arrow*).

The need for MR-compatible instruments for interventional MR imaging has led to a new generation of devices that combine good visualization and safe handling in a magnetic environment. Today a broad range of commonly used MR-compatible interventional equipment is commercially available.

Visualization of Interventional Devices

Another prerequisite for interventional MR imaging is the reliable and sufficient visualization of interventional devices. Density difference is a more challenging problem in MR imaging than in conventional X-ray fluoroscopy. The various methods of instrument visualization in interventional MR imaging can be divided into active and passive methods. Passive visualization is more commonly used and easier to achieve.

Passive Visualization

Passive methods enable instrument visualization on conventionally acquired MR images. This means that instruments will be recognized on MR images without additional equipment, recalculation, or post-processing. The techniques that are employed for passive visualization can be subdivided into three groups based on:

- decrease of MR signal intensity
- susceptibility to artifacts between the interventional instrument and the surrounding tissue
- use of contrast media to increase the initial MR signal intensity.

In the passive visualization of instruments, the interventionalist is continuously confronted with the following problem: the loss of signal or the artifact produced by the instrument needs to be sufficient to precisely localize the position but not so strong as to otherwise influence image quality and prevent precise instrument localization [5]. Hence, it is possible that a fine needle of 0.7 mm can generate an artifact of almost 8 mm in diameter at a maximum angle of 90° related to the static magnetic field (when using gradient echo imaging) and on the other hand it will become almost invisible if placed parallel to the orientation of the magnetic field [6] (Fig. 19.7).

The method of passive visualization – loss of signal – is based on the displacement of surrounding tissue by the solid instrument. The contrast between the signal extinction of the needle and the signal produced by the surrounding tissue will allow the indirect visualization of the instrument on the MR image. With this method the quality of visualization is markedly dependent on the resolution of the acquired MR image. The majority of pertinent procedures require fast interventional MR imaging. To achieve this it necessary to sacrifice resolution, which inevitably leads to decreased contrast. To increase speed, slice thickness is increased as their number is decreased, which leads to decreased resolution.

Passive visualization is appropriate for certain instruments, e.g., needles of caliber >20 gauge. However, this method is not advised in laparoscopic interventions or in interventions at the thoracic level, when the needle needs to cross the air-filled chest where no MR signal is naturally produced.

Another artifact mechanism commonly used in interventional MR imaging is produced by the difference of magnetic susceptibility between two distinct objects in the human body, the principal example being when air and tissue are in contact (Fig. 19.8). This difference in susceptibility produces local inhomogeneities in the static magnetic field that can be visualized. In interventional MR imaging this type of artifact is frequently used to visualize instruments in percutaneous interventions such as biopsies. Initially, this phenomenon was studied during biopsy under MR-imaging guidance [7, 8] and is now also applied in vascular interventions to visualize catheters and guide wires [9, 10].

A third alternative for visualizing instruments is to increase their signal intensity in comparison to the environment by filling it with contrast medium. The contrast medium reduces the longitudinal relaxation time T1, which results in higher signal intensity. On MR images with a short repetition time, the instrument will appear bright compared to adjacent tissue (Fig. 19.9). In this method the concentration of the contrast medium is very important in order to avoid a $T2^*$ effect causing a dephasing that leads to a disadvantageous loss of signal. This technique is especially useful in vascular interventions that require catheter visualization. The most obvious disadvantage is the large diameter of the instruments needed for contrast medium injection.

Several other factors also are important in passive visualization. One is the composition of the alloy employed. As previously described, a standard steel needle (ferromagnetic) generates very large distortions in the magnetic field and will produce a "black hole" on the MR image. A pure titanium needle will be quite visible but will have the disadvantage of being too flexible, lacking the rigidity needed for good needle placement. Another important factor is the type of sequence used for visualization. As the gradient echo sequences are more sensitive to heterogeneity of the magnetic field than spin-echo sequences, needle artifacts will be amplified and increasingly apparent. Lastly, the strength of the magnetic field and the diameter of the instrument represent additional factors influencing the passive visualization of instruments.

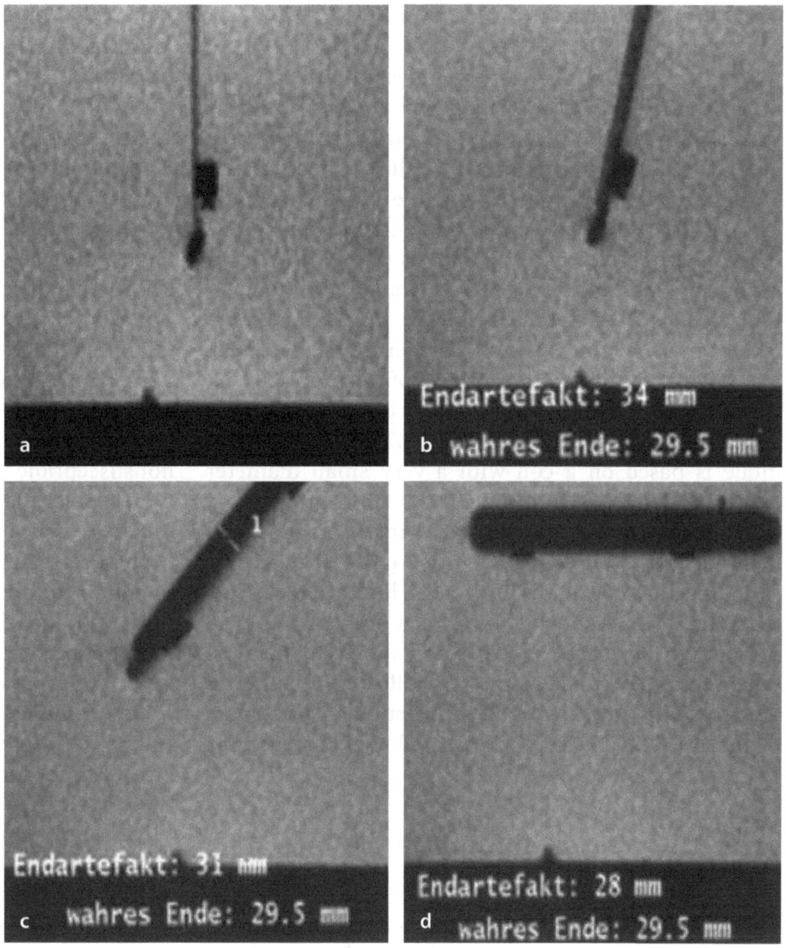

Fig. 19.7 a–d. Four MR images of a 13 gauge needle with different angles to the static magnetic field B_0: **a** 0°, **b** 14°, **c** 44°, **d** 90°. The needle artifact steadily increases width from 1.5 to 6 mm with relation to B_0

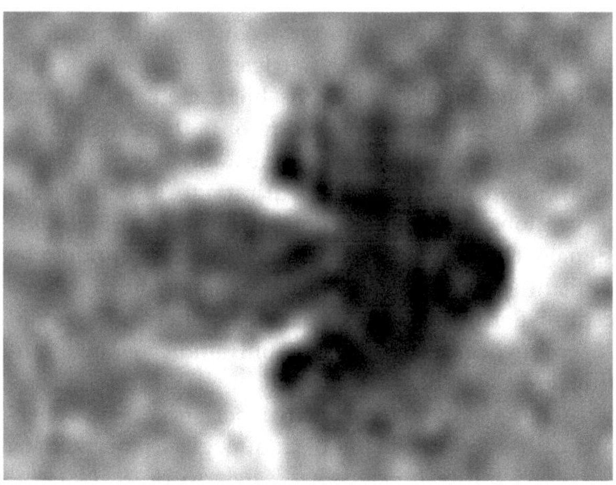

Fig. 19.8. Susceptibility artifact of an 18 gauge needle. The artifact is due to the inhomogeneity in the magnetic field

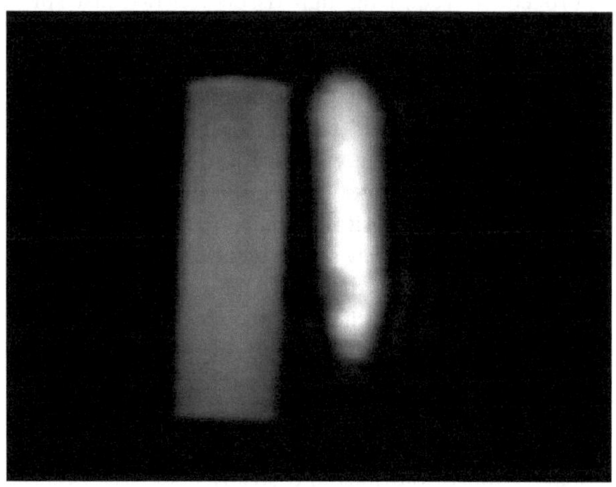

Fig. 19.9. Catheter balloon (4/40 mm) filled with a solution of gadolinium-DTPA (1:80) visualized with a balanced T1-weighted gradient-echo sequence (*right*). On the *left* a syringe for reference.

Active Visualization

Active visualization of instruments is a more complex process that requires a MR signal emitted or detected by the instrument itself. Two methods are currently used: the "MR-tracking" technique where the applied signal is detected by the instrument and the more frequently used "MR-profiling" technique in which a mini-RF coil that emits nonselective RF pulses is placed on the instrument. "MR-tracking" technique allows an acquisition frequency of about 20 images per second for a given target volume [11, 12]. The instrument can be identified according to the position of the mini-RF coil, which allows the MR scanner software to place the slice exactly on the instrument. The "MR-profiling" technique is based on a coil with a very small diameter that is implemented in flexible (catheter or guide wire) or rigid (needle) instruments. The instrument can be identified by a MR signal superimposed on the corresponding anatomical MR image. The limitation of these methods is heating inside the human body due to local production of energy [13, 14] and the complexity of the system. Nevertheless, the possibility of identifying the position of the complete instrument has come to make this technique an essential tool for vascular MR imaging interventions.

MR Imaging Techniques

Important factors to be considered in the choice of suitable MR sequences are the spatial resolution, the duration of image acquisition, and the signal-to-noise ratio. In procedures requiring high-tissue-contrast fast-spin-echo sequences (RARE, FSE, TSE, or LoLo) with an average acquisition time of more than 10 seconds per image may be used. However, in fast spin-echo sequences temporal resolution needs to be sacrificed in order to achieve excellent tissue visualization. When using fast gradient echo sequences (2d-FLASH, FAT, 2D-FISP, or True-FISP) the opposite is true. Gradient echo sequences only need a few seconds for image acquisition but image quality is decreased and artifacts appear amplified. Gradient echo 2D sequences will be less sensitive to motion artifacts than the gradient echo 3D sequences. High-speed double-echo diffusion sequences with acquisition times of a few tens of milliseconds (with reading in a TR of the 256 lines necessary for a space good resolution) and steady-state free precession (SSFP) sequences also known from cardiac cine MR imaging (FISP, FIESTA) have proved to be excellent sequences for ultra-fast MR image acquisition. In addition, SSFP sequences permit fast rebuilding and display of the acquired MR images necessary for MR fluoroscopy. With dedicated MR scanners acquisition of 30 MR images per second at matrices of 256×256 were reported [15]. Nevertheless fluoroscopic near-real-time MR imaging is also possible on a low field MR scanner (0.2 Tesla).

Patient Monitoring

Patient monitoring during interventions is a fundamental principle and of course is essential for interventional MR imaging. Most important cardiovascular and respiratory vital parameters must always be accessible during interventional MR imaging. Certain procedures require neuroleptic analgesia or general anesthesia, which can only be performed with special MR-compatible equipment. Today, complete MR-compatible systems not susceptible to magnetic influences are commercially available allowing complete monitoring in an MR imaging environment [16, 17].

In the treatment of pain using interventional MR imaging, the majority of the procedures can be performed under local or neuroleptic analgesia where monitoring of peripheral pulses, blood pressure, and blood oxygenation is sufficient.

Contraindications for diagnostic MR imaging of course remain valid for interventional MR imaging. Most common contraindications for MR imaging are the presence of Swan-Ganz catheters, metallic cardiac valves, and implantable cardioverter/defibrillators, in which the electromagnetic field can induce dysfunction or damage. Most non-ferromagnetic biological cardiac valves are MR compatible and thus do not preclude MR imaging.

In general, orthopedic prostheses are non-ferromagnetic and do not cause problems in magnetic fields lower than 0.5 Tesla. Certain tattoo or cosmetic products containing ferromagnetic particles can also influence MR signals. Finally, it is advisable to be careful in patients with metallic surgical clips or in those with history of a recent colostomy or jejunostomy.

A known problem in patient monitoring during interventions is the distortion of electrocardiographic signals. Therefore, under certain conditions it might be difficult to diagnose myocardial ischemia during a procedure. For this reason, in our department a history of severe myocardial infarction contraindicates interventional MR imaging.

In summary, only a skilled, experienced, and synergistically working team of radiologists, anesthetists, surgeons and technicians can safely work in interventional MR imaging. The simple replacement of an MR compatible battery with a battery containing ferromagnetic parts can, for example, lead to a fatal interruption of an MR intervention.

Interventional MR Imaging in Pain Therapy

Acute and chronic lumbar back pain with or without prolapsed intervertebral discs are a major problem of public health in the developed countries. Radicular symptoms caused by a dislocation of an intervertebral disk, pseudo-radicular syndromes due to articular disorders, and the localized pain due to inflammation of the sacroiliac joints represent the most common painful pathology. The number of surgically treated patients has increased considerably over the last twenty years. Unfortunately, most of these patients did not regain the ability to work after surgery. Percutaneous techniques on the other hand, which by definition are minimally invasive, may prove more effective in spinal pain disorders. Before the availability of computer tomography at the end of 1980 these procedures were performed by manual palpation. In 1989, Grönemeyer et al. reported their first experiments of MR imaging-guided infiltrations using a low-field MR scanner [18].

Microtherapy of Prolapsed Intervertebral Discs

The first experience of percutaneous nucleotomies was reported by Hijikata in 1975 [19]. Further ablation instruments with a diameter of almost 1 cm were developed. These were placed under X-ray fluoroscopy by using trocars. Since 1988, MR scan has been used for guidance. In addition MR-compatible automatic nucleotomy systems were developed for MR systems with horizontal access. The first laser nucleotomies were done with Ho (holmium) or Nd-Yag (neodymium/yttrium/aluminum/garnet) lasers.

Indication for the percutaneous treatment of a medial or lateral disc prolapse is ineffective standard therapy of six weeks. Contraindications are prominent disc herniation and sequestration or fragmentation of the intervertebral disc. For MR-guided therapy the patients are placed in the MR scanner in a prone or lateral position. The skin entry point is determined by skin markers or more quickly by the operator's finger using MR fluoroscopy as implemented by a balanced T1-weighted sequence in transverse orientation. The planned track for the therapy needle is superior to nerve roots. After sterile draping and wide disinfection, an 18 to 21 gauge therapy needle (Somatex, Teltow, Germany or MRI-Devices Daum, Schwerin, Germany) are placed under MR-fluoroscopy guidance. Local anesthetic (1–2 ml of lidocaine 1%) is administered through the needle and correct position of the needle tip is verified by injection into the disc of diluted contrast medium (gadolinium DTPA). Parameters of MR fluoroscopy may be three slices with an interval of 0.3 mm. The correct position of the needle tip is in the middle of the disc, verified three dimensionally by multiplanar transversal, sagittal, and coronal MR images. The laser nucleotomy is carried out through the therapy needle using an Nd-YAG laser (MBB, Munich, Germany; 10 Watts, impulses of 1 second duration and fibers of 0.4 mm) or a double laser consisting of an Nd-Yag and Ho-Yag laser (Micromed, Bochum, Germany). Maximum number of impulses should be 1,500 (above 1.5 kJ). The process is monitored with fast-gradient echo-sequence MR images every 20 impulses. In the event of adverse effects such as excess heat, the application must be interrupted for a few minutes. A maximum of 180 impulses may be advised [20]. Finally, in order to reduce inflammatory reaction, a local injection of 40 mg of triamcinolone is administered after laser nucleotomy. In the absence of complications, the patients can be treated in an outpatient setting and be able to leave the hospital after 3 hours' observation.

In a study comparing standard percutaneous nucleotomy (N = 110) [21] with nucleotomies carried out with a Nd-Yag laser (N = 116) [22] in patients with lumbar disc prolapse, Seibel and Grönemeyer could not show significant differences in the clinical outcome between these two methods, but laser nucleotomy was considered the easier technique. By using laser ablation, nearly 80% of patients benefited from the percutaneous treatment with a complete reduction of pain. The neurological signs improved in 92% of the cases. One patient in each group developed an infectious spondylodiscitis and 25% of the patients reported symptoms of radicular irritation persisting for 3 to 5 weeks after the intervention.

Facet Joint Block

Low back pain without ischialgia is often caused by osteoarthritis of the intervertebral joints (facet joints, zygapophyseal joints). A diagnostic block of the affected facet joints consists of the para-articular infiltration of 1–5 ml of a local anesthetic (ropivacaine; Naropin, AstraZeneca, Wedel, Germany). The procedure should always be performed bilaterally at the level of the lower lumbar segment, and some authors recommend the simultaneous infiltration of the upper segment [23, 24]. It is necessary to distinguish two techniques: the intra-articular block and the blockade of the medial ramus of the dorsal nerve located dorsolateral to the intervertebral joint.

In general, facet joint blocks are indicated in the presence of low back pain without radicular irritation and resistance to conventional therapy (consisting of anti-inflammatory drugs, analgesics, and physiotherapy). Local infections, coagulation disorders, neoplasia, and inflammatory lesions of the vertebral bodies are contraindications for the intervention. Facet joint blocks are not recommended for major neurological deficits

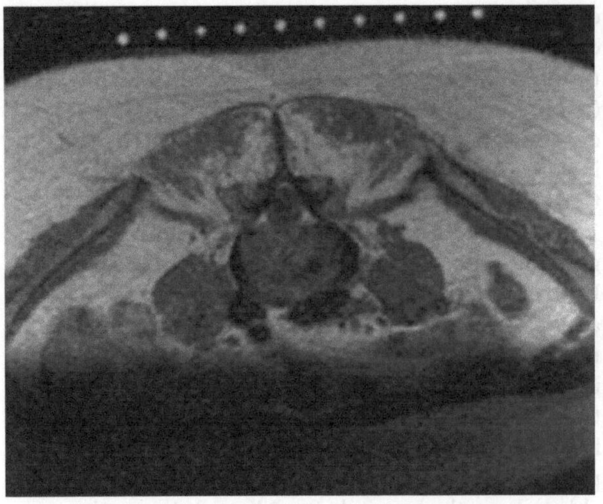

Fig. 19.10. Placement of a epicutaneous contrast grid (TargoGrid, Daum) for determining skin entry points and planning the needle track to facilitate an accurate facet joint block. The plastic grid is filled with a solution of water and gadolinium-DTPA, shown as epicutaneous hyperintense points on a T1-weighted MR image

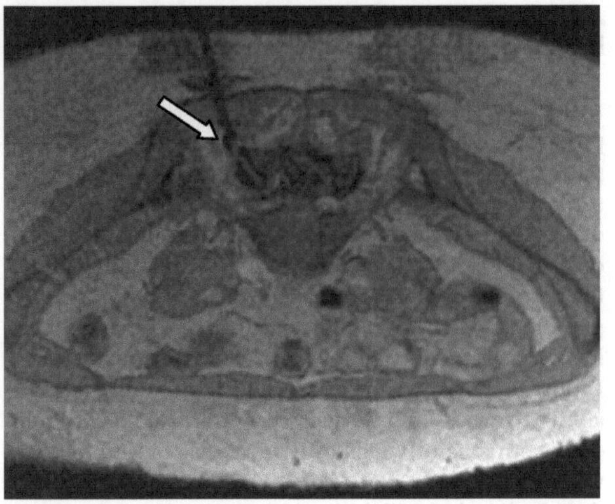

Fig. 19.11. Correctly placed therapy needle (18 gauge) for a diagnostic facet joint block (*white arrow*). A standard anesthetic is administered

clearly localized to a certain dermatome. A disc prolapse does not contraindicate a facet joint blockade.

For facet joint blockade the patient is positioned in a stable and comfortable ventrolateral position. After localization of the level of the facet joints using T1-weighted spin-echo sequences, our procedure is to place a contrast-water filled grid (TargoGrid, MRI-Devices Daum) on the skin in order to plan the level and the angle of the puncture (Fig. 19.10). Following the wide and careful disinfection of the puncture site, an 18 gauge needle (MRI Edition 2000, Somatex) is placed under MR-fluoroscopic guidance. The infiltration is carried out approximately 1 cm dorsolateral to the facet joint (Fig. 19.11).

If pain clearly improves a definitive neurolysis, e.g., with alcohol, can be performed. The first surgical neurolysis of the facet joints were reported by Rees in 1971 [25], followed by electrocoagulation a few years later. Other approaches are cryotherapy and (more promising) radio-frequency ablation [26]. Percutaneous neurolysis is achieved by the local injection of 1–2 ml of ethanol (96–98%) in combination with a local anesthetic. In order to avoid complications to the nerve root due to the diffusion of ethanol [27], it is possible to monitor diffusion of the solution by adding 1 ml of diluted gadolinium-DTPA (1:80; Fig. 19.12). Similar to the diagnostic block, the denervation is performed on at least one pair of facet joints. In our experience, this procedure produces good results in nearly 70% of the patients. It is known that in a certain number of patients regression of the pain occurs within a period of 3 weeks after the diagnostic measure, without further treatment. Therefore, in our institution a denervation is

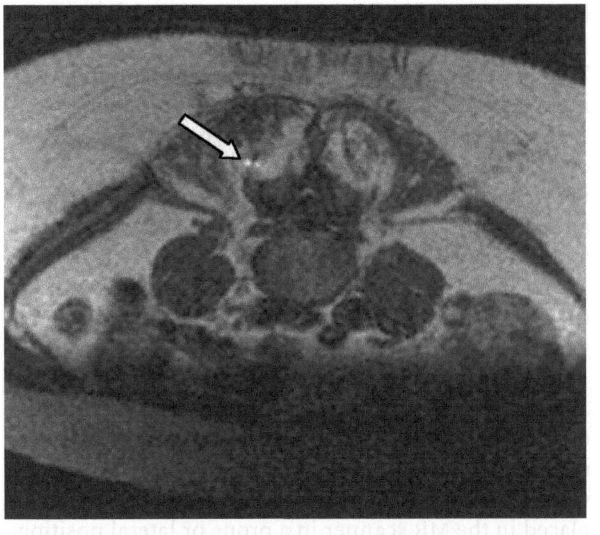

Fig. 19.12. T1-weighted spin-echo MR image demonstrating diffusion of a diluted gadolinium-DTPA solution (1:80) dorsolateral to the facet joint

done only after 3 weeks have elapsed following the diagnostic procedure.

In the case of no response from the para-articular diagnostic block, an intra-articular infiltration of the facet joints can be considered. The intra-articular intervention is carried out in manner similar to the para-articular infiltration: localization of the facet joint using a T1-weighted spin- echo sequence, marking of the skin entry points, careful disinfection and percutaneous intra-articular placement of a 19.5 gauge needle into the facet joint. To ensure accurate needle placement, serial MR images are required. To reduce the time of intervention, we use fast single-slice MR sequences or MR fluoroscopy in non-obese patients. Following correct placement, 1 ml of a steroid–anesthetic mixture (triamcinolone 40 mg – ropivacaine 0.5%) may be injected.

Periradicular Infiltrations

Periradicular infiltrations can be performed extraforaminal or intraforaminal extradural. In interventional MR imaging, extraforaminal nerve root infiltration is preferred in order to avoid an accidental puncture of the dural sac and injection into the spinal canal.

Common indications are compression due to prolapsed intervertebral discs, stenoses of the spinal canal, intervertebral foramina, or of the recess between the dorsal wall of the vertebra and the lateral foramen and finally surgical failures. Back in the 1980s the procedure was carried out under fluoroscopic guidance [28] and periradicular infiltrations were performed under CT guidance. In 1995 Grönemeyer et al. performed such an intervention under MR imaging [29].

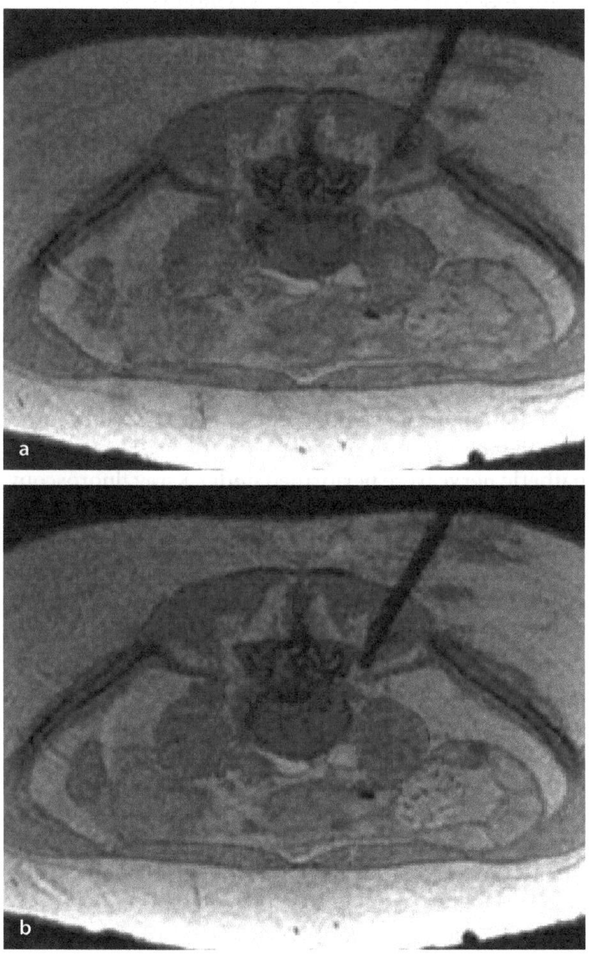

Fig. 19.13a,b. Series of MR images demonstrating the MR-fluoroscopy-guided placement of a therapy needle close to the L5 nerve root

For MR-imaging-guided procedures in our institution we use 18 gauge needles with a length 10 cm (MRI-Devices Daum or Somatex). The placement of the needle is performed either with MR fluoroscopy or with serial MR imaging in step-by-step imaging technique (Fig. 19.13). The puncture is carried out on the level that has been localized at the inferior third of the total intervertebral space, using a lateral needle approach. As the needle tip can precisely be localized with MR imaging, a test injection using a diluted gadolinium solution does not seem necessary to us. Following the verification of the correct needle position, a steroid/anesthetic mixture (Triamcinolone 40 mg, Ropivacaine 0.5%) is injected. The intervention can be repeated 3 or 4 times at intervals of 4 to 6 weeks. On a series of 370 patients treated with use of an MR scanner, after the first infiltration improvement of symptoms was observed only in 15% of the patients. But 72% improved after four successfully performed infiltrations [30].

Complications of periradicular infiltrations are rare and consist mainly of nonbacterial spondylodiscitis with spontaneous remission. Patients with acute gastric ulcers are not candidates for the procedure.

Sacroiliac Joint Infiltrations

The sacroiliac joints are a frequent source of low back pain. In fact, these joints are considered to be the origin in 25% of patients presenting with low back pain. Like the facet joints, the articular capsule and the joint itself are often responsible for pain of degenerative origin. The joints receive sensory fibers from the dorsal rami of the nervous roots L4 to S3. Contrary to pain originating from facet joints, pain originating from the sacroiliac joints may be unilateral. If patients present with distally radiating pain, the radicular signs are often missing.

In general, infiltration of the sacroiliac joints is indicated in patients with persisting pain despite conventional triple therapy (non-steroidal anti-inflammatory drugs, analgesics, and physiotherapy) for a period of at least three months. The efficacy of steroid injections with X-ray fluoroscopy or computertomography-guided procedures [31, 32] has already been reported with improvements lasting for periods of at least 9 months. These promising results were confirmed in a double blind steroid-versus-placebo study by Maugars et al. [33]. The first results of MR imaging-guided infiltration of the sacroiliac joints were described in 2000 [3, 34]. Clinical response was deemed good to excellent in eight of 10 patients with a subjective improvement for a mean of 13.5 ± 5.4 months (time range, 5–19 months). The

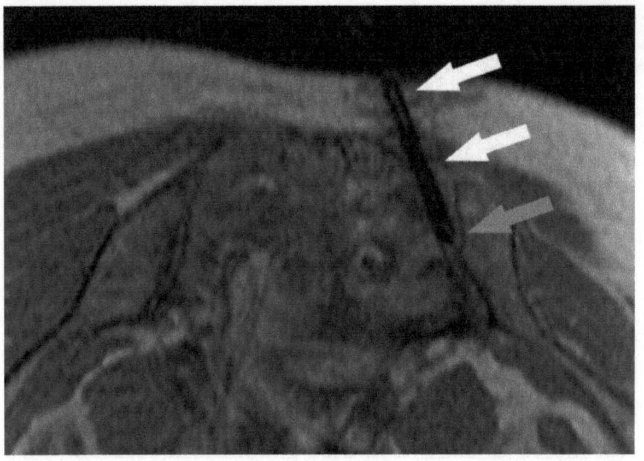

Fig. 19.14. MR-imaging-guided infiltration of the sacroiliac joints with the needle tip (*gray arrow*; approximately 15 mm) located in the articular space

overall pain reduction and remission time was at least as good as achieved with CT or fluoroscopic techniques.

In this procedure MR-imaging guidance has undeniable advantages. It allows precise localization of the subchondral bone marrow edema and subsequent needle placement at the level of the determined inflammation, thus leading to an accurate infiltration of the inflamed area. Especially in the treatment of generally young patients (the average age of the patients in our series was 26.4 years), another advantage is the absence of ionizing radiation

In our institution intra-articular MR-imaging-guided sacroiliac joint infiltrations are performed with patients in prone position using a flexible single-loop circular RF coil with a diameter of 35 or 45 cm. MR-imaging evaluation of the subchondral bone marrow edema is performed using an inversion recovery MR sequence (TIRM sequence). Following the epicutaneous placement of a visible grid (TargoGrid, Daum) a T1-weighted spin-echo sequence is used for the anatomic planning of the puncture. The determined skin entry points are marked with nifedipine capsules (Adalat 5, Bayer AG, Leverkusen, Germany) or with the "finger-pointing" technique. After careful disinfection of the puncture site, 5 ml of a local anesthetic (lidocaine) is subcutaneously and extra-articularly instilled. Placement of the titanium-nickel needle (0.9 mm × 100 mm; Edition 2000, Somatex) is navigated either with a fast-gradient echo sequence with image acquisition every 10 to 21 seconds or with MR fluoroscopy (True-FISP sequence). For verification of the intra-articular localization of the needle tip, perpendicular-gradient echo MR sequences with axial orientation to the needle are used (Fig. 19.14). In obese patients if corrections of the orientation of the needle are necessary, the patient must be pulled out of the MR scanner. Following the verification of the correct position of the needle tip, 40 mg of triamcinolone (1 ml) are slowly injected. To evaluate morphologic changes all patients are examined using a closed 1.5-Tesla MR scanner (Magnetom Vision, Siemens) prior to MR-imaging-guided infiltration of the sacroiliac joints (on average 7 days prior to intervention in our experience) and three months following the procedure.

Clear improvement of the painful symptoms was observed in nearly 80% of the 92 treated patients after the first infiltration, which was performed bilaterally in the majority of cases. Patients without response following the first infiltration did benefit from a second injection in 75% of cases. Drug therapy could be reduced gradually in 50% of cases. Continuation of physiotherapeutic treatment, however, is advised in order to promote further improvement. Noteworthy is that spondylarthopathy subgroups Undifferentiated Spondylarthropathy and Ankylosing Spondylitis showed significantly different results. While response rate was comparable in the two subgroups, patients with undifferentiated spondylarthropathy had a greater benefit from the intervention because pain reduction and remission time was significantly higher and recurrence rate significantly lower for them than for ankylosing spondylitis patients. Since undifferentiated spondylarthropathy today can be considered an [35] early form of ankylosing spondylitis, patients displaying the pertinent clinical features should be treated as early as possible.

Lumbar Sympatholysis

For more than 20 years lumbar sympatholysis has been an established treatment of peripheral pain in patients with occlusive arterial diseases. Other indications are hyperhydrosis, dystrophic reflexes, and the pain caused by irritation of the sympathetic trunk. In former times the ethanol injection necessary for the lysis of the sympathetic nerve were performed under X-ray fluoroscopy or even without radiological control, which was not surprisingly associated with a considerable number of abdominal complications. Today this intervention is generally performed under imaging guidance [36, 37].

For MR-imaging-guided sympatholysis, the patient is placed in a ventrolateral position in the MR scanner [37]. Initially, transverse T1-weighted gradient-echo MR images are acquired at levels L3 through L5. After identifying the ureters, the precise location of the sympathetic nerve trunk and sympathetic ganglia (in the triangle between the vertebral bodies and the median edge of the psoas muscle) is determined. In order to estimate the angulation of the needle and length of the needle track, a virtual track can be drawn on the transverse MR image at the MR workstation. After careful disinfection of the puncture sites, local anesthetics are instilled at the determined skin entry points. A long therapy needle (150 mm, 20 gauge, Micromed, Bochum,

Germany) is introduced using free-hand technique. After approximately 3/4 of the insertion, the patient is pulled back into the MR scanner to complete needle placement under serial MR imaging (True-FISP sequence) control. Following a negative aspiration test, 10 ml of a mixture of bupivacaine (Carbostesin 0.25%, Astra Chemicals, Wedel, Germany) and 0.1 ml gadolinium-DTPA is injected The injection is monitored using transverse MR fluoroscopy. Owing to the insufficient visualization of the needle tip in some cases, a preliminary test injection of contrast medium is strongly advised. During the intervention the interventionalist can follow the procedure on an in-room monitor and, if indicated, the position of the needle can be modified. The predictive test using contrast medium and visualized by MR imaging is followed by the injection of 6 to 10 ml ethanol (concentration: 96%) for complete sympatholysis (Fig. 19.15). Another option is the placement of a flexible catheter in the triangle of the sympathetic trunk and use an infusion pump to achieve a continuous injection of an anesthetic agent (Ropivacaine 0.5% or Bupivacaine 0.25%).

Immediately after the procedure, the lower limbs of the majority of the patients are hyperemic, but in our study of 93 patients no complications were observed. In a larger series of patients, sensory deficits of the genitofemoral nerve were reported in 5 to 18%, and sexual disorders were reported in 2 to 9% of the patients treated by sympathicolysis [37]. A disadvantage of MR-imaging-guided sympathicolysis is the sophisticated nature of the technique. For example, a 150 mm long needle will easily be "lost" on transverse MR images if patient movement occurs. The readjustment of the image plane on the needle requires additional MR images leading to additional needle time. If the intervention is performed by an experienced interventionalist, in our experience laser systems for navigation do not contribute to faster interventions. Such systems seem rather to prolong interventions because of the several stages necessary to initialize the different steps of the procedure.

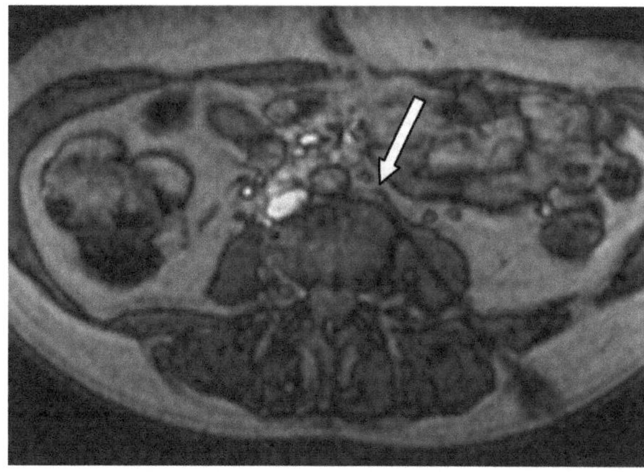

Fig. 19.15. MR-imaging-guided sympatholysis in a patient with pain in the lower limbs. The needle tip (*white arrow*) is located in the triangle of the sympathetic trunk (image rotated)

Summary

Dedicated interventional MR scanners allow good patient access for the accomplishment of the majority of the percutaneous interventions currently performed under X-ray fluoroscopy or computer tomography. Interventional MR imaging is a trade-off between ideal patient access and sufficient imaging quality, especially when using low-field MR scanners. New open high-field MR scanners with a short magnet and a large bore (e.g., Espree, Siemens) appear to promise interventional MR imaging that offers sufficient patient access, excellent high-field MR image quality, plus the integration of new MR-imaging techniques. Due to the development of MR-compatible devices almost all instruments needed for pain therapy are commercially available. With the increasingly powerful hardware and the known advantages of interventional MR imaging, this technique seems bound to become a standard technique in the interventional radiology of tomorrow.

References

1. Lewin JS, Nour SG, Duerk JL (2000) Magnetic resonance image-guided biopsy and aspiration. Top Magn Reson Imaging 11:173–183
2. Cleary K, Anderson J, Brazaitis M, Devey G, DiGioia A, Freedman M et al (2000) Final report of the technical requirements for image-guided spine procedures Workshop, 17–20 April 1999, Ellicott City, Maryland, USA. Comput Aided Surg 5:180–215
3. Pereira PL, Gunaydin I, Trubenbach J, Dammann F, Remy CT, Kotter I et al (2000) Interventional MR imaging for injection of sacroiliac joints in patients with sacroiliitis. AJR Am J Roentgenol 175:265–266
4. Schenck JF, Jolesz FA, Roemer PB, Cline HE, Lorensen WE, Kikinis R et al (1995) Superconducting open-configuration MR imaging system for image-guided therapy. Radiology 195:805–814
5. Koechli VD, McKinnon GC, Hofmann E, von Schulthess GK (1994) Vascular interventions guided by ultrafast MR imaging: evaluation of different materials. Magn Res Med 31:309–314
6. Lewin JS, Duerk JL, Jain VR, Petersilge CA, Chao CP, Haaga JR (1996) Needle localization in MR-guided biopsy and aspiration: effects of field strength, sequence design, and magnetic field orientation. AJR Am J Roentgenol 166:1337–1345
7. Frahm C, Gehl HB, Weiss HD, Rossberg WA (1996) Technique of MRT-guided core biopsy in the abdomen using an open low-field scanner: feasibility and initial clinical results. Rofo 164:62–67
8. Silverman SG, Collick BD, Figueira MR, Khorasani R, Adams DF, Newman RW et al (1995) Interactive MR-guided biopsy in an open-configuration MR imaging system. Radiology 197:175–181
9. Bakker CJ, Hoogeveen RM, Hurtak WF, van Vaals JJ, Viergever MA, Mali WP (1997) MR-guided endovascular interventions: susceptibility-based catheter and near-real-time imaging technique. Radiology 202:273–276

10. Wacker FK, Reither K, Branding G, Wendt M, Wolf KJ (1999) Magnetic resonance-guided vascular catheterization: feasibility using a passive tracking technique at 0.2 Telsa in a pig model. J Magn Reson Imaging 10:841–844
11. Araki T, Aoki S, Ishigame K, Kumagai H, Nanbu A, Hori M et al (2002) MR-guided intravascular catheter manipulation: feasibility of both active and passive tracking in experimental study and initial clinical applications. Radiat Med 20:1–8
12. Bock M, Volz S, Zuhlsdorff S, Umathum R, Fink C, Hallscheidt P et al (2004) MR-guided intravascular procedures: real-time parameter control and automated slice positioning with active tracking coils. J Magn Reson Imaging 19:580–589
13. Schaefer DJ, Bourland JD, Nyenhuis JA (2000) Review of patient safety in time-varying gradient fields. J Magn Reson Imaging 12:20–29
14. Wildermuth S, Dumoulin CL, Pfammatter T, Maier SE, Hofmann E, Debatin JF (1998) MR-guided percutaneous angioplasty: assessment of tracking safety, catheter handling and functionality. Cardiovasc Intervent Radiol 21:404–410
15. Gmitro AF, Ehsani AR, Berchem TA, Snell RJ (1996) A real-time reconstruction system for magnetic resonance imaging. Magn Reson Med 35:734–740
16. Kanal E, Shellock FG (1992) Patient monitoring during clinical MR imaging. Radiology 185:623–629
17. Boesch C (1995) Patient life support and monitoring facilities for whole body MRI. In: Grant DM, Harris RK (eds) Encyclopedia of nuclear magnetic resonance. Whiley, Chichester, pp 3467–3475
18. Gronemeyer DH, Kaufmann L, Rothschild PA, Seibel RMM (1989) Neue Möglichkeiten und Gesichtspunkte der Low-Field Kernspintomographie. Radiol Diagnost 30:519–527
19. Hijikata S (1989) Percutaneous discectomy: a new concept technique and 12 years experience. Clin Orthop 238:9–23
20. Gronemeyer DH, Buschkamp H, Braun M, Schirp S, Weinsheimer PA, Gevargez A (2003) Image-guided percutaneous laser disk decompression for herniated lumbar disks: a 4-year follow-up in 200 patients. J Clin Laser Med Surg 21:131–138
21. Seibel RM, Gronemeyer DH, Sorensen RA (1992) Percutaneous nucleotomy with CT and fluoroscopic guidance. J Vasc Interv Radiol 3:571–576
22. Gronemeyer DH (1993) Atraumatic CT-controlled percutaneous laser nucleotomy. Min Inv Ther 2:247–251
23. Maldjian C, Mesgarzadeh M, Tehranzadeh J (1998) Diagnostic and therapeutic features of facet and sacroiliac joint injection. Anatomy, pathophysiology, and technique. Radiol Clin North Am 36:497–508
24. Tuite MJ (2004) Facet joint and sacroiliac joint injection. Semin Roentgenol 39:37–51
25. Rees WS (1975) Multiple bilateral percutaneous rhizolysis. Med J Aust 26:536–537
26. Dreyfuss P, Halbrook B, Pauza K, Joshi A, McLarty J, Bogduk N (2000) Efficacy and validity of radiofrequency neurotomy for chronic lumbar zygapophyseal joint pain. Spine 25:1270–1277
27. Lora J, Long MD (1976) So called facet denervation in the management of intractable back pain. Spine 1:121–126
28. El-Khoury GY, Ehara S, Weinstein JN, Montgomery WJ, Kathol MH (1988) Epidural steroid injection: a procedure ideally performed with fluoroscopic control. Radiology 168:554–557
29. Melzer A, Seibel RM (1999) MRI-guided treatment of degenerative spinal diseases. Min Invas Ther Allied Technol 8:327–335
30. Seibel RM, Gronemeyer DH, Grumme TH (1990) New treatment of the spinal column diseases using interventional radiological techniques. In: Seibel RM (ed) Interventional computed tomography. Blackwell, Oxford, pp 95–97
31. Bollow M, Braun J, Taupitz M, Haberle J, Reibhauer BH, Paris S, et al (1996) CT-guided intraarticular corticosteroid injection into the sacroiliac joints in patients with spondyloarthropathy: indication and follow-up with contrast-enhanced MRI. J Comput Assist Tomogr 20:512–521
32. Maugars Y, Mathis C, Vilon P, Prost A (1992) Corticosteroid injection of the sacroiliac joint in patients with seronegative spondylarthropathy. Arthritis Rheum 35:564–568
33. Maugars Y, Mathis C, Berthelot JM, Charlier C, Prost A (1996) Assessment of the efficacy of sacroiliac corticosteroid injections in spondylarthropathies: a double-blind study. Br J Rheumatol 35:767–770
34. Pereira PL, Gunaydin I, Duda SH, Trubenbach J, Remy CT, Kotter I et al (2000) Corticosteroid injections of the sacroiliac joint during magnetic resonance: preliminary results. J Radiol 81:223–226
35. Bollow M (2002) Magnetic resonance imaging in ankylosing spondylitis (Marie-Struempell-Bechterew disease). Rofo Fortschr Geb Rontgenstr Neuen Bildgeb Verfahr 174:1489–1499
36. Horma BH, Lucas A, Marin F, Duvauferrier R, Rolland Y (2004) Evaluation of the efficacy of CT guided thoracic sympatholysis to treat palmar hyperhidrosis. J Radiol 85:21–24
37. Konig CW, Schott UG, Pereira PL, Trubenbach J, Schneider W, Claussen CD et al (2002) MR-guided lumbar sympathicolysis. Eur Radiol 12:1388–1393

Treating Painful Osseous Metastases by Internal Radiation Therapy

20

Hatem Boulahdour, Sébastien Klingelschmitt

Introduction

Among frequent consequences – e.g. neurological problems, pathologic fractures, osseous tumefaction, and hypercalcemia – painful bones are the most common indicator of osseous metastases (occurring in approximately 79% of cases). Pain has an extremely negative impact in oncology because patients tend to associate the severity of their condition with the intensity of pain. It is estimated that 40–50% of patients at all stages of cancer suffer pain.

The subjective nature of pain merits a clinical approach based on an overall evaluation of the patient and not merely the illness itself. This implies thoroughly investigating the cause of pain, whether it come from a tumor, or perhaps even therapy. The medical approach adopted in treating the cancer patient very often amounts to evaluating the intensity of pain experienced. The objective of the various therapeutic methods is to treat pain and also to prevent fractures, maintain activity and mobility in order to prolong longevity when possible. or at least improve the quality of life. Numerous studies have shown that such pain is inadequately treated in 30% of cases.

There are specific treatments available for both skeletal metastases and symptomatic treatment of pain. The latter includes surgery, external beam radiation, and chemotherapy, all aiming to reduce pain from osseous metastases by destruction or reduction of tumor mass.

External localized radiation is effective when the number of painful areas is low. Studies have shown that 70% of patients who have had relief from radiation therapy did not go on to develop pain in the radiated area. Its clinical utility is more limited at the dissemination stage because it is then necessary to use the hemicorporal radiation method, which has shown high rate of morbidity despite quite a good success rate.

The symptomatic treatment of metastatic pain includes drug treatment such as antalgics and adjuvants such as corticoids, and invasive methods such as interruption of pain pathways and analgesic electro-stimulation. which tend to reinforce physiological inhibition.

For multiple metastases, antalgic palliative radiation with the aid of systematically administered radiopharmaceuticals appears to be a very useful therapeutic approach. The objective here is to relieve pain by destroying secondary tumor cells in bones. But there is no simple relationship between tumor destruction and pain relief, and so the mechanism of the antalgic effect of ionizing radiation (gamma or electronic rays) is not completely clear. At least part of the effect would seem to come from reduction, not only of the size of the tumor, but also of the surrounding inflammatory reaction. Thus periosteal tension, a major cause of painful bones, is reduced.

Agents used in internal radiation therapy must exclusively target osseous metastases. Osseous metabolism markers are used which are, however, nonspecific to osseous metastases. They are concentrated in zones where osteoblastic metabolism activity is increased. Therefore, osteolytic (osteoclastic) metastases cannot be treated in this manner. Attempt must be made to reduce nonspecific radiopharmaceutical fixation as much as possible. Optimum physical characteristics of the radioisotope used must be ensured, notably a very short ray emission distance. Radiopharmaceuticals must further be non-toxic, of low cost, and composed of a readily available radioelement.

Various markers have been proposed in the treatment of osseous metastases: phosphorus 32, iodine 131 linked to a phosphonate, yttrium 90, tin-117 m DTPA (diethylenetriamine pentacetic acid), rhenium 186 HEDP (hydro-ethylidene diphosphonate), strontium 89, and samarium 153 EDTMP (ethylene-diamine-tetramethylene-phosphonate). Only the latter two possess optimum physical and pharmacological characteristics. The antalgic efficiency of strontium 89 varies between 66–82% for doses of 1.1–1.5 MBq/kg. This agent appears to be a useful adjuvant treatment when coupled with localized external radiation therapy since it has been shown to significantly delay the appearance of new painful bone sites. In any case, due to its long radioactive half-life (50 days) dose rate is low. Myelotoxicity is prolonged, delaying the possibility of myelosuppressive treatment (other radiation therapy or chemotherapy). (We have kept our supply of samarium 153 EDTMP because it is the element with which we are most familiar.)

Agents and Indications

As far back as 1986, Goeckeler *et al.* presented samarium 153 as a radioisotope that can be used for therapeutic purposes in bone. It emits beta rays with the following three maximum energies: 810 KeV (20%), 710 KeV (50%), 640 KeV (30%). Beta particles providing the therapeutic effect have a short trajectory within tissue (1.7 mm maximum in bone). Due to its radioactive half-life of 46.27 hours, samarium 153 can be administered at a relatively high rate, allowing a significantly increased dose rate over a short time span when secondary osseous tension occurs.

Samarium 153 is linked to the diphosphonate ligand EDTMP (or lexidronam). This is an osteophilic complex; a chelating agent from the tetraphosphate family with a high affinity for bone tissue, comparable to agents used in osseous scintigraphy. The favorable pharmacokinetic characteristics of this ligand, when used in conjunction with samarium 153, make metabolic radiation therapy of osseous metastases possible.

Samarium 153 EDTMP targets osteoblastic lesions with high binding ratio for both tumoral bone/normal bone and tumor/soft tissue (5/1 and 6/1 respectively). Samarium is indicated in the treatment of pain from osseous metastases in all types of cancer. Due to its cost however, it is indicated only after the failure of conventional therapies (drug and radiation therapy). Its indication after drug treatment is usually due to failure of major antalgics (necessitating a large dose) or to negative side effects of the treatment. It is called for following radiation therapy when the treatment of sites of pain is no longer possible or when painful areas are so numerous as to require an overly large radiation field. The wide indication of this radiopharmaceutical in the treatment of metastases of all types of cancer, and not just prostate cancer (for which strontium 89 is only used) must be stressed.

Contraindications

Samarium 153 EDTMP is contraindicated in patients with a known hypersensitivity to EDTMP or to phosphonate derivatives, in pregnant women, and in patients who have undergone chemotherapy or hemicorporal external radiation therapy within the previous 6 weeks (due to myelosuppression). Samarium 153 EDTMP is only used as a palliative treatment and must not be used in conjunction with chemotherapy because of the risk of aggravating myelotoxicity. A low uptake on bone scintigraphy using bisphosphonates indicates that samarium 151 EDTMP treatment should be avoided.

Methods

The precise activity of samarium is calculated according to the patient's weight (37 MBq/kg or 1 mCi/kg). On the date of administration the patient is put on a 500 ml IV drip of physiological saline. A slow injection of samarium is performed into the catheter. Following this, a further 500 ml of saline is administered. The patient is kept for 5–6 hours for collection of radioactive urine in an appropriately adapted container.

Complications, Side Effects, Surveillance

Immediate Toxicity

Approximately 8% of patients experience a transient increase in bone pain, known as a "paradoxical reaction," shortly after the injection. This side effect usually occurs within 72 hours of the injection and is generally moderate and brief, lasting approximately 48 hours. It usually helped by analgesics. Other side effects include asthenia, nausea, vomiting, diarrhea, peripheral swelling, headaches, hypertension, vertigo, muscle tiredness, confusion and sweating. To date, no study has demonstrated that samarium 153 EDTMP is causative. There have been rare cases of bone marrow compression, disseminated intravascular coagulation, and stroke; a possible relationship between these complications and the underlying illness cannot be ruled out. In cases of spinal column metastases, an increased risk of spinal cord compression cannot be excluded.

Secondary Toxicity

Secondary toxicity is exclusively due to myelotoxicity. Two controlled studies highlighted this toxicity, which manifests itself by a reduction in leukocyte numbers of 49–51, of platelet levels by 43–45%, and a commensurate decrease in hemoglobin levels. Myelosuppression is moderate in 90% of treated patients. The number of leukocytes and platelets have been found to drop to their lowest levels 3–5 weeks following treatment. This myelosuppression has been experienced as reversible, however, with platelet, leukocyte and hemoglobin levels returning to normal 8 weeks after treatment. The relationship between treatment and a reduction in hemoglobin levels remains debatable. Indeed, levels were only marginally lower in the treated group of patients than in the untreated group. Indeed, hemoglobin levels are often quite low in these patients to begin with, and thus the role of samarium 153 EDTMP in the development of anemia is difficult to evaluate.

Results

Analysis of efficiency focused on response to treatment and response to antalgic treatment. The differences observed among the different studies may result from the choice of analytic criteria and patient randomization. Figure 20.1 is of a successfully treated case.

Pain Relief Evaluation

Pain relief is classified as complete, partial, or non-existent. Complete pain relief corresponds to a complete absence of pain without any intermediate increase; the partial response corresponds to a reduction in pain without any further increase. Complete relief was achieved in 37.5% of patients and partial relief in 40.3%, meaning that a measure of purpose was served in 77.8%. The median delay between the injection and the start pain relief was 12 days (3–35 days). The average duration of pain relief was 2.6 months (0.5–12 months). Other studies have reported similar results.

Evaluation of Response to Antalgic Treatment

Treatment is classified in terms of levels:

- 0: no pain treatment necessary
- I: non-opioid antalgics +/– adjuvant
- II: low-dose opiates +/– adjuvant
- III: strong opiates (morphine and derivatives) + non opiate antalgics +/– adjuvant.

Reduction in analgesic dosage levels was observed in 32% of cases and a reduction by one or more therapeutic levels was noted in another 44.4% of cases. The overall positive response rate was thus 76.4%. Other studies have reported similar response rates.

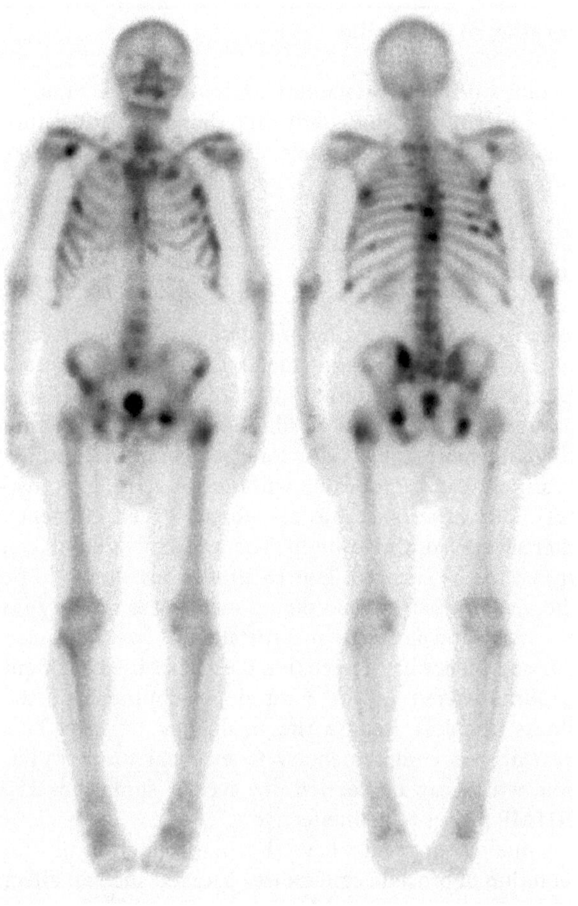

Fig. 20.1. The case of a 63-year-old male suffering from prostate cancer for four years and undergoing hormone-resistance treatment for 8 months. Four months previously he began to experience pain in the pelvis, dorsal spine, and rib areas, unrelieved by nonopioid antalgics and only partially relieved by opioids. This pain became debilitating, curtailing the patient's activities and obliging him to spend 50% of the day in bed. An osseous scintigraphy highlighted several areas of osseous markers' hyperfixation leading to the suspicion of bony metastases, especially in the left sacroiliac joint, the dorsal spinal column, and the ribs. Treatment by samarium 173 EDTMP was performed. The procedure was a complete success with total pain relief after one week. Blood test results showed a slight drop in hemoglobin and white blood cell levels, which did not require a transfusion. The effectiveness of this treatment allowed the patient to resume some activities and the pain relief lasted for four months. Anterior and posterior views are seen

Effectiveness in the Treatment of Primary Cancer

Different types of cancer have been evaluated according to their response to this treatment.

Therapeutic Efficiency Against Pain

In prostate cancer 79.1% of patients showed complete or partial relief from pain. In breast cancer the figure was 76.1%, and in other cancer types 72.7%.

Therapeutic Efficiency of Antalgic Treatment

In prostate cancer 58.3% of patients dropped one or more therapeutic level in their analgesic treatment (good or very good response). A moderate response was observed in a further 10 patients (20.9%). The positive response rate in antalgic treatment is 79.2%

Duration of Pain Relief

In our study the maximum duration of the antalgic effect was 12 months, confirming data in the literature that generally reports an interval ranging from 2 weeks to 16 months.

Conclusion

Internal radiation treatment has shown to be effective in treating pain from bone metastases. Results are often dramatic, with a moderate and predictable toxicity that is (most importantly) reversible after 8 weeks. Duration of antalgic effects can be as long as 12 months, and the treatment can be repeated without reducing effectiveness. Our experience has shown preserved efficiency after several administrations. The integrity of blood cell lines must be ensured. This treatment has shown to be effective in treating pain due to metastases in all types of cancer and not only in prostate and breast cancer. Our experience has shown that the earlier the treatment is administered in the natural development of the illness, the less intense the medullary toxicity. This treatment is complementary to external beam radiation, which can be carried out even if samarium 153 EDTMP proves to be ineffective.

Some of our results have shown a reduction in PSA secretion in prostate cancer; we observed such an effect approximately one month after treatment. A possible curative therapeutic action on metastases is suggested. Indeed, research has already commenced on the use of samarium 153 EDTMP for curative purposes.

References

1. Twycross R, Zenz M (1983) Use of oral morphine in incurable pain. Anaesthesist 32:279–283
2. Lewington VJ (1996) Cancer therapy using bone-seeking isotopes. Phys Med Biol 41:2027–2042
3. Tong EC, Finkelstein P (1973) The treatment of prostatic bone metastases with parathormone and radioactive phosphorus. J Urol 109:71–75
4. Eisenhut M, Berberich R, Kimmig B, Oberhausen E (1986) Iodine-131-labeled diphosphonates for palliative treatment of bone metastases: II. Preliminary clinical results with iodine-131 BDP3. J Nucl Med 27:1255–1261
5. Eisenhut M, Fritz P, Kimmig B, Wingen F, Krempien B (1986) Iodine-131-labeled diphosphonates for the palliative treatment of bone metastases–III. Considerations of interaction, binding and absorbed dose. Int J Rad Appl Instrum 37:741–747
6. Kutzner J, Dahnert W, Schreyer T, Grimm W, Brod KH, Becker M (1981) [Treatment of pains from bone metastases with 90Y (author's transl)]. Nuklearmedizin 20:229–235
7. Atkins HL, Mausner LF, Srivastava SC, Meinken GE, Cabahug CJ, D'Alessandro T (1995) Tin-117m(4+)-DTPA for palliation of pain from osseous metastases: a pilot study. J Nucl Med 36:725–729
8. Maxon HR, 3rd, Thomas SR, Hertzberg VS, Schroder LE, Englaro EE, Samaratunga R, Scher HI, Moulton JS, Deutsch EA, Deutsch KF et al (1992) Rhenium-186 hydroxyethylidene diphosphonate for the treatment of painful osseous metastases. Semin Nucl Med 22:33–40
9. Porter AT, McEwan AJ, Powe JE, Reid R, McGowan DG, Lukka H, Sathyanarayana JR, Yakemchuk VN, Thomas GM, Erlich LE et al (1993) Results of a randomized phase-III trial to evaluate the efficacy of strontium-89 adjuvant to local field external beam irradiation in the management of endocrine resistant metastatic prostate cancer. Int J Radiat Oncol Biol Phys 25:805–813
10. Goeckeler WF, Troutner DE, Volkert WA, Edwards B, Simon J, Wilson (1986) 153Sm radiotherapeutic bone agents. Int J Rad Appl Instrum 13:479–482
11. Goeckeler WF, Edwards B, Volkert WA, Holmes RA, Simon J, Wilson D (1987) Skeletal localization of samarium-153 chelates: potential therapeutic bone agents. J Nucl Med 28: 495–504
12. Eary JF, Collins C, Stabin M, Vernon C, Petersdorf S, Baker M, Hartnett S, Ferency S, Addison SJ, Appelbaum F et al (1993) Samarium-153-EDTMP biodistribution and dosimetry estimation. J Nucl Med 34:1031–1036
13. Serafini AN (1994) Current status of systemic intravenous radiopharmaceuticals for the treatment of painful metastatic bone disease. Int J Radiat Oncol Biol Phys 30:1187–1194
14. Serafini AN, Houston SJ, Resche I, Quick DP, Grund FM, Ell PJ, Bertrand A, Ahmann FR, Orihuela E, Reid RH, Lerski RA, Collier BD, McKillop JH, Purnell GL, Pecking AP, Thomas FD, Harrison KA (1998) Palliation of pain associated with metastatic bone cancer using samarium-153 lexidronam: a double-blind placebo-controlled clinical trial. J Clin Oncol 16:1574–1581
15. Resche I, Chatal JF, Pecking A, Ell P, Duchesne G, Rubens R, Fogelman I, Houston S, Fauser A, Fischer M, Wilkins D (1997) A dose-controlled study of 153Sm- ethylenediaminetetramethylenephosphonate (EDTMP) in the treatment of patients with painful bone metastases. Eur J Cancer 33:1583–91
16. Klingelschmitt S, Boulahdour H, Blagosklonov O, Rudenko B, Aubry R, Bidet A-C, Bosset J-F, Cardot J-C (2002) Traitement des métastases osseuses douloureuses par Quadramet : Expérience rétrospective chez 77 patients sur 2 ans. Médecine nucléaire 26(9):461–469
17. Boulahdour H, Benmelha Z, Aubry R, Klingelschmitt S, Rudenko B, Loboguerrero A, Cardot J-C (2001) Traitement antalgique des métastases osseuses : apport de la radiothérapie métabolique. Séance "Radiologie thérapeutique non invasive", JFR, Paris, 20–24 octobre. Communication orale
18. Lovera C, Massardo T, Galleguillos MC, Gonzalez P, Comparini B, Yanez M, Fodor M, Gil MC, Araya G, Tomicic M (1998) [Analgesic response and secondary effects in patients with osteoblastic metastasis, treated with Samarium 153 ethylenediaminotetramethylenephosphate]. Rev Med Chil 126:963–971
19. Ahonen A, Joensuu H, Hiltunen J, Hannelin M, Heikkila J, Jakobsson M, Jurvelin J, Kairemo K, Kumpulainen E, Kulmala J et al (1994) Samarium-153-EDTMP in bone metastases. J Nucl Biol Med 38:123–127

Suggested Readings

Bonica JJ (1990) The management of pain. Lea & Febiger editor, Philadelphia, London (The "Bedside Bible")

Seibel RM, Gronemeyer DHW (1990) Interventional computed tomography. Blackwell Scientific Publications Inc., Massachusetts, USA

Waldman SD (1998) Atlas of interventional pain management. WB Saunders Company, Philadelphia, Pennsylvania, USA

Subject Index

MIX
Papier aus verantwortungsvollen Quellen
Paper from responsible sources
FSC® C105338

If you have any concerns about our products,
you can contact us on
ProductSafety@springernature.com

In case Publisher is established outside the EU,
the EU authorized representative is:
Springer Nature Customer Service Center GmbH
Europaplatz 3, 69115 Heidelberg, Germany

Printed by Libri Plureos GmbH
in Hamburg, Germany